Women's Cancers

Women's Cancers

Edited by

Alison Keen and Elaine Lennan

Foreword by Professor Stan Kaye

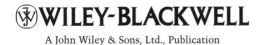

WILEY-BLACKWELL

A John Wiley & Sons, Ltd., Publication

This edition first published 2011
© 2011 by Blackwell Publishing Ltd

Wiley-Blackwell is an imprint of John Wiley & Sons, formed by the merger of Wiley's global Scientific, Technical and Medical business with Blackwell Publishing.

Registered Office
John Wiley & Sons, Ltd, The Atrium, Southern Gate, Chichester, West Sussex, PO19 8SQ, UK

Editorial Offices
9600 Garsington Road, Oxford, OX4 2DQ, UK
The Atrium, Southern Gate, Chichester, West Sussex, PO19 8SQ, UK
2121 State Avenue, Ames, Iowa 50014-8300, USA

For details of our global editorial offices, for customer services and for information about how to apply for permission to reuse the copyright material in this book, please see our website at www.wiley.com/wiley-blackwell.

The right of the author to be identified as the author of this work has been asserted in accordance with the UK Copyright, Designs and Patents Act 1988.

Library of Congress Cataloging-in-Publication Data

Women's cancers / [edited by] Alison Keen and Elaine Lennan.
    p.   cm.
  Includes bibliographical references and index.
  ISBN 978-1-4051-8851-7 (pbk.)
  1. Cancer in women.   2. Breast–Cancer.   3. Generative organs, Female–Cancer.
I. Keen, Alison.   II. Lennan, Elaine.
  RC281.W65W67 2011
  616.99′40082–dc22
                                          2010048018

A catalogue record for this book is available from the British Library.

This book is published in the following electronic formats: ePDF 9781444340129; ePub 9781444340136

Set in 10/12.5pt Times by SPi Publisher Services, Pondicherry, India
Printed and bound in Malaysia by Vivar Printing Sdn Bhd

1   2011

Contents

Contributors

C. Basu, MBBS, DGO, MRCOG
Consultant, Reproductive Medicine, Wessex Fertility Centre, Southampton, UK

Ellen Bull, MSC, BSc(Hons), DPSN, RGN
Director of Nursing and Patient Experience, Royal Surrey County Hospital Foundation, Guildford, Surrey, UK

Gillian Crawford, RGN, MSc, BA(Hons), ENB 237
Principal Genetic Counsellor, University of Southampton/Wessex Clinical Genetics Service, Princess Anne Hospital, Southampton, UK

Carol L. Davis
Lead Consultant Palliative Medicine and Team Leader Hospital Palliative Care Team, Southampton University Hospitals Trust, Southampton General Hospital, Southampton, UK

Karen Donelly-Cairns, RGN, Dip N(Lond), Dip HE(Womens Health), BA(Hons), MSc
Sexual Medicine, MSc Advanced Practice, Advanced Nurse Practitioner, Senior Clinical Nurses Office, St Mary's Hospital, Manchester, UK

Alison Farmer, RN, PhD
Patient/Lecturer in Psychology, The University of Southampton, Southampton, UK

Louisa G. Gordon, PhD
Health Economist, Queensland Institute of Medical Research, Brisbane, Queensland, Australia

Martin Gore, MBBS, PhD, FRCP
Professor of Cancer Medicine, Department of Medicine, Royal Marsden NHS Foundation Trust, London, UK

Jane Grant, MSc, SRN, RSCN
Palliative Care Clinical Nurse Specialist, Southampton University Hospitals Trust, Southampton General Hospital, Southampton, UK

Kate Gregory, MBBS, FRCP, MB
Medical Oncologist, Gynaecological Oncology, Department of Medicine, Nelson Hospital, Nelson, New Zealand

Victoria Harmer, RN, BSc(Hons), Dip(br ca), MBA, AKC
Clinical Nurse Specialist Breast Care, Breast Care Unit, Imperial College Healthcare NHS Trust, London, UK

Michelle L. Harrison
Research Fellow, Royal Marsden NHS Foundation Trust, London, UK

Beccy Hoddinott Isaac, BSc Econ(Hons), RGNDip, NDip, OncN
Clinical Nurse Specialist, Gynaecological Oncology, Southampton University Hospitals Trust, Princess Anne Hospital, Southampton, UK

Rachel Howitt, FRCPath
Consultant Histo/Cytopathologist, Newcastle Upon Tyne Hospitals NHS Trust, Newcastle-Upon-Tyne, UK

Susan Ingamells, MD, PhD, DRCOG, MRCOG
Consultant, Reproductive Medicine, Wessex Fertility Centre, Southampton, UK

Alison Keen, RGN, MSc
Clinical Nurse Specialist, Gynaecological Oncology, Southampton University Hospitals Trust, Princess Anne Hospital, Southampton, UK

Elaine Lennan, RN, MSc, PhD
Consultant Cancer Nurse, Southampton University Hospitals Trust, Southampton General Hospital, Southampton, UK

Katherine McCarthy
Specialist Registrar, Colorectal Unit, Royal Bournemouth Hospital, Bournemouth, UK

Ken Metcalf, MD, FRCS(ed), FRCOG
Consultant, Gynaecologiacal Oncology, Princess Anne Hospital, Southampton University Hospitals Trust, Southampton, UK

Ana Montes, LMS, PhD
Consultant in Medical Oncology, Guy's Hospital, London, UK

Christina M. Nagle, PhD
Postdoctoral Research Fellow, NHMRC Public Health Research Fellow, Queensland Institute of Medical Research, Cancer and Population Studies Group, Herston, Queensland, Australia

Maureen Royston-Lee, BSc(Hons), MSc(Occup. Psych), MSc(Couns. Psych)
*Chartered Counselling Psychologist, Head of Patient Information and Support,
London, UK*

Neeta Singh, FRCPath
*Consultant Cyto/Histopathologist, Southampton University Hospitals Trust,
Southampton General Hospital, Southampton, UK*

Sandra Tinkler, FRCP
*Consultant, Clinical Oncology, Southampton University Hospitals Trust, Southampton
General Hospital, Southampton, UK*

J. Tucker, MbChB, MRCPOG, MFFP
Consultant, Sexual and Reproductive Health, Wessex Fertility Centre, Southampton, UK

A. Umranikar, MRCOG, MFFP
*Specialist Registrar, Obstetrics and Gynaecology, Princess Anne Hospital, Southampton
University Hospitals Trust, Southampton, UK*

Penelope M. Webb, DPhil
*Senior Research Fellow, Queensland Institute of Medical Research, Brisbane,
Queensland, Australia*

Robert Woolas, MBBS, MD, FRCS, FRCOG
*Consultant, Gynaecological Oncology, Department of Gynaecology, Queen Alexandra
Hospital, Portsmouth, UK*

Lisa Young, MSc(ACP Cancer Care), BNS(Hons), Onc cert., DPSN, RGN
*Clinical Nurse Specialist, Gynaecological Oncology, Southampton University
Hospitals Trust, Princess Anne Hospital, Southampton, UK*

Noeleen Young, RN
Chair of Ovacome, Ovacome, London, UK

Foreword

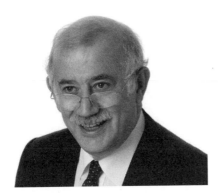

The cancers which specifically affect women are breast and gynaecological cancers, and in both cases much has changed over the past 5–10 years. Scientists now have a much better understanding of the basic mechanisms causing these cancers to develop, and with this has come the development of new and promising forms of treatment, called targeted therapy. Treatment results are beginning to improve, but still have some way to go. Patients with breast and gynaecological cancers, as well as their families, have to contend with a large number of difficult and challenging issues; to help them to do this it is vital that their carers are fully informed in all areas.

This textbook is designed to meet those needs, and the editors and authors are to be congratulated on providing a comprehensive, highly readable and up-to-date resource, suitable for a wide range of health care professionals, as well as patients and families. The editors have assembled an experienced team of experts from across the relevant disciplines, and the public can be assured that this is indeed an authoritative piece of work. No doubt the patients' experiences described throughout the book will strike a chord with many, and the perspective which this provides epitomizes the holistic approach of the editors. As treatments are improving, more women are living with cancer than ever before; this continues to present a wide range of problems that need to be addressed, and these are comprehensively covered in several chapters.

In recent years, a major change in the public's attitude to cancer has taken place. Formerly a taboo subject, it is now discussed widely and openly in a wide range of situations. For various reasons, women's cancers generally receive most attention, and in an era of ever-increasing dissemination of knowledge, it is all the more important that information that is available is accurate and provided in the appropriate context. With this in mind, this textbook is extremely timely and most welcome.

Professor Stan Kaye
Professor of Medical Oncology
Royal Marsden Hospital, London

Introduction

This book is dedicated to the women that the authors have met over many years in their roles as Clinical Nurse Specialist in Gynaecological Cancer and Consultant Nurse. Whilst much of the understanding of the physiological and psychological effects of women's cancer has been gained through the study of theory, the most complete and in-depth understanding comes from sitting alongside women at diagnosis, through various treatments, and in the anxiety-ridden periods between 'follow-up' appointments. Women and their families have trusted us enough to share their fears, celebrated the success of treatments and discussed intimate issues that often go unsaid in the course of 'normal' life. The varying ways in which people react and cope with the often seemingly unbearable stresses of living with cancer never cease to astound and amaze. Whilst advanced communication skills training, years of nursing practice, and life experience, offer a framework for supporting and helping people whose lives are suddenly in crisis and surrounded by uncertainty, these are not the key elements in enabling a therapeutic relationship. It is the authors' philosophy that the relationship is a two-way experience based on mutual respect, trust and kindness. Much of the book, whilst grounded in theory, is an exploration of the experience of living with cancer, based on years of profound and privileged communication. Women known to the authors, who have offered to contribute to the book, have given many of the quotes, have written their accounts and stories, and some of the accounts are taken from the authors' research. All contributors have kindly given permission for their words to be published.

The aim of the book is to provide a comprehensive and meaningful picture of women's cancers, including epidemiology, histopathology, normal anatomy and physiology, staging, genetic predisposition, sexual function, fertility, the treatment and management of women's cancers, survivorship, and palliative care. The readership who are likely to gain most from the text will be any health care professional who is working in a cancer care setting with particular relevance to women's cancers, or health care workers in community practice, who wish to update. The authors are an eclectic mix of carefully selected specialists in their field, who have researched and written from current clinical experience and have demonstrated their motivation and expertise by their contribution. The book demonstrates their wealth of experience and expertise and the chapters reflect this well.

Chapter 1 is an exploration of the history of women in relation to health and cancer. The following Chapter 2 on epidemiology gives a comprehensive account of cancer prevalence. Chapter 3 is a comprehensive section on histopathology and staging of breast and gynaecological cancers, and includes a section on the importance of the histopathologist in the Multi-disciplinary Cancer Team. It outlines the staging frameworks used for specific cancers and the relationship between staging and prognosis. The significance of tumour markers is detailed in Chapter 4, with the meaning of markers to women highlighted by a patient. Chapter 5 on genetics covers susceptibility to female cancers and the process of genetic testing, inherited predisposition and the psychological impact of genetics testing. Strategies to manage increased risk are discussed and illustrated succinctly by a woman's own story. This will become increasingly important over the next decade. In Chapter 6, lifestyle and prevention provides a detailed account of risk factors associated with cancer development. It examines lifestyle choices and the public health messages aimed at public awareness. Site specific Chapters 7 to 13 also include risk factors, presentation and incidence, and discuss the importance of histopathological staging in determining the treatment plan. Future research and therapies are summarised at the conclusion of each of these chapters. The impact of cancer and treatments on fertility is comprehensively described in Chapter 14, which includes modern fertility preservation techniques and the effect of pregnancy on cancer. A book on women's cancers could not be complete without Chapter 15, providing information on normal sexual function and how cancer and treatment affects these. Assessment tools and therapeutic interventions are also included. Chapter 16, on rehabilitation and survivorship, covers aspects of living beyond cancer treatments and the many policies and strategies available to patients and carers to enable self management and support. Palliative care is the obvious choice for the concluding Chapter 17, which explains the relevant organisational aspects and explores the many facets of total care, including psychological, social, cultural and spiritual care. The section on symptom control gives guidance on common cancer related symptoms, with particular reference to breast and gynaecological cancer.

The impact of a cancer diagnosis on a woman and her loved ones cannot be underestimated. Relationships change and there is often the need to re-evaluate interactions with family and friends. The challenges to contend with include adapting to the diagnosis, coping with the effects of treatment, adjusting from active treatment to follow-up, and living with the uncertainty of recurrence. However, given the right amount of care and support can mean that the patient and her family can cope with the total disruption in their lives. The health care professionals' holistic aim should be to help people to manage their distress, keep them well informed, provide supportive care, guide and help them through the health care system, provide specialist support in symptom control, nutritional help, psychological care, and practical support to maintain independence. Support groups, patient advocacy agencies, patients' own voices and contribution to health boards and health care teams and cancer charities are engaging with health care providers to enable collaboration in the planning of future cancer care services.

A woman with ovarian cancer observed:

One of the greatest struggles in the battle against cancer is to realise that 'the essential self' endures. Despite so much else getting in the way – so many fears, so much discomfort and pain, so many reasons to give up. Yet there are the reasons for keeping going: the hope, the love of family and friends, the support of caregivers, and the desire to live and feel like myself again. In the midst of it all it is easy to feel lost and to be identified as a number, an operation, and CT images. The bald woman looking back at me in the mirror was alien, a constant reminder of the losses that I had experienced.

To enable people to regain a sense of self is one of the many challenges of cancer care; of course, the means of achieving this are complex. But a good starting point is to face each individual new patient as an opportunity in 'getting it right'; to give time and respect, to listen and inform and to treat with unconditional positive regard. At the end of treatment, carers need to ensure that care continues by providing services that offer rehabilitation and survivorship and by having awareness that the end of treatment is often a new beginning.

Alison Keen

Chapter 1

The History of Women in Relation to Health and Cancer

Victoria Harmer and Maureen Royston-Lee

Women and health

Throughout history, women have been considered the weaker sex. Health surveys repeatedly illustrate that females have higher rates of illness, disability days and health service utilization than do males (Verbrugge 1979). This is in spite of women giving priority to fulfilling their work responsibilities over their discomfort (Amin and Bentley 2002); indeed those with employment or who have an ill child are significantly less likely to cut down on their activity because of symptoms (Woods and Hulka 1979).

Women and mental illness

Women are commonly believed to be more susceptible to emotional breakdowns and mental illness, as they are deemed to be not as psychologically durable as men.

The notion of nymphomania developed during the second half of the seventeenth century. A third of all patients in Victorian asylums apparently suffered from this condition. Described as an irresistible desire for sexual intercourse and a female pathology of over-stimulated genitals, it was associated with a loss of sanity. It was believed that without treatment these women would become raving maniacs, robbed of their minds. Cures for nymphomania included separation from men, induced vomiting, cold douches over the head, bloodletting, warm douches over the breasts, solitary confinement, leeches, straight-jackets, bland diets and occasionally clitorectomies.

Spinsters and lesbians were also considered a threat to society during the nineteenth century. Any women, who went outside the social norm and made their own decisions, were thought to be mentally ill, as doctors claimed being without male interaction over the long term would result in irritability, anaemia, tiredness and fussing. Again women were admitted to the asylum or forced into marriage, as it was assumed their condition could be cured by repeated sexual interaction with men.

During the mid-nineteenth century came the idea of the 'wandering womb'. Madness was associated with menstruation, pregnancy and the menopause, and the womb was

Women's Cancers, First Edition. Edited by Alison Keen and Elaine Lennan.
© 2011 Blackwell Publishing Ltd. Published 2011 by Blackwell Publishing Ltd.

thought to wander throughout the body acting like an enormous sponge, sucking life from vulnerable women (Ussher 1991). Thus women became more synonymous with madness and generally thought to be emotional and unstable.

In developed countries such as Britain, women are more likely than men to be admitted to hospital for psychiatric treatment, and both first-time and total admissions to psychiatric hospitals are dominated by women (Miles 1988; DH 1995; Payne 1995). Women are also more likely to be treated by general practitioners and community psychiatric teams for mental health problems. Whilst women and men are equally represented amongst admissions for schizophrenia, women are twice as likely to be admitted due to depression and anxiety (Payne 1995; DH 1995). Older women and women from minority ethnic groups are the most likely to be given a psychiatric diagnosis and to receive treatment for that condition (Doyal 1998).

Eating disorders

Anorexia is an eating disorder and a mental health condition that usually develops over time, most commonly starting in the mid-teens. In teenagers and young adults, the condition affects about 1 in 250 females and 1 in 2000 males (DH 2008a).

Anorexia was officially recognised as a disease in 1873 (Wiederman 1996), and flourished throughout the nineteenth century as women wanted to accentuate their femininity. The physical and spiritual ideal of anorexia became a status symbol for women, showing them to be middle to upper class, as working-class women could not afford to become anorexic as they needed to eat in order to work. Once more, treatment was by admission to an asylum, where the women could rest and be excessively fed.

Breast cancer in ancient Egypt and Greece

Breast cancer was first 'discovered' by the ancient Egyptians over 3500 years ago. In 460 BC, Hippocrates, the father of Western medicine, described breast cancer as a disease of one of the 'humours' in the body. There were four 'humours', blood, phlegm, yellow bile and black bile. Hippocrates suggested that cancer was a result of an excess of black bile or 'melanchole'. The breast, if left untreated, would become black and hard and would eventually break open and black fluid would ooze from it.

In 200 AD, Hippocrates' successor, Galen, also described cancer in terms of 'excessive black bile', but he felt that some tumours were more serious than others. The treatment available for breast cancer at the time of Galen included opium, castor oil, liquorice and sulphur. Surgery was not an option as it was felt that the cancer would reappear at the site of the surgery or elsewhere in the body (Garrison 1966).

For the next 2000 years, physicians considered breast cancer as a systemic disease, as the dark bile was thought to travel around the entire body, causing tumours in other organs.

It was not until 1680 that a French physician, Francois de la Boe Sylvius, began to challenge the notion of breast cancer as a 'humoural' disease. He felt that cancer was caused by a chemical process that resulted in lymphatic fluids becoming acrid instead of acidic (Olson 2002).

An interesting hypothesis was put forward by Bernardino Ramazzini in 1713, who noted the higher than normal occurrence of breast cancer in nuns, and concluded that the origin of breast cancer was sexual. The absence of sexual activity in nuns was thought to affect the reproductive organs, including the breast, which started to decay resulting in cancer (Olson 2002)!

There were of course other theories that did not involve sex, including depression, which constricted the blood vessels and trapped coagulated blood, again resulting in breast cancer. Another theory postulated that the cause lay in a sedentary life, causing bodily fluids to become sluggish.

The eighteenth century onwards: breast cancer and surgery

There was no shortage of theories but there was a major shift in opinion amongst eighteenth-century physicians who began to see breast cancer as a more localised disease. The implications of this were enormous, as it meant that surgery now had a significant part to play in the treatment. In 1757, Henri Le Dran, argued that surgery could actually cure breast cancer, provided that it also included the removal of the infected axillary lymph nodes.

By the mid-nineteenth century, breast cancer was accepted as a localised disease and surgery was the treatment of choice. This view was enhanced by the vast improvements in anaesthesia, antiseptic procedures, blood transfusion and the public trust in medicine. William Halstead, an American surgeon, emerged as the leader in the field of breast surgery, when he pioneered the Halstead Mastectomy that became the 'gold standard' for the next 100 years (Olson 2002). This was a radical mastectomy that involved removal of the breast, axillary nodes and both chest muscles in a single block procedure. Halstead performed hundreds of radical mastectomies but the procedure was not without severe side effects. Women had to cope with a poor cosmetic result, including a deformed chest wall and hollow areas under the collar bone, chronic pain and lymphoedema due to the removal of the lymph glands. Halstead felt that this was a small price to pay, as the women's average age was 'nearly fifty-five years and they are no longer active members of society' (Olson 2002).

Twentieth-century breast surgery

A major advancement in the treatment of breast cancer was made by the Scottish surgeon, George Beatson, in 1895. He discovered that when he removed the ovaries from his patients, their breast cancers shrunk significantly. This resulted in many surgeons carrying out oophorectomy routinely, which resulted in debilitating side effects, as they were unaware that not all breast tumours had oestrogen receptors.

Fast forward to 1976, when Bernard Fisher published results indicating that breast conserving surgery, followed by radiotherapy or chemotherapy, were just as effective as radical mastectomy, and often even more so (Hellman 1993).

Gynaecological cancers

In the nineteenth century, cancer was seen predominately as a 'woman's disease'. This notion was based on the prevalence of cancer in the breast and uterus and the incidence of cancer being three times higher in women than in men (Walshe 1846).

Walshe felt that women were at greater risk of getting cancer because of their biological role in reproduction and the menopause. His contemporaries believed that problems of nutrition due to repeated pregnancies made women more prone to cancer.

By the mid-nineteenth-century, physicians began to take the view that cancer was more a systemic disease, with a hereditary component making it incurable. The hereditary issue is interesting, as it carried with it a stigma and evoked undesirable qualities that meant people's lives were adversely affected socially, economically and emotionally. There was also the notion that predisposing causes could also be acquired as well as inherited. These included temperament and immoral habits! Cervical cancer was associated with excessive sexual activity and breast cancer was associated with trauma.

The treatment of women's cancers in the first half of the nineteenth century was somewhat harsh. There was a brief period when gynaecological cancers were treated surgically by amputation of the cervix but thankfully that 'fashion', which carried a high mortality rate, was short-lived. In the second half of the nineteenth century, there was a new understanding that these cancers were more of a local disease and surgical techniques improved accordingly.

In 1896, leading obstetrician, William Japp Sinclair (1896), believed that there was a strong connection between poor social conditions and the development of cancer (Sinclair 1902). Cervical cancer was usually associated with lack of personal hygiene, venereal disease and the recurrent lacerations and infections caused by multiparity and poor obstetric care.

In the late 1880s, there was a belief that the origins of cancer existed outside the body. Germs and parasites were detected in cancer cells and this led to controversy at the time. In 1902, a general practitioner remarked that 'the loose and open arrangement of the nether garments of the majority of women would naturally favour access to the generative organs of the infective micro-organism' (Brand 1902). It would appear that the medical profession had 'it in for' women, and the vast majority of medical doctors at the time would have been men.

Nineteenth century onwards

By the end of the nineteenth century, a new risk factor liable to cause gynaecological cancer emerged, that of unclean male genitalia (Mort 1987). The social purity movement, comprising feminists, medics and nonconformist Protestants, were involved in reshaping the nation's morals and took a view that male sexuality was a source of 'moral pollution'. There was a drive to denounce the 'double standards' of sexuality that existed between men and women. Within this context, a major public health hazard was identified, that of men's foreskins, where germs were harboured and led to cervical cancer. Doctors made a connection between the low incidence of cervical cancer, as well as syphilis and gonorrhoea, amongst the Jews (Darby 2003).

The end of the nineteenth century saw surgery as the treatment of choice for gynaecological cancers, and some of the major developments in surgical procedures occurred in gynae-cology. At this time in Britain, maternal health and infant mortality emerged as major public concerns, as there were huge gaps between the rich and poor in terms of morbidity. There was a drive to improve the health of the nation to provide a strong workforce and armed forces. It was against this background that cancer of the cervix began to emerge as a major focus and public health concern.

Cervical screening

The initiative to educate women in the early recognition of cervical cancer was first discussed at a meeting of the British Medical Association in 1907. The big question for doctors was how to get the message across to the uneducated masses. It was deemed inappropriate to place advertisements in newspapers, because of the taboo nature of the subject. References to the 'morbid and lurid aspects' of cervical cancer, such as abnormal bleeding and vaginal discharges, were deemed 'too shocking for the sensibilities of the public' (Childe 1914).

Midwives and health visitors became involved with instructing women on the early signs of the disease and they were instrumental in emphasising the importance of seek-ing medical advice from professionals rather than 'healers'. Upper middle-class ladies were taken on board to instruct the 'unreading and unthinking' members of the public (Childe 1923).

The BMA created an advice leaflet about early detection of cervical cancer for midwives and general practitioners, to give out to women following childbirth. The message was very clear: early detection saves lives.

Screening as a tool for cancer

Survival from cancer depends on the type and the stage at which it is treated; prognosis is invariably better for those treated at an early stage. Evidence illustrates that many cancers are potentially avoidable, and could be prevented or diagnosed earlier using knowledge that is already available. The purpose of screening is for early detection of cancer and to interrupt its natural course, preventing it from progressing and causing death (Austoker 1995).

Breast cancer is the most common cancer for women in the UK and one where there is much information. The Forrest Report (Forrest 1986) showed favourable evidence against the criteria required to establish a screening programme. Thus in 1988 the National Health Service Breast Screening Programme was set up in the UK, aiming to reduce mortality from breast cancer by 25% in the population screened. Certainly, in all randomised trials of women aged 50 and over, mortality from breast cancer is reduced in those offered screening compared with unscreened controls.

Health services were already providing regular smear tests in the mid-1960s, although women at greatest risk were not necessarily being tested and follow-up procedures for those with a positive test were inefficient (DH 2008b). However, in 1988, the Department of Health established a computerised call and recall system and their first external quality assessment schemes for laboratories.

These programmes are quality assured and regularly reviewed to monitor standards, and to ensure that more sophisticated screening practices are introduced as technology and knowledge develop.

A more recent development in cancer screening is the NHS Bowel Cancer Screening Programme; launched in 2006, it is the first screening programme to target both men and women (DH 2008b).

Breast screening attendance – are their differences based on ethnicity?

Using the methodology of focus groups, Scanlon (2004) identified that Asian and Arab women share common themes with white British socially disadvantaged women, for example poor general knowledge about breast cancer. However, the Asian and Arab women's ideas were based on historical and cultural practices and beliefs. A lack of breast awareness information in different languages and formats was therefore required.

Another study (Scanlon and Wood 2005) highlighted that Black and Minority Ethnic (BME) women had less knowledge about breast cancer, its symptoms and risk factors, when compared to the general population. BME women were less likely to be breast aware and 43% stated they did not know what to look for. This group of women also reported a lower uptake of breast screening. Therefore, it appears that they are at a higher risk of letting symptoms go unnoticed. Ironically black women are three times more likely to have triple negative tumours (tumours negative for HER2, oestrogen or progesterone receptors); a characteristic associated with a poorer prognosis (Stead et al. 2009). Thus the group most likely to experience aggressive tumours are the ones less likely to have these tumours identified early.

Breast screening attendance – other variables

Partner gender is not associated with any barriers to screening and women who partner with women, women who partner with only men, and women who partner with women and men have comparable attendance records (Clark et al. 2009). As expected, academic women have a strong relationship between breast screening and a health promoting lifestyle (Oran et al. 2008).

Health promotion/education/screening

Health promotion strategies are not focused on a specific health problem, more on enabling a person to increase the control over and to improve their health. Health promotion activities demand participation and it is only through achieving this, that they can be successful.

Health education is involved with the communication of information concerning underlying conditions that impact on health. It comprises of constructed opportunities for learning, and improving and disseminating knowledge conducive to health. Both these concepts are vital channels when promoting breast or cervical screening and in trying to boost attendance numbers. These methods target the 'well person' and attempt to engage them in taking responsibility for their own health.

Health care professionals need to act as an effective resource for people, championing the idea of a healthy lifestyle, which can hopefully only increase the public's personal responsibility for their own health, resulting in them attending screening, and being more susceptible in adopting better lifestyle choices (Harmer 2009).

References

Amin, A. and Bentley, M.E. (2002) The influence of gender on rural women's illness experience and health-seeking strategies for gynaecological symptoms. *Journal of Health Management* **4(2)**, 229–249.

Austoker, J. (1995) *Cancer Prevention in Primary Care*. London: BMJ Publishing Group.

Brand, A.T. (1902) The etiology of cancer. *British Medical Journal* **2**, 238–42.

Childe. C.P. (1914) Cancer, public authorities, and the public. *British Medical Journal* **1**, 643–5.

Childe, C.P. (1923) The need for public education in the control of cancer. *British Medical Journal* **1**, 509–10.

Clark, M.A., Rogers, M.L., Armstrong, G.F. et al. (2009) Comprehensive cancer screening amongst unmarried women aged 40–75 years: results from the cancer screening project for women. *Journal of Women's Health* **18(4)**, 451–9.

Darby. R. (2003) Where doctors differ: the debate on circumcision as a protection against syphilis, in *Social History of Medicine* **16(1)**, 57–78.

Department of Health (1995) *Mental Health in England*. London: Government Statistical Service.

Department of Health (2008a) Anorexia Nervosa http://www.nhs.uk/conditions/Anorexia-nervosa/Pages/Introduction.aspx (accessed 22 February 2010).

Department of Health (2008b) *NHS Cancer Screening Programmes. Breast and Cervical Screening: the first 20 years*. London: Department of Health.

Doyle, L. (1998) *Women and Health Services*. Philadelphia: Open University Press.

Forrest, A.P.M. (1986) *Breast Cancer Screening: Report to the Health Ministers of England, Wales, Scotland and Northern Ireland*. London: HMSO

Garrison, F. (1966) *History of Medicine*. Philadelphia PA: W.B. Saunders Company.

Harmer, V. (2009) Promotion, education and breast screening. *British Journal of Healthcare Management* **15(8)**, S22–6.

Hellman. S. (1993) Dogma and inquisition in medicine. *Cancer* **71(1)**, 2430–3.

Miles, A. (1988) *Women and Mental Illness*. Hemel Hempstead: Harvester Wheatsheaf.

Mort, F. (1987) *Dangerous Sexualities: Medico-Moral Politics in England since 1830*. New York: Routledge & Kagan Paul.

Olson, K. (2002) *Bathsheba's Breast: Women, Cancer and History*. Baltimore MD: John Hopkins Press.

Oran, N.T., Can, H.O., Senuzan, F. and Aylaz, R.D. (2008) Health promotion lifestyle and cancer screening behaviour: a survey amongst academician women. *Asian Pacific Journal of Cancer Prevention* **9(3)**, 515–18.

Payne, S. (1995) The rationing of psychiatric beds: changing trends in sex-ratios in admission to psychiatric hospital. *Health and Social Care in the Community* **3(5)**, 289–300.

Scanlon, K. (2004) *An investigation into breast cancer related knowledge, beliefs and attitudes amongst women from black and minority ethnic groups living in London and Sheffield: a qualitative study.* London: Breast Cancer Care.

Scanlon, K and Wood, A. (2005) Breast cancer awareness in Britain: are there differences based on ethnicity? *Diversity in Health and Social Care* **2(3)**, 211–21(11)

Sinclair, W.J. (1902) Carcinoma in women, chiefly in its clinical aspects. *British Medical Journal* **2**, 321–7.

Stead, L.A. et al. (2009) Triple-negative breast cancer are increased in black women regardless of age or body mass index. *BMC Breast Cancer Research* **11**, R18 doi:10.1186/bcr2242

Ussher, J.A. (1991) *Women's Madness: Misogyny or Mental Illness?* New York: Harvester Wheatsheaf.

Verbrugge, L.M. (1979) Female illness rates and illness behaviours: testing hypotheses about sex differences in health. *Women and Health* **4(1)**, 61–79.

Walshe, W.H. (1946) *The Nature and Treatment of Cancer.* London: Taylor & Walton, pp. 152–3.

Wiederman, M.W. (1996) Women, sex and food: a review of research on eating disorders and sexuality. *The Journal of Sex Research* **33(4)**, 301–11.

Woods, N.F. and Hulka, B.S. (1979) Symptom reports and illness behaviour amongst employed women and homemakers. *Journal of Community Health* **5(1)**, 36–45.

Chapter 2

The Epidemiology of Women's Cancers

Louisa G. Gordon, Christina M. Nagle
and Penelope M. Webb

Learning points

At the end of this chapter the reader will have an understanding of:
- The global impact, i.e. social, epidemiological and economic, of women's cancers
- The trends in incidence of women's cancers across the world
- The differences in disease burden across populations

Introduction

Worldwide, more than 2 million women every year are diagnosed with cancers of the breast and female genital tract, including the ovary, fallopian tube, uterus, cervix, vulva and vagina, and 860,000 women die from their disease (Ferlay et al. 2004). Four of these cancers, namely those of the breast, cervix, ovary and uterus, are amongst the top ten most common cancers in women (Figure 2.1), although there is considerable geographical variation in their relative frequency (Ferlay et al. 2004). Worldwide, and in less developed regions, cervical cancer is the second most common cancer in women after breast cancer, whilst ovarian and uterine cancers occur much less frequently. In contrast, cervical cancer is relatively less common in more developed regions, but ovarian and uterine cancers are much more common. The incidence of cancers at other gynaecological sites, including the vulva and vagina, is low in all areas of the world (Ferlay et al. 2004).

In addition to affecting large numbers of women, management of breast and gynaecological cancers imposes a substantial economic burden on health systems, and these cancers account for a significant proportion of the total cancer budget in many countries (Chirikos 2001; Radice et al. 2003). With the rising incidence of these cancers in most developed countries, the associated costs to health systems will continue to increase (Chirikos 2001; Radice and Redaelli 2003). Although clinical staff are often removed from the broader economic impact of their everyday clinical decisions, these cannot be ignored because patients are increasingly required to pay for a proportion of their medical

Women's Cancers, First Edition. Edited by Alison Keen and Elaine Lennan.
© 2011 Blackwell Publishing Ltd. Published 2011 by Blackwell Publishing Ltd.

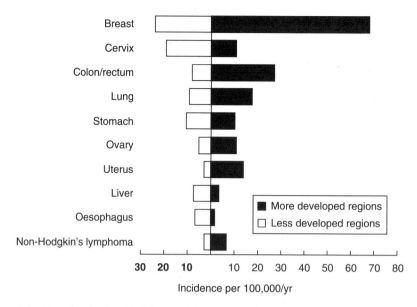

Figure 2.1   Age-standardised incidence of the ten most common cancers in women worldwide, by level of economic development (drawn from Ferlay et al. (2004)).

care, expenditures need to be prioritised to determine the most reasonable use of limited health care funds and it may be important to be aware of the broader context in which new treatment decisions are made (Shih and Halpern 2008).

Beyond the economic burden to the health system, women with breast and gynaecological cancers and their families are often confronted with a number of financial outlays (expenses related to side effects, medications and clinic visits) at a time when they may also need to forego employment and income, potentially resulting in financial distress (Chirikos 2001). Other important personal costs to women faced with these particular cancers may include difficulties associated with treatment-related menopause, feelings of loss of femininity and motherhood, sexual difficulties, lymphoedema, impaired body image and low self-esteem.

In the following sections we discuss the epidemiologic, social and economic features of breast cancer and the most common gynaecological malignancies. Unless otherwise specified, incidence and mortality rates are presented per 100,000 women per year, standardised to the world population.

Breast cancer

Worldwide, one in ten new cancers diagnosed is a cancer of the female breast. It is the most commonly occurring cancer in women in both developed and less developing regions, and in 2002 over 1 million new cases were diagnosed (Ferlay et al. 2004). Breast cancer is also the most important primary cause of death amongst women globally. The estimated number of deaths from breast cancer in 2002 was just over 410,000 worldwide

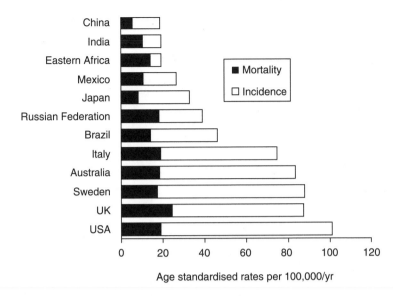

Figure 2.2   Age-standardised incidence and mortality rates for breast cancer in selected countries in 2002 (drawn from Ferlay et al. (2004)).

(Ferlay et al. 2004). There is marked geographical variation in incidence and mortality, with at least a 10-fold variation in incidence rates worldwide. Figure 2.2 shows the international variability in breast cancer incidence and mortality rates in selected populations (Ferlay et al. 2004). The incidence is low (~20/100,000) in most countries from eastern Africa, China and other Asian countries, except Japan. The highest rates are recorded in North America, parts of South America, northwestern Europe including the UK and Australia (80–100/100,000). In part, the high incidence rates in more developed regions may reflect the presence of screening programmes that detect early invasive cancers (Vainio and Bianchini 2007).

Time trends show that over the past few decades the incidence of breast cancer has increased in most countries and regions of the world (Figure 2.3) (Parkin et al. 2005). The most rapid rises have been seen in less developed regions, where breast cancer risk has historically been low (Boyle and Levin 2008; Bray et al. 2004; Curado et al. 2007). In more developed regions the rate of increase in breast cancer incidence rates has slowed in recent years, and these trends parallel decreases in use of menopausal hormone therapy and increases in screening practices (Canfell et al. 2008; Glass et al. 2007; Parkin 2009). Breast cancer mortality rates in most of America, Europe and Australia were fairly stable between 1960 and 1990, but have since shown appreciable declines (Bosetti et al. 2008; Gatta et al. 2006; Smith et al. 1998). Despite the lack of sufficiently long-term time-series cancer data, available evidence seems to indicate that in less developed countries there have been increases in mortality, particularly in recent birth cohorts (Yang et al. 2003; Parkin et al. 2003).

The incidence of breast cancer increases linearly with age up to menopause (Figure 2.4), after which time the rate slows, probably as a consequence of diminishing levels of circulating oestrogens (Boyle and Levin 2008). In less developed countries with low incidence

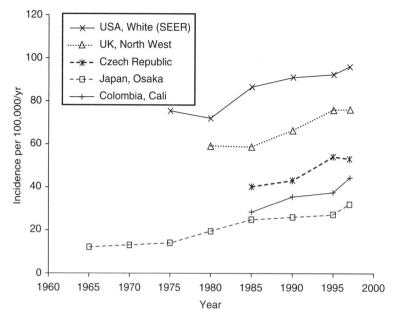

Figure 2.3   Trends in incidence of breast cancer in five selected countries 1965–1997 (rates age standardised to the world population) (drawn from Parkin et al. (2005)).

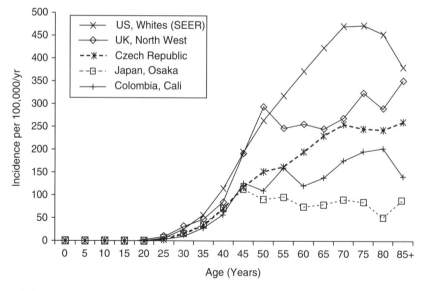

Figure 2.4   Incidence of breast cancer by age in five selected populations, 1997 (drawn from Parkin et al. (2005)).

rates, the age-specific incidence curve may be flat, or even fall in those over 50 (Bray et al. 2004). This is a result of the increasing incidence in younger generations of women, rather than a real decline in risk with increasing age (Moolgavkar et al. 1979).

The Cancer Survival in Five Continents study (CONCORD) showed that relative survival at 5 years ranges from over 80% in North America, Japan, Sweden and Australia, to less than 60% in Brazil and Slovakia, to below 40% in Algeria (Coleman et al. 2008). Survival following breast cancer is highly correlated with stage at diagnosis. In a recent analysis of Surveillance, Epidemiology and End Results (SEER) data from the US, the 5-year survival for women with early stage breast tumours was 100% compared to 71% amongst women with locally advanced tumours (Sant et al. 2004). In low- to middle-income countries, the overall worse breast cancer survival is largely due to women presenting with more advanced disease which, coupled with limited diagnosis and treatment capabilities, leads to particularly poor outcomes (Boyle and Levin 2008).

Because of its high incidence and relatively good prognosis, breast cancer is the most prevalent cancer in the world today and there are an estimated 4.4 million women alive who have had a diagnosis of breast cancer within the last 5 years (Hewitt et al. 1999). It has been predicted that by the end of the year 2010, there will have been 2.9 million breast cancer survivors in the US alone, equalling 1.85% of the female population (De Angelis et al. 2009).

Worldwide, the total economic burden of breast cancer was reported to be around US$400 billion in 2001, or 20–30% of the total cost of cancer care (Radice and Redaelli 2003). In the US alone, the total health system cost of breast cancer was estimated at US$56.4 billion. This includes direct costs for physician visits, diagnosis, surgery, drug and radiation therapy costs and home health care visits. A further $100 billion was attributed to indirect costs arising from lost productivity. In the UK, the mean cost of treating primary breast cancer in 2004 was £15,470 (with an upper estimate of £23,355) and the cost of treating recurrent disease was £11,701 (upper estimate £15,950) (Karnon et al. 2007). The average total costs of treating one woman with breast cancer aggregated over 5 years were estimated at up to £36,804. However, these estimates are all likely to be underestimates of current costs, because they do not reflect use of newer more expensive drugs, such as Anastrazole or Letrozole, that are widely used today (Karnon et al. 2007). Although there is considerable variation in costs across countries, due to different treatment approaches and the different health care systems themselves, several studies agree that costs are higher in the first year of the disease (due to high surgery and hospitalisation costs) and for women with advanced disease at diagnosis, whilst costs are lower for women diagnosed at older ages (Radice and Redaelli 2003; Karnon et al. 2007; Taplin et al. 1995; Will et al. 2000).

Mammography screening has consistently been shown to have economic and survival benefits in many developed countries and at least 22 countries either have existing national screening programmes or are currently piloting them (Shapiro et al. 1998). The impact of a national screening programme is a reduction in the overall treatment costs for breast cancer, because screening increases the proportion of cancers detected at an early stage (Kenny et al. 2000). However, it is recognised that a cost-effective screening programme requires high participation rates, a relatively high-risk population (older age) and minimal screening frequency (De Koning 2000). These factors may all differ across individual countries.

Newer technologies include those for diagnosis (e.g. magnetic-resonance imaging), surgery (e.g. sentinel lymph node biopsy), adjuvant care (e.g. chemotherapy and pharmaceutical

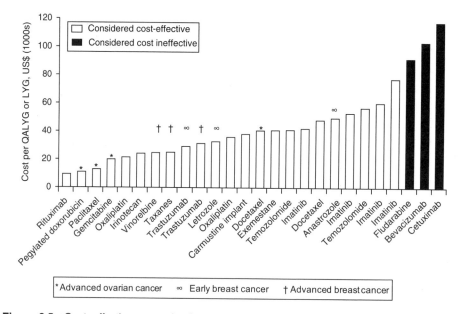

Figure 2.5 Cost–effectiveness ratios for oncology drugs for specific conditions appraised by National Institute of Clinical Research (UK). Reprinted and adapted from The Lancet Oncology, Vol. 8, Rawlins M, Paying for modern cancer care: a global perspective, 749–751. Copyright (2007), with permission from Elsevier.

agents), rehabilitation support services and genetic testing and counselling services (Sevilla et al. 2002; Capelli et al. 2001). These technologies are often expensive and make government reimbursement decisions very challenging when health budgets are fixed. For example, in the US, magnetic-resonance imaging screening for breast cancer is US$1,000 per image and ten times the cost of screening mammography; a positron emission tomography scan for cancer staging costs US$1,800; and trastuzumab (Herceptin) treatment for HER2–positive breast cancer costs US$50,000 per patient per year (Shih and Helpern 2008). In the developing world, the costs of these enhanced services and therapeutics (Figure 2.5) are mostly prohibitive, thus until solutions can be found to increase the equity of access to these modern treatments, individuals in poorer countries will not reap their benefits (Rawlins 2007).

The economic impact to individuals and families affected by breast cancer is less well-known. A diagnosis of advanced disease requiring more expensive medications (Grunfeld et al. 2004), treatment with hormone therapy, incomplete health insurance resulting in a gap between costs and insurance payments, and greater travelling distances to the treating hospital (Clark 1998; Lauzier et al. 2005), all increase the out-of-pocket costs for a woman diagnosed with breast cancer. Whilst the need for many women to reduce their working hours during treatment (Grunfeld et al. 2004; Bradley et al. 2002; Butler and Howarth 1999; Maunsell et al. 2004) and loss in income appear to be short-term, as women resume normal activities over time (Bradley et al. 2002; Santariano and DeLaorenze. 1996), a small proportion of women report having to take early retirement (≈10%), experience difficulties when returning to work, and/or refusal of insurances (Hensley et al. 2005; Stewart et al. 2001) as a result of their cancer. In general, unemployment rates appear to be slightly higher in breast cancer survivors compared with their age-matched peers without cancer (35.6 vs 31.7%), with similar patterns seen in both Europe and the US (de Boer et al. 2009).

Cancer of the cervix

Cervical cancer is one of the most important global public health problems. In 2002, an estimated 493,000 new cases were diagnosed, 273,000 women died from their disease and there were approximately 1.4 million cervical cancer survivors worldwide (Ferlay et al. 2004; Boyle and Levin 2008). This cancer accounts for 8% of the global burden of cancer amongst women and it is the secondmost common cancer amongst women worldwide (Boyle and Levin 2008). There is enormous geographical variation in the incidence of cervical cancer, with more than a 20-fold difference between the highest and lowest rates worldwide (Ferlay et al. 2004) (Figure 2.6). The highest rates are seen in parts of Africa, South America and India, where age standardised incidence rates exceed 30/100,000/year, with much lower rates seen in China, UK, Australia and the US (Ferlay et al. 2004). There is also considerable racial variation within countries, with much higher rates seen amongst black and Hispanic women in the US, compared to white women (Ferlay et al. 2004; Parkin et al. 2005). Cancer of the cervix occurs predominantly in younger women. In Caucasian populations, the peak incidence can be as young as 35–45 years of age, whereas in developing countries, it occurs approximately 20 years later (Figure 2.7) (Ferlay et al. 2004; Parkin et al. 2005).

The estimated age-adjusted cervical cancer mortality rates range from 2–5/100,000 in more developed regions, to 10–30/100,000 in less developed regions (Figure 2.6) (Ferlay et al. 2004). Clinical stage at diagnosis is the single most important predictor of survival and survival rates also decline with increasing age (Boyle and Levin 2008). Five-year

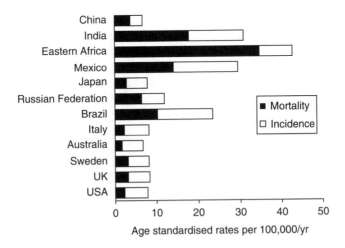

Figure 2.6 Age-standardised incidence and mortality rates for cervical cancer in 12 selected countries in 2002 (drawn from Ferlay et al. (2004)).

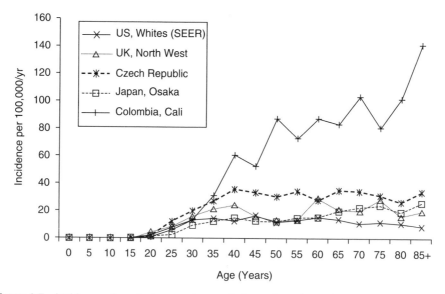

Figure 2.7   Incidence of cervical cancer by age in five selected populations, 1997 (drawn from Parkin et al. (2005)).

survival rates for cervical cancer are as high as 88% for localised disease, but drop to only 13% for metastatic disease (Bielska-Lasota et al. 2007). Because of widespread cervical cancer screening in countries such as the UK, almost two-thirds of cervical cancers are diagnosed at an early stage and, as a consequence, overall 5-year survival rates are around 60% (Bielska-Lasota et al. 2007).

In more developed regions with effective cervical cancer screening programmes, incidence and mortality rates for cervical cancer have fallen over recent decades (Figure 2.8) (Parkin et al. 2005). Mortality rates have also fallen. The most recent data from the UK show that cervical cancer mortality rates in 2006 were nearly 70% lower than they were 30 years earlier (Cancer Research UK 2008).

The direct medical cost associated with cervical cancer in the US has been estimated to be in the range of US$300–400 million annually (2004 dollars; equivalent to $335–$447 million in 2009) (Insinga et al. 2005, 2008). The 2006 costs of treating a woman with cervical cancer increase with the stage of disease at diagnosis and are estimated to range from €19,630–27,244 in the UK, Canadian $11,915–25,759 in Canada and US$25,430–43,593 in the US (Insigna et al. 2008; Rogoza et al. 2008). In the past ten years, significant progress has been made into the prevention of cervical cancer (Franco and Drummond 2008) and the potential health and economic implications of adopting the two cervical cancer vaccines that are currently available (Gardasil® and Ceravix®) are being modelled in many developed countries. Models from the UK and North America (Ferko et al. 2008) predict that vaccination will substantially reduce the incidence of and thus mortality from cervical cancer, as well as the incidence of pre-cancerous lesions and genital warts. Costs of screening will also be reduced. The models suggest that it is most cost-effective to vaccinate 12-year-old girls; the cost-effectiveness of the vaccine improves with herd protection, and is partly determined by the vaccine's expected duration of effectiveness.

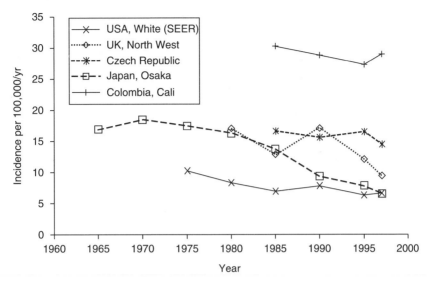

Figure 2.8 Trends in incidence of cervical cancer in five selected countries 1965–1997 (drawn from Parkin et al. (2005)).

The vaccination remains cost-effective in combination with current cervical cancer screening and under different screening programme starting ages and frequency (Rogoza et al. 2008; Ferko et al. 2008). However, it is still unclear whether vaccinating boys in addition to girls is a cost-effective strategy. Despite the predicted benefits of vaccination, reductions in both the incidence of cervical cancer and the associated economic burden will not be realised for several decades, when the teenagers being vaccinated reach the age range when cervical cancer is most common (Ferko et al. 2008).

Cancer of the endometrium

Worldwide, uterine cancer is the seventh most common cancer in women, but it is the fourth most commonly occurring cancer in females in more developed countries after breast, lung and colorectal cancers (Boyle and Levin 2008). This cancer was responsible for 3.9% of all new cancer cases in females in 2002, but it caused only 1.7% of deaths (Ferlay et al; 2004, Boyle and Levin 2008). There is considerable geographical variation in the incidence of uterine cancer (Figure 2.9) (Ferlay et al. 2004). The highest rates are seen in Western Europe, North America and Australia, with consistently lower rates in Africa and Asia (Ferlay et al. 2004; Boyle and Levin 2008). This geographical variation is in direct contrast to what we see for cervical cancer. There is also regional variation within racial groups. Incidence rates in black and Asian women living in the US are much higher than those amongst their racial counterparts in other countries, but are still not as high as US Caucasians (Parkin et al. 2005). Wide differences in the incidence of endometrial cancer between urban and rural areas in the same country, as well as studies from groups that have migrated from low- to high-incidence areas, suggest that environmental factors

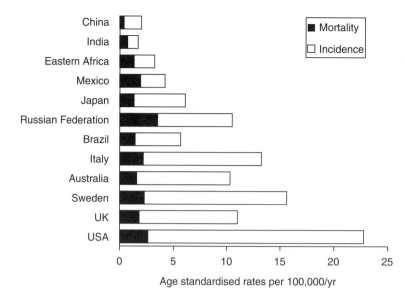

Figure 2.9 Age-standardised incidence and mortality rates for corpus uteri in 12 selected countries in 2002 (drawn from Ferlay et al. (2004)).

play a major role in the aetiology of this disease (Boyle and Levin 2008). However, it is important to note that population rates do not allow for the proportion of women who have had a hysterectomy and thus are no longer at risk of endometrial cancer. Comparisons between geographical areas or over time can thus be complicated if the populations being compared have very different hysterectomy rates (Luoto et al. 2004).

Endometrial cancer predominantly occurs in postmenopausal women. More than 90% of cases occur in women who are older than 50 years, with the highest incidence reached after 65 years (Figure 2.10) (Parkin et al. 2005). Amongst US women, the incidence of uterine cancer showed a marked increase in the early 1970s, which coincided with a marked increase in the prescription of hormone replacement therapy (HRT), particularly unopposed oestrogens (Weiss et al. 1976). The subsequent decline in use of HRT with oestrogens in the US was followed by a fall in the early 1980s back to previous levels (Devesa et al. 1995). Since the mid-1980s, the incidence rate has remained reasonably steady in most developed regions (Figure 2.11); however, the increasing age of the populations is going to lead to greater numbers of new cases and deaths. The number of new cases of endometrial cancer in England is predicted to increase by 53% between 2001 and 2020 (Moller et al. 2007). Increasing incidence rates in postmenopausal women have recently been observed in the Nordic countries, and parts of Eastern and Southern Europe (Bray et al. 2005). Rates in low incidence areas appear to be increasing slightly (Parkin et al. 2005), and this is possibly linked to changes in reproductive behaviour and the prevalence of obesity. Survival from this cancer is much better than for the other gynaecological cancers. Five-year survival rates are around 76% in both the UK (Cooper et al. 2008) and Europe (Sant et al. 2009) and are reported to be as high as 85% in the US, but they do vary by stage at diagnosis and race (Rieslag et al. 2005). Five-year survival rates in white women in the US are up to 96% for localized disease but drop to 25% for women

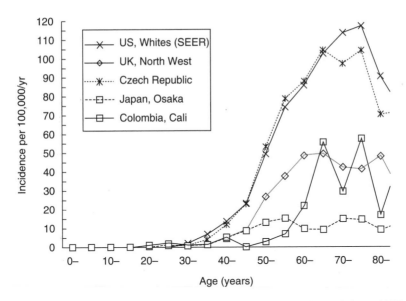

Figure 2.10 Incidence of corpus uteri cancer by age in five selected populations, 1997 (drawn from Parkin et al. (2005)).

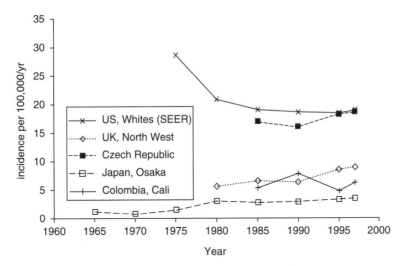

Figure 2.11 Trends in incidence of corpus uteri cancer in five selected countries 1965–1997 (drawn from Parkin et al. (2005)).

with metastatic disease at diagnosis. The comparable rates for black women are 84 and 14%. Approximately three-quarters of uterine cancers in white women and half of those in black women are diagnosed at an early stage (Rieslag et al. 2005).

Like breast cancer, endometrial cancer is typically diagnosed at an early stage and is therefore effectively and cost-effectively treated by surgical intervention to maximise survival outcomes in women. Most women diagnosed with endometrial cancer undergo a hysterectomy and bilateral salpingo-oophorectomy and the average cost of treating a woman surgically in the US in 2007 was US$16,273. Additional treatment costs for women with distant metastases included $7,895 for external beam radiation and $19,462 for a 6-cycle chemotherapy regimen of paclitaxel, adriamycin and cisplatin (Havrilesky et al. 2009) These costs vary depending on individual characteristics, age and complications (e.g. febrile neutropenia, vomiting and diarrhoea) (Ashih et al. 1999). The optimal choice of adjuvant therapy for women without distant metastases is still being investigated (Havrilesky et al. 2009).

Around 30% of women who have surgery for endometrial cancer also have their lymph nodes removed for staging purposes (Havrilesky et al. 2009). The role of surgical staging, which involves pelvic lymph node dissection, possible para-aortic node dissection, cytology and biopsies, for early stage endometrial cancer is the subject of some debate, as these assessments lack accuracy, increase treatment costs and have not been shown to confer any survival benefit (Frederick and Straughn 2009). However, they do inform the choice of adjuvant therapy, with staged women receiving more appropriate radiation therapy or monitoring as necessary (Frederick and Straughn. 2009). Surgical staging occurs more frequently in the US than in Canada or the UK (Bijen et al. 2009; Kwon et al. 2007). Recent developments in surgery, which use less invasive procedures such as laparoscopy or robotic surgery, can increase operating times but have advantages of reducing blood loss, hospital days and complication rates and thus may be cost-effective (Bell et al. 2008). Use of CT or PET scans to detect nodal disease has been found to have very limited value at high cost (Bansal et al. 2008). Similarly, the use of pap testing, clinical examination and radiology for routine surveillance of asymptomatic women to detect early recurrences has not been shown to improve survival rates and thus does not appear to be effective (Bristoe et al. 2006; Morice et al. 2001; Tjalma et al. 2004).

The personal cost to women diagnosed with endometrial cancer who are treated with surgery may include ongoing problems such as urinary incontinence, sexual difficulties, lower-leg lymphoedema and pain (Skjeldestad et al. 2009). Problems associated with surgical and adjuvant treatment can be substantial and adversely affect quality of life and may be exacerbated if a woman has co-existing obesity or diabetes (Bijen et al. 2009). With the general movement towards less-invasive surgical techniques such as laparoscopy, these personal costs to women should be minimised in the future; thereby enabling a quicker return to daily activities (Bijen et al. 2009).

Cancer of the ovary

Ovarian cancer is the sixth most common cancer in women and the seventh most common cause of cancer death. In 2002, the estimated number of new cases of ovarian cancer worldwide was over 204,000, with 125,000 deaths (Ferlay et al. 2004). Although 5-year survival rates can be as high as 93% for localised disease, they drop to only 31% for distant disease (Rieslag et al. 2005). There is currently no good screening test for ovarian cancer and almost two-thirds of cancers are not diagnosed until they have spread beyond the pelvis and, as a result, the overall 5-year survival rate for ovarian cancer is only about 45% (Rieslag et al. 2005).

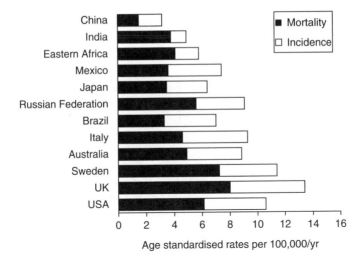

Figure 2.12   Age-standardised incidence and mortality rates for ovarian cancer in 12 selected countries in 2002 (drawn from Ferlay et al. (2004)).

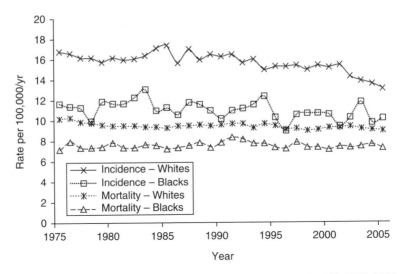

Figure 2.13   Trends in incidence and mortality of ovarian cancer in the US 1975–2000 (rates standardised to the 2000 US population, drawn from Ries et al. (2008)).

Compared to the other major gynaecologic cancers, there is less geographical variation in the incidence of ovarian cancer (Figure 2.12) (Ferlay et al. 2004). Somewhat higher rates are seen in the UK, Northern Europe, Australia and the US (approximately 10–12/100,000), with lower rates in Asia, China and central Africa (Ferlay et al. 2004). Within the US, rates are higher amongst white women than amongst black women (Rieslag et al. 2005). Also, in contrast to cervical and uterine cancer, both incidence of and mortality from ovarian cancer in the US have remained fairly constant over the last 25 years (Figure 2.13) (Rieslag et al. 2005). The increasing age of the populations in more

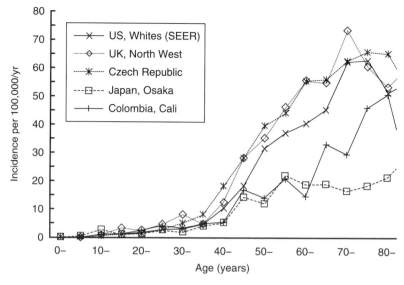

Figure 2.14　Incidence of ovarian cancer by age in five selected populations, 1997 (drawn from Parkin et al. (2005)).

developed regions will, however, lead to greater numbers of new cases and deaths from ovarian cancer each year. For example, the number of new cases of ovarian cancer in the UK is predicted to increase by 24% between 2001 and 2020, and the main reason is the increasing numbers of middle-aged and older women that will make up the population in future (Moller et al. 2007).

Ovarian cancer is rare below the age of 40 years (Figure 2.14) (Parkin et al. 2004) and the majority of tumours that occur in young women are germ cell cancers, including dysgerminomas and teratomas. These tumours account for less than 5% of all ovarian cancers in developed countries (Curado et al. 2007) and, although they are relatively more common in African, Central American and Asian populations (5–15% of ovarian cancers), this may be a consequence of the lower overall incidence of ovarian cancer in these regions.

There has recently been a rapid growth in the number of studies investigating the optimal treatment for and economic impact of ovarian cancer (Main et al. 2006; Rocconi et al. 2006; Bristow et al. 2007; Case et al. 2007; Fung-Kee-Fung et al. 2008; Havrilesky et al. 2007; Pignata et al. 2009). Women with ovarian cancer typically receive surgery and, unless they have very early stage disease, first-line chemotherapy using a platinum-based agent. Currently, the standard treatment is usually paclitaxel plus carboplatin, incurring an overall cost of £8,841 per treatment course (£2,003) (Main et al. 2006). Many women experience serious side effects from chemotherapy, such as myelosuppression or high levels of toxicity causing nausea, vomiting, neutropoenia and anaemia, amongst others (Fung-kee-Fung et al. 2008). The true cost of chemotherapy treatment therefore includes costs for treating adverse effects (i.e. neutropoenia, thrombocytopenia, anaemia, diarrhoea, nausea/vomiting, stomatitis/pharyngitis at Grade 3 or 4 levels), in addition to drug acquisition and administration. The costs for adverse events are particularly dominated by the costs of associated hospitalisations (Main et al. 2006). In 2001, following treatment for ovarian cancer, average additional costs were US$4,908 per women with side effects, US$11,830 for neutropoenia and US$7,550 for thrombocy-topoenia (Calhoun et al. 2001). In addition, the costs of ovarian cancer relating to lost or decreased ability to work are thought to be significant (Szucs et al. 2003; Max et al. 2003).

As up to 80% of ovarian tumours recur (McGuire et al. 1996), women with platinum-sensitive disease are often treated with repeated lines of multiple-agent platinum-based chemotherapy (Fung-Kee-Fung et al. 2008; National Health and Medical Research Council 2004) in an attempt to achieve stable disease. A study in the US found that whilst second-line therapy for platinum-sensitive tumours was cost-effective, regard-less of which chemotherapy agents were used, additional courses of therapy did not appear to provide significant benefits relative to the additional costs, even when costs associated with managing side effects of the therapy were excluded (Case et al. 2007). The rapidly changing and more expensive chemotherapy options, such as gemcitabine or topotecan, for ovarian cancer are driving medical costs upwards, thus published estimates of the total medical costs of treating ovarian cancer (Max et al. 2003) are unlikely to reflect resource use in current clinical practice (Szucs et al. 2003). Clinical trials are still underway to assess other new chemotherapy agents for women with advanced ovarian cancer (Pignata et al. 2009). These new agents have the dual promise of extending life without toxic side effects, but can cost US$50,000–70,000 per patient per line (Rocconi et al. 2006; McKoy et al. 2007). New prophylactic anti-emetic drugs administered to avoid chemotherapy-induced nausea and vomiting further add to the economic burden of ovarian cancer (Stewart et al. 1999), as they are offered in combination with existing regimes. Once an ovarian cancer has recurred, it is mostly regarded as incurable, thus the impact of treatment on quality of life is also paramount in economic assessments of new chemotherapy agents. As new chemotherapy agents emerge, it is crucial for reimbursement bodies to know which options offer the best value for money.

Two large population-based trials are currently underway, involving many thousands of women from the UK (Menon et al. 2009) and US (Partridge et al. 2009), and whilst they show that screening using Ca 125 and transvaginal ultrasound is feasible and acceptable to women aged over 50 years, information regarding the potential benefits, if any, on subsequent mortality and the cost-effectiveness of screening is still pending.

In a climate of rapidly-changing medical treatments for ovarian cancer, the personal impact to the women and her family remain substantial. given the overall poor prog-nosis of this disease. Women experience frequent clinical appointments, ongoing tests and examinations and often a bloated abdomen arising from the build-up of fluid (ascites) caused by the cancer. Chemotherapy treatment is particularly demanding for women and families affected by ovarian cancer, with commonly occurring side effects such as tiredness, loss of hair, nausea, constipation, pain and fevers (Fung-Kee-Fung et al. 2008). Treatment for ovarian cancer may affect a woman's fertility and mean she can no longer have children. Supportive palliative caregivers are especially impor-tant to help families and women adjust and manage symptoms and issues at the end-of-life.

Cancers of the vulva and vagina

Vulva cancer is a rare malignancy, accounting for 3–5% of gynaecological cancers. Approximately 90% of vulva cancers are squamous cell in origin, and the remaining 10% include melanomas, sarcomas, basal cell carcinomas and adenocarcinomas (Ghurani and Penalver 2001). The literature suggests that 40% of all vulva cancers can be attributed to human papillomavirus (HPV) infection (Parkin and Bray 2006). In 2002, this cancer accounted for 26,800 new cases worldwide, of which 15,700 occurred in developed countries (Sankaranarayanan and Ferley 2006). The incidence of vulva cancer in the UK is approximately 2.3 (per 100,000/year) (CRUK 2008), and in the US rates are around 1.5 in whites and 1.2 in blacks (Curodo et al. 2007). Rates range from 0.3 (per 100,000/year) in parts of Asia and Africa, to approximately 1.6 in parts of central and South America, and Europe (Curado et al. 2007). In contrast to many other cancers, the incidence of vulva cancer (both invasive and *in situ*) in the US is significantly lower in black, Hispanic and Asian and Pacific Islander women than white and non-Hispanic women (Saraiya et al. 2008). Vulva cancer is predominantly a disease of older women; it is very rare in young women under 25 years of age. As Figure 2.15 shows, rates in the UK are less than 1/100,000 amongst women aged 25–44, then rise to about 3 per 100,000 women aged 45–64, and peak at 13.5 per 100,000 at 65+ years (CRUK 2008).

Trends show that in the US the incidence of vulva carcinoma *in situ* has risen over the last 30–40 years, but the rate of invasive cancer has remained relatively stable (Figure 2.16) (Judson et al. 2006). Similar patterns have been observed in Europe (Joura et al. 2000), particularly amongst women younger than 50 years of age. These increases correlate with increases in HPV infection (Judson et al. 2006; Joura et al. 2000). Although, overall rates of invasive vulva cancer appear to have changed less over the same period, increases have again been reported amongst younger women (Joura et al. 2000). Compared to the other gynaecologic cancers, the prognosis for vulva cancer is relatively good, with 5-year survival

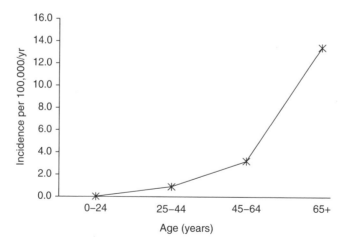

Figure 2.15 Age-specific average incidence rates for vulva cancer in the UK, 2001–2005 (drawn from Cancer Research UK (2008)).

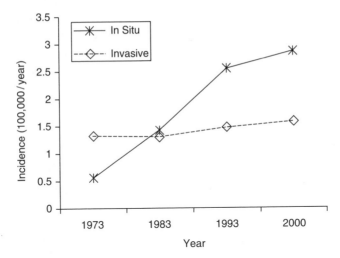

Figure 2.16   Changes in incidence of invasive and in-situ vulva cancer in the US, 1973–2000 (drawn from Judson et al. (2006)).

rates in the US of approximately 86% (Saraiya et al. 2008). However, survival is strongly influenced by age, race and the stage of the disease at diagnosis (Saraiya et al. 2008).

Primary vaginal cancer is very rare, accounting for only 1–2% of all gynaecological malignancies. Studies have shown that vaginal cancer, particularly the most common type squamous cell carcinomas (SCC), share many of the same risk factors as cervical cancer, including persistent human papillomavirus (HPV) infection (Daling et al. 2002; Brinton et al. 1990; Carter et al. 2001). It has been reported that approximately 40% of vaginal cancers could be attributed to HPV, and HPV type 16 has been detected in 50–64% of high grade intraepithelial lesions (Sroden et al. 2006; Hampl et al. 2006; Parkin and Bray 2006). In 2002, approximately 13,200 women were diagnosed with vaginal cancer worldwide and approximately 9000 of these cases occurred in less developed regions (Curado et al. 2007; Sankaranarayanan and Ferlay 2006). Rates vary from 0.2/100,000 females in Western Asia, 0.5/100,000 in North America to 0.7/100,000 in Southern Asia and the South America (Curado et al. 2007). In the UK, around 240 new cases of vaginal cancer were diagnosed in 2005, and the incidence rate was approximately 0.6 (per 100,000/year) (CRUK 2008). The rates of vaginal cancer increase with age. In a recent US-based study of 6800 women diagnosed with primary vaginal cancer between 1998 and 2003, incidence rates for *in-situ* SCC peaked at age 70 years, whereas rates for invasive SCC increased continuously with advancing age (Wu et al. 2008). This study also found that, compared to white women, rates of invasive vaginal SCC were 72% higher amongst black women, whereas the rate amongst Asian and Pacific Islander women was 34% lower (Wu et al. 2008). The incidence of vaginal cancer in Britain, Europe and the US has remained relatively stable over the last 20 years (CRUK 2008; Rieslag et al. 2005).

Each year in the UK, there are approximately 100 deaths from vaginal cancer. The age-standardised death rate is 0.2/100,000, and this rate has been declining steadily since the early 1970s when the mortality rate was 0.4/100,000 (CRUK 2008). In the UK, survival data are only available for cancers of the vagina and vulva combined, but recent results from the US show that the overall 5-year relative survival rate for vaginal SCC between 1996 and 2003 was 64% (Wu et al. 2008). Survival rates varied by stage, being 96% for *in-situ* cancers, but only 42% for late-stage (regional and distant) cancers. Survival rates also varied markedly by race, ethnicity and age, with black, Asian, Pacific Islander and older women faring worse (Wu et al. 2008).

Due to the lower incidence relative to other gynaecological cancers, the total medical costs of treating vulva and vaginal cancers are the lowest relative to all gynaecological cancers (Insinga et al. 2008). In 2003, the direct annual costs to the US health system were $25 million for vaginal cancers and $40 million for vulva cancers (Insinga et al. 2008). The cost for treating 1 woman over 3 years was $21,963 for vaginal cancer and $10,913 for vulva cancer (Insinga et al. 2008). Costs per case were higher by 2- to 4-fold with increased age and in women who died during the 4-year follow-up time-frame (Insinga et al. 2008).

Personal concerns to women affected by vulva and vaginal cancers are similar to those for gynaecological cancers in general, such as fear of the cancer spreading, uncertainty about the future, treatment-related menopause, feelings of loss of femininity and motherhood, and sexual difficulties. However, many women with vulva cancer have reported lower limb lymphoedema and therefore functional and body image issues may be particularly distressing for these women (Beesley et al. 2007).

Conclusion

Breast and gynaecological cancers are a major cause of morbidity and mortality amongst women, with more than 2 million women diagnosed with and 860,000 dying from one of these cancers every year. Breast cancer is the most common cancer in women around the world. It is followed by cervical cancer in less developed countries, whilst uterine and ovarian cancers are relatively more common in more developed countries. Together they account for a high proportion of cancer costs and also place a huge burden on the women themselves and their families. A diagnosis of one of these cancers commonly means aggressive surgery, often followed by chemotherapy and/or radiotherapy with inevitable consequences for a woman's quality of life. In addition, the out-of-pocket expenses incurred by women for ongoing treatment during the course of the disease should not be underestimated as an added source of family distress and burden.

Reflective points

- How does the incidence of women's cancers vary across the world?
- Think about a patient with a gynaecological malignancy and outline the economic burden to the patient and the organisation from diagnosis to completion of standard treatment.

References

Ashih, H., Gustilo-Ashby, T., Myers, E.R. et al. (1999) Cost-effectiveness of treatment of early stage endometrial cancer. *Gynaecology Oncology* **74(2)**, 208–16.

Bansal, N., Herzog, T.J., Brunner-Brown, A. et al. (2008) The utility and cost effectiveness of preoperative computed tomography for patients with uterine malignancies. *Gynaecology Oncology* **111(2)**, 208–12.

Beesley, V., Janda, M., Eakin, E., Obermair, A. and Battistutta, D. (2007) Lymphedema after gynecological cancer treatment: prevalence, correlates, and supportive care needs. *Cancer* **109(12)**, 2607–14.

Bell, M.C., Torgerson, J., Seshadri-Kreaden, U., Suttle, A.W. and Hunt, S. (2008) Comparison of outcomes and cost for endometrial cancer staging via traditional laparotomy, standard laparoscopy and robotic techniques. *Gynaecology Oncology* **111(3)**, 407–11.

Bielska-Lasota, M., Inghelmann, R., van de Poll-Franse, L. and Capocaccia, R. (2007) Trends in cervical cancer survival in Europe, 1983–1994: a population-based study. *Gynaecology Oncology* **105(3)**, 609–19.

Bijen, C.B., Briet, J.M., de Bock, G.H., Arts, H.J., Bergsma-Kadijk, J.A., Mourits, M.J. (2009) Total laparoscopic hysterectomy versus abdominal hysterectomy in the treatment of patients with early stage endometrial cancer: a randomized multi center study. *BMC Cancer* **9(23)**, 23.

Bosetti, C., Bertuccio, P., Levi, F., Lucchini, F., Negri, E. and La Vecchia, C. (2008) Cancer mortality in the European Union, 1970–2003, with a join point analysis. *Annals of Oncology* **19(4)**, 631–40.

Boyle, P. and Levin, B. (2008) *World Cancer Report 2008*.

Bradley, C.J., Bednarek, H.L. and Neumark, D. (2002) Breast Cancer and Women's Labor Supply. *Health Services Research* **37(5)**, 1309–28.

Bradley, C.J., Bednarek, H.L. and Neumark, D. (2002) Breast cancer survival, work, and earnings. *Journal of Health Economics* **21(5)**, 757–79.

Bray, F., McCarron, P. and Parkin, D.M. (2004) The changing global patterns of female breast cancer incidence and mortality. *Breast Cancer Research* **6(6)**, 229–39.

Bray, F., Loos, A.H., Oostindier, M. and Weiderpass, E. (2005) Geographic and temporal variations in cancer of the corpus uteri: incidence and mortality in pre- and post-menopausal women in Europe. *International Journal of Cancer* **117(1)**, 123–31.

Brinton, L.A., Nasca, P.C., Mallin, K. et al. (1990) Case-control study of *in situ* and invasive carcinoma of the vagina. *Gynaecology Oncology* **38(1)**, 49–54.

Bristow, R.E., Santillan, A., Salani, R. et al. (2007) Intraperitoneal cisplatin and paclitaxel versus intravenous carboplatin and paclitaxel chemotherapy for Stage III ovarian cancer: a cost-effectiveness analysis. *Gynaecology Oncology* **106(3)**, 476–81.

Bristow, R.E., Purinton, S.C., Santillan, A., Diaz-Montes, T.P., Gardner, G.J. and Giuntoli, R.L. (2006) Cost-effectiveness of routine vaginal cytology for endometrial cancer surveillance. *Gynaecology Oncology* **103(2)**, 709–13.

Butler, J.B. and Howarth, A.L. (1999) *Out-of-pocket Expenses Incurred by Women for Diagnosis and Treatment of Breast Cancer in Australia*. Sydney: NHMRC National Breast Cancer Centre, 1 October 1999, Contract No. 20/1/2000.

Calhoun, E.A., Chang, C.H., Welshman, E.E., Fishman, D.A., Lurain, J.R. and Bennett, C.L. (2001) Evaluating the total costs of chemotherapy-induced toxicity: results from a pilot study with ovarian cancer patients. *Oncologist* **6(5)**, 441–5.

Cancer Research UK(2008). *CancerStats Incidence-UK*. Available from: http://info.cancerresearchuk.org/cancerstats/incidence

Canfell, K., Banks, E., Moa, A.M. and Beral, V. (2008) Decrease in breast cancer incidence following a rapid fall in use of hormone replacement therapy in Australia. *Medical Journal of Australia* **188**(11), 641–4.

Capelli, M., Surh, L., Humphreys, L. et al. (2001) Measuring women's preferences for breast cancer treatments and BRCA1/BRCA2 testing. *Quality of Life Research* **10**(7), 595–607.

Carter, J.J., Madeleine, M.M., Shera, K. et al. (2001) Human papillomavirus 16 and 18 L1 serology compared across anogenital cancer sites. *Cancer Research* **61**(5), 1934–40.

Case, A.S., Rocconi, R.P., Partridge, E.E. and Straughn, J.M. (2007) A cost-effectiveness analysis of chemotherapy for patients with recurrent platinum-sensitive epithelial ovarian cancer. *Gynaecology Oncology* **105**(1), 223–7.

Chirikos, T.N. (2001) Economic impact of the growing population of breast cancer survivors. *Cancer Control* **8**(2), 177–83.

Clarke, P.M. (1998) Cost-benefit analysis and mammographic screening: a travel cost approach. *Journal of Health Economics* **17**(6), 767–87.

Coleman, M.P., Quaresma, M., Berrino, F. et al. (2008) Cancer survival in five continents: a worldwide population-based study (CONCORD). *Lancet Oncology* **9**(8), 730–56.

Cooper, N., Quinn, M.J., Rachet, B., Mitry, E. and Coleman, M.P. (2008) Survival from cancer of the uterus in England and Wales up to 2001. *British Journal of Cancer* **99**(Suppl 1), S65–7.

Curado, M.P., Edwards, B., Shin, H.R. et al. (2007) *Cancer Incidence in Five Continents*, Vol. IX, IARC *Scientific Publications*, No. 160.

Daling, J.R., Madeleine, M.M., Schwartz, S.M. et al. (2002) A population-based study of squamous cell vaginal cancer: HPV and cofactors. *Gynaecology Oncology* **84**(2), 263–70.

De Angelis, R., Tavilla, A., Verdecchia, A. et al. (2009) Breast cancer survivors in the United States: geographic Variability and Time Trends, 2005–2015. *Cancer* **115**(9), 1954–66.

de Boer, A.G., Taskila, T., Ojajarvi, A., van Dijk, F.J. and Verbeek, J.H. (2009) Cancer survivors and unemployment: a meta-analysis and meta-regression. *Journal of the American Medical Association* **301**(7), 753–62.

De Koning, H.J. (2000) Breast cancer screening; cost-effective in practice? *European Journal of Radiology* **33**(1), 32–7.

Devesa, S.S., Blot, W.J., Stone, B.J., Miller, B.A., Tarone, R.E. and Fraumeni, J.F. (1995) Recent cancer trends in the United States. *Journal of National Cancer Institute* **87**(3), 175–82.

Ferko, N., Postma, M., Gallivan, S., Kruzikas, D. and Drummond. M (2008) Evolution of the health economics of cervical cancer vaccination. *Vaccine* **26 Suppl 5**(26), F3–15.

Ferlay, J., Bray, F., Pisani, P. and Parkin, D.M. GLOBOCAN 2002 (2004): *Cancer Incidence, Mortality and Prevalence Worldwide*. Lyon: IARC Press, Available from: http://www-dep.iarc.fr/

Franco, E.L. and Drummond, M.F. (2008) Cost-effectiveness analysis: an essential tool to inform public health policy in cervical cancer prevention. *Vaccine* **26**(Suppl 5), F1–2.

Frederick, P.J. and Straughn, J.M. (2009) The role of comprehensive surgical staging in patients with endometrial cancer. *Cancer Control* **16**(1), 23–9.

Fung-Kee-Fung, M., Oliver, T., Elit, L., Oza, A., Hirte, H.W. and Bryson, P. (2008) Optimal chemotherapy treatment for women with recurrent ovarian cancer. *Current Oncology* **14**(5), 195–208.

Gatta, G., Ciccolallo, L., Kunkler, I. et al. (2006) Survival from rare cancer in adults: a population-based study. *Lancet Oncology* **7**(2), 132–40.

Ghurani, G.B. and Penalver, M.A. (2001) An update on vulvar cancer. *American Journal of Obstetric Gynecology.* **85**(2), 294–9.

Glass, A.G., Lacey, J.V., Carreon, J.D. and Hoover, R.N. (2006) Breast cancer incidence, 1980–2006: combined roles of menopausal hormone therapy, screening mammography, and estrogen receptor status. *Journal of National Cancer Institute* **99**(15), 1152–61.

Grunfeld, E., Coyle, D., Whelan, T. et al. (2004) Family caregiver burden: results of a longitudinal study of breast cancer patients and their principal caregivers. *Canadian Medical Association Journal* **170(12)**, 1795–801; (2001) **185(2)**, 294–9.

Hampl, M., Sarajuuri, H., Wentzensen, N., Bender, H.G. and Kueppers, V. (2006) Effect of human papillomavirus vaccines on vulvar, vaginal, and anal intraepithelial lesions and vulvar cancer. *Obstetric Gynecology* **108(6)**, 1361–8.

Havrilesky, L.J., Maxwell, G.L., Chan, J.K. and Myers, E.R. (2009) Cost effectiveness of a test to detect metastases for endometrial cancer. *Gynaecology Oncology* **12(3)**, 526–30.

Havrilesky, L.J., Secord, A.A., Kulasingam, S. and Myers, E. (2007) Management of platinum-sensitive recurrent ovarian cancer: a cost-effectiveness analysis. *Gynaecology Oncology* **107(2)**, 211–8.

Hensley, M.L., Dowell, J., Herndon, J.E. et al. (2005) Economic outcomes of breast cancer survivorship: CALGB study 79804. *Breast Cancer Research Treatment* **91(2)**, 153–61.

Hewitt, M., Breen, N. and Devesa, S. (1999) Cancer prevalence and survivorship issues: analyses of the 1992 National Health Interview Survey. *Journal of National Cancer Institute* **91(17)**, 1480–6.

Insinga, R.P., Dasbach, E.J. and Elbasha, E.H. (2005) Assessing the annual economic burden of preventing and treating anogenital human papillomavirus-related disease in the US: analytic framework and review of the literature. *Pharmacoeconomics* **23(11)**, 1107–22.

Insinga, R.P., Ye, X., Singhal, K. and Carides, G.W. (2008) Healthcare resource use and costs associated with cervical, vaginal and vulvar cancers in a large US health plan. *Gynaecology Oncology* **111(2)**, 188–96.

Joura, E.A., Losch, A., Haider-Angeler, M.G., Breitenecker, G. and Leodolter, S. (2000) Trends in vulvar neoplasia. Increasing incidence of vulvar intraepithelial neoplasia and squamous cell carcinoma of the vulva in young women. *Journal of Reproductive Medicine* **45(8)**, 613–5.

Judson, P.L., Habermann, E.B., Baxter, N.N., Durham, S.B. and Virnig, B.A. (2006) Trends in the incidence of invasive and *in situ* vulvar carcinoma. *Obstetric Gynecology* **107(5)**, 1018–22.

Karnon, J., Kerr, G.R., Jack, W., Papo, N.L. and Cameron, D.A. (2007) Health care costs for the treatment of breast cancer recurrent events: estimates from a UK-based patient-level analysis. *British Journal of Cancer* **97(4)**, 479–85.

Kenny, P., King, L.M., Shiell, A. et al. (2000) Early stage breast cancer: costs and quality of life one year after treatment by mastectomy or conservative surgery and radiation therapy. *The Breast* **9**, 37–44.

Kwon, J.S., Carey, M.S., Goldie, S.J. and Kim, J.J. (2007) Cost-effectiveness analysis of treatment strategies for Stage I and II endometrial cancer. *Journal of Obstetric Gynaecology of Canada* **29(2)**, 131–9.

Lauzier, S., Maunsell, E., De Koninck, M., Drolet, M., Hebert-Croteau, N., Robert, J. (2005) Conceptualization and sources of costs from breast cancer: findings from patient and caregiver focus groups. *Psychooncology* **14(5)**, 35–60.

Luoto, R., Raitanen, J., Pukkala, E. and Anttila, A. (2004) Effect of hysterectomy on incidence trends of endometrial and cervical cancer in Finland 1953–2010. *British Journal of Cancer* **90(9)**, 1756–9.

Main, C., Bojke, L., Griffin, S. et al. (2006) Topotecan, pegylated liposomal doxorubicin hydrochloride and paclitaxel for second-line or subsequent treatment of advanced ovarian cancer: a systematic review and economic evaluation. *Health Technology Assessment* **10(9)**, 1–132, iii–iv.

Maunsell, E., Drolet, M., Brisson, J., Brisson, C., Masse, B. and Deschenes, L. (2004) Work situation after breast cancer: results from a population-based study. *Journal of National Cancer Institute* **15: 96(24)**, 1813–22.

Max, W., Rice, D.P., Sung, H.Y., Michel, M., Breuer, W. and Zhang, X. (2003) The economic burden of gynecologic cancers in California, 1998. *Gynaecology Oncology* **88(2)**, 96–103.

McGuire, W.P., Hoskins, W.J., Brady, M.F. et al. (1996) Cyclophosphamide and cisplatin compared with paclitaxel and cisplatin in patients with stage III and stage IV ovarian cancer. *New England Journal of Medicine* **334(1)**, 1–6.

McKoy, J.M., Fitzner, K.A., Edwards, B.J. et al. (2007) Cost considerations in the management of cancer in the older patient. *Oncology* **21(7)**, 851–7.

Menon, U., Gentry-Maharaj, A., Hallett, R. et al. (2009) Sensitivity and specificity of multimodal and ultrasound screening for ovarian cancer, and stage distribution of detected cancers: results of the prevalence screen of the UK Collaborative Trial of Ovarian Cancer Screening (UKCTOCS). *Lancet Oncology* **10**, 10.

Moller, H., Fairley, L., Coupland, V. et al. (2007) The future burden of cancer in England: incidence and numbers of new patients in 2020. *British Journal of Cancer* **96(9)**, 1484–8.

Moolgavkar, S.H., Stevens, R.G. and Lee, J.A. (1979) Effect of age on incidence of breast cancer in females. *Journal of National Cancer Institute* **62(3)**, 493–501.

Morice, P., Levy-Piedbois, C., Ajaj, S. et al. (2001) Value and cost evaluation of routine follow-up for patients with clinical stage I/II endometrial cancer. *European Journal of Cancer* **37(8)**, 985–90.

NHMRC National Health and Medical Research Council (2004) *Clinical Practice Guidelines for the Management of Women with Epithelial Ovarian Cancer*. Canberra: Commonwealth Government.

Parkin, D.M. and Bray, F. (2006) Chapter 2: The burden of HPV-related cancers. *Vaccine* **24(Suppl 3)**, S3/11–25.

Parkin, D.M., Whelan, S.L., Ferlay, J. and Storm, H. (2005) *Cancer Incidence in Five Continents*. Lyon: IARC Press. Available from: http://www-dep.iarc.fr/

Parkin, D.M. (2009) Is the recent fall in incidence of post-menopausal breast cancer in UK related to changes in use of hormone replacement therapy? *European Journal of Cancer* February 11.

Parkin, D.M., Ferlay, J., Hamdi-Cherif, M. et al. (2003) *Cancer in Africa: Epidemiology and Prevention*. Lyon: IARC.

Parkin, D.M. (2006) The global health burden of infection-associated cancers in the year 2002. *International Journal of Cancer* **118(12)**, 3030–44.

Partridge, E., Kreimer, A.R., Greenleem, R.T. et al. (2009) Results from four rounds of ovarian cancer screening in a randomized trial. *Obstetric Gynaecology* **113(4)**, 775–82.

Pignata, S., Scambia, G., Savarese, A. et al. (2009) Carboplatin and pegylated liposomal doxorubicin for advanced ovarian cancer: preliminary activity results of the MITO-2 phase III trial. *Oncology* **76(1)**, 49–54.

Radice, D. and Redaelli, A. (2003) Breast cancer management: quality-of-life and cost considerations. *Pharmacoeconomics* **21(6)**, 383–96.

Rawlins, M. (2007) Paying for modern cancer care: a global perspective. *Lancet Oncology* **8(9)**, 749–51.

Rieslag, L.A.G., Melbert, D., Krapcho, M. et al. (2005) *SEER Cancer Statistics Review, 1975–2005*. Available from: http://seer.cancer.gov/csr/1975_2005.

Rocconi, R.P., Case, A.S., Straughn, J.M., Estes, J.M. and Partridge, E.E. (2006) Role of chemo-therapy for patients with recurrent platinum-resistant advanced epithelial ovarian cancer: A cost-effectiveness analysis. *Cancer* **107(3)**, 536–43.

Rogoza, R.M., Ferko, N., Bentley, J. et al. (2008) Optimization of primary and secondary cervical cancer prevention strategies in an era of cervical cancer vaccination: a multi-regional health economic analysis. *Vaccine* **26(Suppl 5)**, F46–58.

Sankaranarayanan, R. and Ferlay, J. (2006) Worldwide burden of gynaecological cancer: the size of the problem. *Best Practice Research. Clinical Obstetric Gynaecology* **20(2)**, 207–25.

Sant, M., Allemani, C., Santaquilani, M., Knijn, A., Marchesi, F. and Capocaccia, R. (2009) EUROCARE-4. Survival of cancer patients diagnosed in 1995–1999. Results and commentary. *European Journal of Cancer* **45(6)**, 931–91.

Sant, M., Allemani, C., Berrino F. et al. (2004) Breast carcinoma survival in Europe and the United States. *Cancer* **100(4)**, 715–22.

Saraiya, M., Watson, M., Wu, X. et al. (2008) Incidence of *in situ* and invasive vulvar cancer in the US, 1998–2003. *Cancer* **113(10 Suppl)**, 2865–72.

Satariano, W.A. and DeLorenze, G.N. (1996) The likelihood of returning to work after breast cancer. *Public Health Report* **111(3)**, 236–41.

Sevilla, C., Moatti, J-P., Julian-Reynier, C. et al. (2002) Testing for BRCA1 mutations: a cost-effectiveness analysis. *European Journal of Human Genetics* **10(10)**, 599–606.

Shapiro, S., Coleman, E.A., Broeders, M. et al. (1998) Breast cancer screening programmes in 22 countries: current policies, administration and guidelines. International Breast Cancer Screening Network (IBSN) and the European Network of Pilot Projects for Breast Cancer Screening. *International Journal of Epidemiology* **27(5)**, 735–42.

Shih, Y.C. and Halpern, M.T. (2008) Economic evaluations of medical care interventions for cancer patients: how, why, and what does it mean? *CA Cancer Journal of Clin.* **58(4)**, 231–44.

Skjeldestad, F.E. and Rannestad, T. (2009) Urinary incontinence and quality of life in long-term gynecological cancer survivors: a population-based cross-sectional study. *Acta Obstetric Gynaecology Scandinavia* **88(2)**, 192–2.

Smith, C.L., Kricker, A. and Armstrong, B.K. (1998) Breast cancer mortality trends in Australia: 1921–1994. *Medical Journal of Australia* **168(1)**, 11–4. *Obstetric Gynaecology Scandinavia* **88(2)**, 192–9.

Srodon, M., Stoler, M.H., Baber, G.B. and Kurman, R.J. (2006) The distribution of low and high-risk HPV types in vulvar and vaginal intraepithelial neoplasia (VIN and VaIN). *American Journal of Surgical Pathology* **30(12)**, 1513–8.

Stewart, D.E., Cheung, A.M., Duff, S. et al. (2001) Long-term breast cancer survivors: confidentiality, disclosure, effects on work and insurance. *Psychooncology* **10(3)**, 259–63.

Stewart, D.J., Dahrouge, S., Coyle, D. and Evans, W.K. (1999) Costs of treating and preventing nausea and vomiting in patients receiving chemotherapy. *Journal of Clinical Oncology* **17(1)**, 344–51.

Szucs, T.D., Wyss, P. and Dedes, K.J. (2003) Cost-effectiveness studies in ovarian cancer. *International Journal of Gynaecological Cancer* **13(Suppl 2)**, 212–9.

Taplin, S.H., Barlow, W., Urban, N. et al. (1995) Stage, age, comorbidity, and direct costs of colon, prostate, and breast cancer care. *Journal of National Cancer Institute* **87(6)**, 417–26.

Tjalma, W.A., van Dam, P.A., Makar, A.P. and Cruickshank, D.J. (2004) The clinical value and the cost-effectiveness of follow-up in endometrial cancer patients. *International Journal of Gynaecological Cancer* **14(5)**, 931–7.

Vainio, H. and Bianchini, F. (eds) (2007) *Breast Cancer Screening*. Lyon: IARC Press.

Weiss, N.S., Szekely, D.R. and Austin, D.F. (1976) Increasing incidence of endometrial cancer in the United States. *New England Journal of Medicine* **294(23)**, 1259–62.

Will, B.P., Berthelot, J.M., Le Petit, C., Tomiak, E.M., Verma, S. and Evans, W.K. (2000) Estimates of the lifetime costs of breast cancer treatment in Canada. *European Journal of Cancer* **36(6)**, 724–35.

Wu, X., Matanoski, G., Chen, V.W., Saraiya, M., et al. (2008) Descriptive epidemiology of vaginal cancer incidence and survival by race, ethnicity, and age in the United States. *Cancer* **113 (10 Suppl)**, 2873–82.

Yang, L., Parkin, D.M., Li, L. and Chen, Y. (2003) Time trends in cancer mortality in China: 1987–1999. *International Journal of Cancer* **106(5)**, 771–83.□

Chapter 3

Pathology and Staging of Major Types of Gynaecological and Breast Cancers

Neeta Singh and Rachel Howitt

Learning points

At the end of this chapter the reader will have an understanding of:
- The importance of the histopathologist in multidisciplinary team
- The different staging frameworks used for specific cancers
- The relationship between staging and prognosis

Introduction

Histopathology refers to the microscopic examination of tissue in order to study the manifestations of disease. Specifically, in clinical medicine, histopathology refers to the examination of a biopsy or surgical specimen by a pathologist, after the specimen has been processed and histological sections have been mounted onto glass slides. The tissue is prepared using staining techniques to allow the histopathologist to view the cells clearly. From this examination the oncologist can be advised on the extent and nature of the disease and also whether surgical margins are clear. Surgical margins relate to the distance between the tumour and the normal skin as viewed under the microscope. The importance of the histopathology department and the histopathologist cannot be stressed enough. Their careful consideration to the staging of disease offers the oncologist the opportunity to set realistic goals and treatment options. The last decade has seen a specialisation of histopathologists, but they remain in short supply. They are valued and core members of the multidisciplinary team (MDT). This chapter outlines the staging of cancer and offers a link to prognosis.

Women's Cancers, First Edition. Edited by Alison Keen and Elaine Lennan.
© 2011 Blackwell Publishing Ltd. Published 2011 by Blackwell Publishing Ltd.

Cancer of the cervix

The cervix is the lower narrow end of the uterus, which leads to the vagina. Cervical cancer is the second-most common malignancy in women worldwide, after breast cancer, and remains the leading cause of cancer related deaths for women in developing countries. Cervical cancer usually develops slowly over many years. Before carcinoma develops in the cervix, the cells lining the cervix go through precancerous changes known as cervical intraepithelial neoplasia (CIN). These changes, if left untreated, may develop into cancer. In the UK the incidence of cervical cancer has declined steadily since the introduction of the NHS Cervical Screening Programme. Cervical screening aims to detect abnormal cells in cervical smears and provide treatment before the development of cancer. The abnormal epithelium can be eradicated by local measures, such as diathermy large loop excision of the transformation zone (LLETZ).

Cervical cytology is a simple, safe, non-invasive method of detecting precancerous or dyskaryotic cells. In the UK women are screened every 3–5 years from 25–65 years of age.

Symptoms

Early cervical cancer may not show any signs or symptoms. Common symptoms include:

- Abnormal vaginal bleeding, which may be intermenstrual bleeding (IMB), post-coital bleeding (PCB), or post-menopausal bleeding (PMB).
- Unpleasant smelling vaginal discharge
- Discomfort or pain during sexual intercourse (dyspareunia). There are many more common benign conditions that may cause dyspareunia.

Risk factors

Infection with Human Papilloma Virus (HPV) is the most important risk factor in the development of cervical cancer. However, all women with HPV infection do not develop cervical cancer. The virus is sexually transmitted and known to be causative in vulval and cervical condyloma acuminata (genital warts), vulval, vaginal and cervical carcinomas. More than 100 strains of HPV are described, most of which do not cause significant disease in humans. However, some subtypes – 16, 18, 31 and 33 – are confirmed as causative agents in cervical cancer. This group of 'high risk' HPV types have been found in close to 100% of all cervical cancers.

Other possible risk factors include the following:

- Early age at first intercourse
- Multiple sexual partners
- Increased parity
- A male partner with multiple previous sexual partners
- Smoking

- Oral contraceptive use
- Genital infections such as Chlamydia and herpes
- Weakened immune system

Classification

The major histological subtypes of invasive cervical cancer include:

- Squamous cell carcinoma (~85%)
- Adenocarcinoma
- Adenosquamous carcinoma
- Small cell carcinoma
- Neuroendocrine carcinoma

Rarely non-carcinoma malignancies, such as lymphoma and melanoma, may occur in the cervix.

Table 3.1   Staging of cancer of the cervix as Federation of Gynaecology and Obstetrics (FIGO 2009).

Stage 0	Full thickness involvement of the epithelium without invasion into the stroma (carcinoma *in situ*)

Stage I	Limited to the cervix:
	    IA – no visible lesion, diagnosed by microscopy
	        IA1 – stromal invasion <3 mm in depth and 7 mm
	            or less in horizontal spread
	        IA2 – stromal invasion between 3 and 5 mm with horizontal spread
	            of 7 mm or less
	    IB – histologically invasive carcinoma confined to the cervix and greater
	        than stage 1A2.
	        IB1 – clinically visible lesions <4 mm in greatest dimension
	        IB2 – clinically visible lesion of >4 mm in greatest dimension

Stage II	Carcinoma invades beyond the cervix but not onto the pelvic wall. Carcinoma involves the vagina but not the lower third:
	    IIA – without parametrial invasion
	        IIA1 – clinically visible lesion <4 cm in greatest dimension
	        IIA2 – clinically visible lesion of >4 cm in greatest dimension
	    IIB – with obvious parametrial invasion

Stage III	Carcinoma has extended to the pelvic wall/involves the lower third of the vagina and/or causes hydronephrosis or non-functioning kidney:
	    IIIA – tumour involves lower third of the vagina, with no extension
	        to the pelvic wall
	    IIIB – extension to the pelvic wall and/or hydronephrosis and
	        or non-functioning kidney

Stage IV	Carcinoma has extended beyond the true pelvis or has involved the mucosa of the bladder or rectum. This stage also includes those with metastatic dissemination:
	    IVA – spread of the growth to adjacent organs
	    IVB – spread to distant organs

Prognosis and treatment

The outcome or prognosis in invasive cervical cancer depends on two factors:

(1) Extent of local disease (stage)
(2) The presence or absence of deposits in draining lymph nodes.

Other factors of prognostic significance are the histological type of cancer (adenocarcinoma has a poorer prognosis than squamous carcinoma), tumour grade and presence of vascular permeation.

Treatment is based on:

- Stage of the cancer
- Size of the tumour
- The patient's desire to have children
- The patient's age

The treatment options for cervical cancer include surgery, radiotherapy and chemotherapy. Factors that determine the type of treatment include the age of the patient and stage of cancer. These may be used alone or in combination depending on the stage of cancer.

Micro-invasive cancer (stage IA) is usually treated by hysterectomy.

Stage IA2 cancer is treated by total hysterectomy with removal of pelvic lymph nodes (Wertheim's hysterectomy or radical hysterectomy).

For patients who desire to remain fertile, the surgical options include:

- Cone biopsy (LLETZ)
- Laser therapy
- Cold coagulation
- Radical trachelectomy (removal of the cervix, part of the vagina and pelvic lymph nodes)

Stages IB and IIA cancers of less than 4 cm can be treated with radiotherapy alone or radical hysterectomy followed by radiotherapy and or chemotherapy.

Stages IB2 and IIA cancers of more than 4 cm can be treated with radiation therapy and cisplatin-based chemotherapy, hysterectomy with adjuvant radiation or chemotherapy followed by hysterectomy.

Advanced stage tumours (stages IIB–IVA) are treated with radiation therapy and cisplatin-based chemotherapy.

Table 3.2   5-year survival according to the stage of the cervical cancer (Cancer Research UK).

Stage	5-year survival
IA	95%
IB	80–90%
II	75%
III	<50%
IV	<15%

Prevention

National Health Services Cervical Screening Programme (NHSCSP)

The NHSCSP has been successful in considerably reducing the incidence of cervical cancer, by regularly screening women at risk.

All women aged between 25–64 years are offered cervical smears on the NHSCSP. The aim of the programme is to detect abnormal cells (CIN) in smears and provide early treatment before the development of invasive cancer. Women are invited for their first smear at 25 years of age. Screening is every 3 years from 25–49 years and every 5 years from 50–64 years.

CIN is graded as CIN I, CIN 2 or CIN 3, depending on the thickness of the cervical epithelium replaced by atypical cells. Abnormal epithelial changes occur at the cervical transformation zone and may extend to involve the cells of the endocervical canal. In about 10% cases, atypia of the endocervical epithelium is seen, when it is termed cervical glandular intraepithelial neoplasia (CGIN).

HPV vaccine

Immunisation with vaccination against HPV infection is aimed at girls before they become sexually active.

In the UK, HPV vaccination was introduced into the national immunisation programme from September 2008, for girls aged 12–13. This was followed by a 2-year catch-up campaign beginning in autumn 2009. By the end of the catch-up campaign, all girls under 18 were offered the HPV vaccine.

Cancer of the endometrium

Endometrial or uterine cancer is the most common invasive cancer of the female genital tract. At one time it was far less common than cervical cancer, but earlier detection and eradication of CIN and an increase in endometrial cancers in younger women has reversed this ratio. However, in developing countries, it still remains much less common than cervical cancer.

The peak incidence of endometrial cancer is 55–65 years of age. It is uncommon in women younger than 40.

Signs and symptoms

- Abnormal uterine bleeding
- IMB in pre-menopausal women
- Vaginal bleeding in post-menopausal women
- Lower abdominal pain or pelvic cramping
- Thin white or clear discharge in post-menopausal women

Risk factors

- High levels of oestrogen (either as replacement therapy or produced endogenously, e.g. polycystic ovary syndrome)
- Endometrial hyperplasia
- Obesity (increases endogenous oestrogen)
- Diabetes
- Hypertension
- Nulliparity
- Infertility
- Early menarche (onset of menstruation)
- Late menopause (cessation of menstruation)
- Endometrial polyps
- Tamoxifen treatment for breast cancer
- Pelvic radiation therapy

Classification

Most endometrial cancers are adenocarcinomas, originating from the endometrial glands. There are different microscopic subtypes of endometrial carcinoma, including the common endometrioid type, in which the cancer cells grow in a pattern reminiscent of normal endometrium, and the more aggressive papillary serous and clear cell types.

Two pathogenic groups have been identified:

- *Type 1*: These cancers occur most commonly in pre- and peri-menopausal women, often with a history of unopposed oestrogen exposure or endometrial hyperplasia. These are usually low grade, early invasive endometrioid carcinomas and carry a good prognosis.
- *Type 2*: These cancers occur in older post-menopausal women and are not associated with increased exposure to oestrogen. They are typically high-grade endometrioid, papillary serous or clear cell carcinomas, and carry a poor prognosis.

In contrast to endometrial carcinomas, the uncommon endometrial stromal sarcomas are cancers that originate in the non-glandular connective tissue of the endometrium.

Uterine carcinosarcoma or malignant mixed Mullerian tumour is a rare form of uterine cancer, which contains malignant glandular (epithelial) and stromal (sarcomatous) components.

Cases in various stages can be sub-grouped into three grades:

- *Grade 1* – Well differentiated adenocarcinoma with <5% solid growth pattern
- *Grade 2* – Differentiated adenocarcinoma with <50% solid growth pattern
- *Grade 3* – Predominantly solid or entirely undifferentiated carcinoma. Includes papillary serous and clear cell carcinoma.

Table 3.3 Staging of cancer of the endometrium (FIGO 2009).

Stage I	Tumour confined to corpus uteri:
	  IA – no or less than half myometrial invasion
	  IB – tumour involvement equal or more than half the depth
	    of the myometrium

Stage II	Carcinoma invades cervical stroma, but does not extend beyond the uterus

Stage III	Local and regional spread of the tumour:
	  IIIA – tumour invades the stroma of the corpus uteri and/or adenexae
	  IIIB – vaginal and/or parametrial involvement
	  IIIC – metastases to pelvis and/or para-aortic lymph nodes
	    IIIC1 – positive pelvic nodes
	    IIIC2 – positive para-aortic lymph nodes with or without
	      positive pelvic lymph nodes

Stage IV	Invasion of bladder and/or bowel mucosa and/or distant metastases:
	  IVA – tumour invasion of bowel and/ or bladder mucosa
	    IVB – distant metastases, including intra-abdominal and/or inguinal
	      lymph nodes

Prognosis

The prognosis depends on the clinical stage of the disease at the time of diagnosis and its histological grade and type. About 80% women have stage I disease clinically and have well to moderately differentiated endometrioid carcinomas. Surgery alone or in combination with irradiation gives about 90% 5-year survival in stage I (grade 1–2) disease.

The 5-year survival drops to about 75% for grade 3/Stage I and to 50% or less for stages II and III endometrial carcinoma.

Papillary serous and clear cell carcinomas have a propensity for extra-uterine (lymphatic or transtubal) spread, even when confined to the endometrium. Overall, fewer than 50% of patients with these tumours are alive 3 years after diagnosis and 35% after 5 years. If peritoneal cytology and adnexal histological examination are negative, the 5-year survival of stage I disease is approximately 80–85%. The additional advantage of prophylactic radiation and chemotherapy in stage I disease is unclear.

Ovarian neoplasms

Primary tumours of the ovary may originate from any of the normal constituents of the ovary. Accordingly they are divided into those derived from the surface epithelium (70%), those derived from the sex-cord and stromal cells (10%) and those derived from germ cells (20%).

In addition to primary tumours, the ovary is frequently involved in metastatic disease from other sites.

Table 3.4 5-year survival according to the stage of ovarian cancer (Cancer Research UK).

Stage	5-year survival
I	80–85%
II	50%
III	30%
IV	<5%

Table 3.5 Staging of cancer of the ovary (FIGO-Pecorelli et al. 1998).

Stage I	Limited to one or both ovaries: IA – involves one ovary; capsule intact; no tumour on ovarian surface; no malignant cells in ascites or peritoneal washings IB – involves both ovaries; capsule intact; no tumour on ovarian surface; negative washings IC – tumour limited to ovaries with any of the following: capsule ruptured, tumour on ovarian surface, positive washings
Stage II	Pelvic extension or implants: IIA – extension or implants onto uterus or fallopian tube; negative washings IIB – extension or implants onto other pelvic structures; negative washings IIC – pelvic extension or implants with positive peritoneal washings
Stage III	Microscopic peritoneal implants outside the pelvis; or limited to the pelvis with extension to the small bowel or omentum: IIIA – microscopic peritoneal metastasis beyond pelvis IIIB – macroscopic peritoneal metastases beyond pelvis <2 cm in size IIIC – peritoneal metastases beyond pelvis >2 cm or lymph node metastases
Stage IV	Distant metastases to the liver or outside the peritoneal cavity

Although some of the specific tumours have distinctive features and are hormonally active, most are non-functional and tend to produce relatively mild symptoms until they have reached a large size. Malignant tumours have often spread outside the ovary by the time a definitive diagnosis is made. Some of these tumours, principally epithelial tumours, may be bilateral.

The most common symptoms include abdominal pain and distension, abnormal vaginal bleeding, and urinary and gastrointestinal tract symptoms due to compression or invasion by the tumour.

Malignant tumours of the ovary spread locally, particularly to the peritoneum, causing ascites as a common complication.

Risk factors

Risk factors for ovarian cancer are much less clear than for other genital tumours, but nulliparity, family history and heritable mutations play a role in tumour development.

There is a higher frequency of carcinoma in unmarried women and in married women with low parity.

Gonadal dysgenesis in children is associated with a higher risk of ovarian cancer.

Women 40–59 years of age, who have taken oral contraceptives or undergone tubal ligation, have a reduced risk of developing ovarian cancer.

Genetic factors

The breast cancer gene 1 (BRCA1) and breast cancer gene 2 (BRCA2) are most often associated with an increased risk of hereditary breast and ovarian cancer syndrome (HBOC). These are tumour suppressor genes, which code for proteins that suppress tumour formation by limiting cell growth. Mutations in these genes result in loss of ability to restrict tumour growth and, as a result, cancer may develop.

It is estimated that mutations in the BRCA1 gene account for almost 75% of families with hereditary ovarian cancer, and mutations in the BRCA2 gene account for about 15% of families with hereditary ovarian cancer. Women with BRCA1 or BRCA2 genes have a 15–40% lifetime risk of ovarian cancer and 50–85% lifetime risk of breast cancer.

Men with BRCA1 and BRCA2 gene mutations have an increased risk of prostate cancer and breast cancer.

Mutations in the BRCA2 gene are associated with an increased risk of other types of cancer, including melanoma and pancreatic cancer.

Hereditary non-polyposis colorectal cancer (HNPCC), or Lynch syndrome type II, is associated with an increased risk of developing ovarian and endometrial cancer.

Classification

Epithelial cancers

The epithelial ovarian tumours are derived from the surface epithelium, which originates from the embryonic coelomic epithelium. These may differentiate into a variety of tissues:

- Endocervical differentiation – *Mucinous* ovarian tumours
- Tubal differentiation – *Serous* ovarian tumours
- Endometrial differentiation – *Endometrioid* and clear cell carcinoma
- Transitional differentiation – *Brenner* tumour
- *Undifferentiated carcinoma*

On histological examination, epithelial tumours are further classified as benign, borderline (proliferating) or malignant, according to their biological behaviour.

Benign tumours are lined by a single layer of well differentiated and normally oriented epithelial cells. If papillary projections are present, they are of vascularised fibrous stroma lined by a single layer of the same cells.

Borderline tumours are highly proliferative neoplasms. in which the epithelium shows stratification with nuclear atypia. Papillae, if present, show a complex architecture.

The most important defining criteria for this group are the absence of stromal invasion. These lesions have a better prognosis than their invasive counterparts. These tumours have an overall 5-year survival rate of 90% and a 15-year survival rate of 70%. With unilateral borderline tumours, there is a 15% chance of another tumour developing in the contralateral ovary in the following 5–7 years.

Malignant tumours exhibit a more complex growth, with severe nuclear atypia with infiltration or frank effacement of the underlying stroma with solid tumour.

Ca 125 is a high molecular weight glycoprotein expressed by Mullerian epithelium. Its plasma concentration is increased in 80–85% of serous and endometrioid epithelial tumours.

Role of cytology in ovarian cancer

The main role of cytology in the management of ovarian carcinoma is the detection of malignant cells in the peritoneal cavity. Unfortunately, most patients present with stages III or IV disease, with tumours spread outside the pelvis. Peritoneal washing cytology (PWC) is an important component of the FIGO staging: a positive finding modifies stages I and II tumours to stages IC and IIC (Cibas 2003). This technique is useful in initial surgical staging. Serous and endometrioid carcinomas are more often positive than other carcinomas. A high positive rate is related to advanced stage and worse prognosis.

Ascitic fluid cytology is also used in advanced inoperable cancers for confirmation of the presence of malignant cells, prior to commencing chemotherapy.

Prognosis and treatment

Surgical excision of either part of or the whole ovary is the primary form of treatment for benign and borderline epithelial tumours.

Carcinomas require bilateral salpingo-oophorectomy, with total abdominal hysterectomy and omentectomy. It is important to examine the peritoneal cavity during the course of the operation and to biopsy selected sites for proper staging and future therapy. Patients with stage IC and stage II carcinomas are given post-operative chemotherapy. Platinum-based combination chemotherapy is most commonly used and has been shown to enhance survival.

As a result of rapid growth rate and lack of early symptoms, the prognosis of ovarian cancers is poor. The overall survival rate is approximately 35% at 5 years, 28% at 10 years and 15% at 25 years. Factors influencing prognosis are:

- The most important prognostic factor is the presence and extent of spread outside the ovary (FIGO stage)
- Younger patients have a better outcome.
- Patients with BRCA1 mutation seem to have a favourable outcome.
- The presence of ascites is a bad prognostic sign.

- Borderline tumour vs invasive carcinoma. The prognosis for borderline tumours is very good, even in the presence of peritoneal involvement or micro-invasion.
- Tumour grade (degree of differentiation) and type. Clear cell and mucinous tumours behave more aggressively.
- Over expression of Her2/neu proto-oncogene is associated with aggressive behaviour.

Germ cell tumours

About 20% of all ovarian neoplasms are germ cell tumours. Most are benign cystic teratomas, but the remainder, which occur more commonly in children and young adults, have a higher incidence of malignant behaviour. The classification of these tumours is similar to their counterparts occurring in the testis.

Teratoma

These are divided into:

(1) *Mature (benign) cystic teratomas or dermoid cyst* – These are the most common germ cell tumours, accounting for about 10% of all ovarian neoplasms. The ovary is replaced by a cyst lined by skin and skin appendage structures. Teeth, bone, respiratory tract tissue, mature neural tissue, fat and smooth muscle are common types of tissue seen. These lesions are benign, but may be bilateral in 10% cases. About 1% of the dermoids may undergo malignant transformation.

(2) *Immature (malignant) teratoma* – These are rare tumours seen mainly in adolescents. As in benign teratomas they are composed of a variety of tissue embryonal tissue or other types of germ cell tumours may be present, classifying the tumour as 'malignant immature teratoma' or 'mixed malignant germ cell tumour', respectively.

Immature teratomas grow rapidly and frequently penetrate the capsule with local spread or metastases.

(3) *Monodermal or specialised teratomas* – This is a rare group of tumours, the most common of which is struma ovarii composed entirely of mature thyroid tissue. These tumours may produce thyroxine. The other common type of monodermal teratoma is a carcinoid tumour.

(4) *Dysgerminoma* is the ovarian counterpart of the testicular seminoma. These are relatively uncommon tumours and account for about 2% of all ovarian cancers. All dysgerminomas are malignant, but the degree of cytological atypia is variable. Only about one-third are aggressive. Treatment is surgical excision with or without radiotherapy, depending on whether the tumour is confined to the ovary or has penetrated the capsule. The overall survival rate is over 80%.

(5) *Yolk sac tumour* is a rare, highly malignant form of germ cell tumour. Most patients are children or young women presenting with abdominal pain and a rapidly developing pelvic mass. Similar to the yolk sac, the tumour is rich in α-etoprotein (AFP) and α1-antitrypsin. Previously thought to be uniformly fatal within 2 years of diagnosis,

the outcome of these tumours has improved greatly with the use of combination chemotherapy.

Serum levels of AFP are used as a tool for monitoring tumour activity.

(6) *Choriocarcinoma* is a rare form of germ cell tumour composed of trophoblastic cells. Most ovarian choriocarcinomas occur in combination with other germ cell tumours. Pure choriocarcinomas are extremely rare. These are very aggressive tumours with a propensity for vascular invasion and widespread metastasis.

These tumours produce βHCG, which may be used as a tumour marker.

Sex-cord stromal tumours

These ovarian neoplasms are derived from the ovarian stroma, which in turn is derived from the sex cords of the embryonic gonads. Because the undifferentiated gonadal mesenchyme eventually produces structures of specific cell type in both male (Sertoli and Leydig) and female (theca) gonads, tumours resembling all of these cell types can be identified in the ovary. As the normal function of some of these cells is production of oestrogen (theca cells) or androgen (Leydig cells), their corresponding tumours may be feminising or masculinising. The detailed classification of these tumours is complex, and the major groups include:

- *Fibroma/thecoma* – these may show a variable mixture of fibroblasts and theca cells. The presence of theca cells may be responsible for oestrogenic manifestations and may give rise to abnormal uterine bleeding, endometrial hyperplasia or endometrial cancer.
- *Granulosa cell tumour* – this can occur at any age and all cases are potentially malignant. These tumours tend to produce large amounts of oestrogen and may present with precocious sexual development in pre-pubertal girls. In adult women they may be associated with endometrial hyperplasia, cystic disease of the breast and endometrial carcinoma. Occasionally granulosa cell tumours may produce androgens and present with masculinising features.

    Elevated serum levels of inhibin have been associated with granulosa cell tumours. This biomarker may be useful for identifying granulosa and other sex cord stromal tumours, and for monitoring patients undergoing therapy.
- *Sertoli-Leydig cell tumours (androblastomas)* – are very rare tumours, which resemble the cells of the testis at various stages of development. They commonly produce masculinisation, but some may produce oestrogen.

Metastatic tumours

The most common sites of origin of metastatic tumours to the ovary are from the breast and gastrointestinal tract. Krukenberg's tumour is a classical example of metastatic carcinoma from the stomach, which is usually bilateral and composed of mucin secreting signet ring type cells.

Cancer of the vulva

Vulval carcinoma is an uncommon malignant neoplasm accounting for about 4% of all gynaecological cancers. Mean age at presentation is 60–74 years. Eighty-five percent of vulval malignancies are squamous cell carcinomas; the remainder are basal cell carcinoma, melanoma and adenocarcinoma.

Risk factors include number of lifetime sexual partners, cigarette smoking, immunodeficiency and genital granulomatous disease (lymphogranuloma venereum and granuloma inguinale).

On the basis of pathogenesis and clinical presentation, vulval squamous cell carcinoma is divided into two groups.

The first group occurs in younger women and is associated with cancer related (high risk) HPV infection, and frequently co-exists with or is preceded by precancerous change called vulval intraepithelial neoplasia (VIN). These lesions usually present as white or pigmented plaques on the vulva. VIN is frequently multicentric and 10–30% are associated with primary squamous neoplasia in the cervix or vagina.

The second, more common, group occurs in older women, is not HPV related and occurs on a background of squamous cell hyperplasia and lichen sclerosus.

Table 3.6   Staging for cancer of the vulva (FIGO 2009).

Stage 0	Intraepithelial neoplasia (VIN3)
Stage I	Tumour confined to the vulva:
	IA – lesions 2 cm or less in size, confined to vulva or perineum and with stromal invasion of <1 mm, no nodal metastases
	IB – lesions >2 cm in size with stromal invasion >1 mm. Tumour confined to vulva and/or perineum. >2 cm in greatest dimension, confined to vulva or perineum with negative nodes
Stage II	Tumour of any size with extension to adjacent perineal structures (1/3 lower urethra, 1/3 lower vagina, anus) with negative nodes
Stage III	Tumour of any size with or without extension to adjacent perineal structures (1/3 lower urethra, 1/3 lower vagina, anus) with positive inguino-femoral lymph nodes:
	IIIA – with 1 lymph node metastasis of equal to or >5 mm or 1–2 lymph node metastases <5 mm
	IIIB – with 2 or more lymph node metastases equal to or >5 mm or 3 or more lymph node metastases <5 mm
	IIIC – with positive nodes with extracapsular spread
Stage IV	Tumour involves other regional (2/3 upper urethra, 2/3 upper vagina), or distant structures
	IVA – tumour invades any of: upper urethra, bladder mucosa, rectal mucosa, pelvic bone, or Fixed or ulcerated inguino-femoral lymph nodes
	IVB – any distant metastasis including pelvic lymph nodes

Signs and symptoms

Vulval cancer typically develops over a few years and does not cause early symptoms. Presenting symptoms may include:

- A lump or ulceration in the vulva
- Itching or irritation
- Bleeding and discharge
- Dysuria and dyspareunia

Prognosis and treatment

Factors influencing prognosis are the tumour size, extent of local direct invasive spread at the time of diagnosis and presence or absence of lymph node involvement.

The overall reported 5-year survival rate in patients treated for vulval squamous cell carcinoma is 50–75%.

The usual treatment for invasive carcinoma is radical vulvectomy with bilateral inguinal lymph node dissection. Iliac lymphadenectomy and pelvic exenteration are reserved for advanced cases. Conversely, early cases can be treated more conservatively with wide local excision.

Verrucous carcinomas a distinct variety of well-differentiated squamous cell carcinoma, which presents as a large warty growth that is difficult to distinguish from condyloma acuminata (viral wart) on biopsy material. These tumours are slow growing and locally invasive but almost never metastasise.

Cancer of the vagina

Vaginal carcinomas are uncommon tumours, occurring in elderly women and accounting for about 1% of all gynaecological malignancies. Ninety-five percent of these are squamous cell carcinomas, most of which are associated with HPV infection. The greatest risk factor is previous cervical or vulval cancer. Extension of cervical cancer to the vagina should be excluded before diagnosing a primary neoplasm.

Vaginal cancer grows insidiously and may remain asymptomatic, or they may present with irregular spotting or vaginal discharge.

Tumours occur more often in the upper part of the vagina and tend to metastasise to the pelvic lymph nodes; tumours from the lower part of the vagina tend to involve the inguinal lymph nodes.

Table 3.7   Staging of cancer of the vagina (Cancer Research UK).

Stage I	Tumour limited to vaginal wall
Stage II	Tumour involves sub-vaginal tissue, but has not spread to pelvic wall
Stage III	Tumour has extended to pelvic wall
Stage IV	Tumour has extended beyond the true pelvis or involves the mucosa of the bladder or rectum

Vaginal adenocarcinomas are rare but are of importance because of the increased frequency of clear cell adenocarcinoma in young women whose mothers had been treated with diethylstilbestrol (DES) during pregnancy.

Breast cancer pathology

Breast cancer is the most common malignancy in women in the UK. Approximately 45,000 new cases are diagnosed each year and account for 20% of all malignancies. Most patients who develop breast cancer are women over 50 years of age, who have reached the menopause, but breast cancer can develop at any age, and approximately 1 in 100 cases of breast cancer occur in men.

Prevention – NHS Breast Screening Programme

One in nine women will develop breast cancer during their lifetime. However, if the disease can be detected at an early stage there is a good chance of recovery. All women between 50 and 70 years of age are offered breast cancer screening, in the form of a mammogram, every 3 years, as part of the UK NHS Breast Screening Programme. In addition, women with two or more close relatives with breast cancer are eligible for breast mammography, or screening for the genes that increase the risk of breast cancer developing.

Diagnosis – the 'Triple Approach'

The 'Triple Approach' refers to the combination of clinical examination, radiological imaging and pathological assessment by fine needle aspiration cytology and/or needle core biopsy. Equal weighting should be given to each modality so that every case is diagnosed according to the most suspicious opinion.

The surgeon and radiologist assess the significance of the breast abnormality independently and classify their opinion as follows:

- Normal
- Benign
- Probably benign
- Probably malignant
- Malignant

Fine needle aspiration cytology and/or needle core biopsy is then used to further investigate the lesion.

Cytological findings are reported as follows:

- C1 – inadequate
- C2 – benign
- C3 – atypia probably benign
- C4 – suspicious of malignancy
- C5 – malignant

Histological examination of the needle core biopsy forms part of the assessment process for evaluating a breast lesion, but is not intended to provide a definitive diagnosis, although this is possible in the majority of cases. There are five reporting categories, but these are not all equivalent to those used in fine needle aspiration cytology:

- B1 – normal tissue
- B2 – benign lesion
- B3 – lesion of uncertain malignant potential
- B4 – suspicious
- B5 – malignant

These reporting categories are a histological assessment of the lesion. All case should be discussed at a MDT meeting, which allows the lesion to be assessed according to its clinical, radiological and histological appearances, and the appropriate management planned.

Risk factors

Female sex and age

Breast cancer is much more common in women than in men – less than 1% of all breast cancers occur in men.

The risk of cancer developing increases with increasing age. In fact, there is a marked increase between the ages of 40 and 50 years, but the highest incidence is in women aged 60–70 years.

Genetics and family history

First-degree relatives of breast cancer patients have a 1.2–3 times increased risk of breast cancer when compared to the general population. For first-degree relatives of pre-menopausal women with bilateral cancer, this risk is 9 times that of the general population.

A small proportion of all breast cancers (5–10%) are related to specific inherited gene mutations. Mutations of BRCA1 (on chromosome 17) and BRCA2 (on chromosome 13) are associated with an increased risk of both breast and ovarian cancer. The exact role of these genes in carcinogenesis is still being investigated, but they are thought to be involved in DNA repair.

A third gene, TP53, is also associated with an increased risk of breast cancer. Patients with an inherited mutation of this gene have Li-Fraumeni Syndrome, which confers a 25-fold increased risk of developing a variety of cancers before the age of 50.

Exposure to oestrogens

Some breast cancer cells are stimulated by oestrogen and the risk of developing breast cancer is increased in women with an early age at menarche or late age at menopause, as these women have been exposed to oestrogen over a longer period of time. In addition, not having children, or late age at first pregnancy, increases the risk of breast cancer by 2–3 times.

Benign breast disease

A diagnosis of atypical ductal hyperplasia increases the risk of breast cancer by 2–5 times, and lobular carcinoma *in situ* increases the risk by 7–12 times.

Radiation

Irradiation to the chest before the age of 30 years, for example, as treatment for Hodgkin's lymphoma during childhood, increases the risk of breast cancer.

Other risk factors

There are a number of other less established risk factors, such as smoking, alcohol, high fat diet and obesity.

Classification

Breast cancer can be classified as follows:

- Non-invasive:
  - Ductal carcinoma *in situ* (DCIS)
  - Lobular carcinoma *in situ* (LCIS)
- Invasive (relative incidence in brackets):
  - Infiltrating ductal (85%)
  - Infiltrating lobular (10%)
  - Mucinous (2%)
  - Tubular (2%)
  - Medullary (<1%)
  - Papillary (<1%)
  - Others (<1%)

There are many different histological subtypes of invasive breast cancer, the vast majority of which are adenocarcinomas (>99%), and they are classified according to their histological appearance. However, it is now well recognised that most breast carcinomas arise from the terminal-duct lobular unit, and the names given to these tumours are based on their histological appearance, and do not refer to a presumed site of origin. For example, ductal carcinomas do not arise exclusively from ducts; neither do lobular carcinomas arise exclusively from lobules. Furthermore, an invasive carcinoma developing in a patient with previous LCIS can be of ductal subtype and vice versa. In addition, LCIS and DCIS can co-exist with an invasive tumour of any subtype.

Non-invasive carcinoma

A non-invasive (*in situ*) carcinoma shows no evidence of penetration of the basement membrane by tumour cells. This means that the malignant cells are confined within the ducts or acini and have not invaded into the stroma or lymphatic channels. There are two types of *in-situ* carcinoma: ductal carcinoma *in situ* (DCIS), and lobular carcinoma *in situ*

(LCIS). Although they are both thought to arise from the same part of the duct system (specifically, the terminal duct lobular unit), they have different morphological appearances, and very different prognostic and management implications.

Ductal carcinoma in situ

DCIS occurs in both pre- and post-menopausal women, and is most common in the 40–60 age group. Although it may present with a palpable mass, particularly if extensive, or nipple discharge, DCIS is most often detected by mammography as part of the screening programme. The malignant cells within the ducts often become necrotic, and subsequent calcification of the necrotic debris can be detected radiologically as it is radio-opaque.

DCIS is usually unifocal and hence confined to one quadrant of the breast, although larger lesions may be multifocal. Bilateral disease is uncommon. *In-situ* disease may be present in isolation, but more often it is associated with invasive carcinoma.

The prognosis for pure DCIS, where there is no identifiable invasive tumour, is excellent. However, some patients, notably those with extensive high-grade DCIS at initial presentation, may develop recurrent *in-situ* tumour, invasive disease in the same breast or even distant metastases in the absence of any local recurrence. In some cases this can occur many years after the first presentation.

Treatment for pure DCIS is primarily surgical, either by wide local excision or mastectomy if extensive, sometimes with the addition of radiotherapy. Close clinical follow-up, with regular mammography, is necessary to enable early detection of recurrent disease. Where DCIS is associated with an invasive tumour, as is usually the case, treatment options have to take into account both the *in-situ* and invasive components.

Paget's disease of the nipple

Clinically Paget's disease presents as reddening and roughening of the nipple, sometimes with slight erosions, similar to the changes seen in eczema.

It is important to recognise Paget's disease, as it is associated with underlying DCIS in the subareolar region, often with associated invasive carcinoma. Approximately 2% of breast carcinomas show evidence of Paget's disease. Prognosis is based on the underlying carcinoma and is not worsened by the presence of Paget's disease.

Lobular Carcinoma in situ

LCIS occurs mainly in pre-menopausal women, and it is usually detected as an incidental finding. It is often multifocal and frequently bilateral. Unlike DCIS, it is rarely associated with calcification. Up to one-third of patients with pure LCIS, who are treated by biopsy alone, go on to develop an invasive carcinoma, which may arise in either breast, regardless of which breast was involved by LCIS. In addition, approximately one-third of the invasive carcinomas occurring after LCIS will be of lobular subtype. In comparison, only about 10% of cancers arising *de novo* are lobular carcinomas. LCIS is therefore a risk factor for developing breast cancer in either breast, and is also a direct precursor of some cancers.

Treatment for LCIS consists of either close clinical and radiological follow-up of both breasts, or bilateral mastectomy.

Invasive carcinoma

Signs and symptoms

Invasive carcinoma may present symptomatically or through the screening programme.

Symptoms include a palpable mass, which may show tethering to the overlying skin or underlying muscle, nipple discharge, nipple retraction, or enlarged axillary lymph nodes due to metastatic involvement.

The mammographic features of a tumour include architectural distortion, an ill-defined or spiculate (star-like) mass or asymmetrical density. There may also be granular and linear calcifications, especially if there is DCIS present.

Clinical course

Breast carcinomas may spread locally or metastasize to distant sites. Local (direct) spread into the overlying skin presents as skin tethering or ulceration. Infiltration into underlying pectoral muscle presents as an immobile mass tethered to the chest wall.

Lymphatic spread results in regional lymph nodes metastases, most commonly involving the axillary nodes, although internal mammary nodes and supraclavicular nodes may also be involved. Approximately 40–50% of women with symptomatic breast cancer have regional lymph node metastasis at the time of presentation.

Tumours can also spread via the bloodstream to the lungs, bones, liver and brain, or even to the opposite breast. Occasionally breast cancer metastasises to the pleura on the same side as the tumour, resulting in an effusion.

There is a marked variation in the length of time between initial presentation of the primary breast cancer and the development of recurrent or metastatic disease. Some breast tumours never recur; some recur after a few years, whilst others may show no evidence of clinical recurrence until 15 years or more after the original diagnosis. The tumour might recur at the site of the initial excision or as distant metastases.

Management

Surgical excision is the treatment of choice for the vast majority of breast cancers, either by wide local excision for smaller tumours (usually <3 cm) or mastectomy, combined with axillary lymph node surgery. The number of lymph nodes removed will depend on preoperative clinical and radiological assessment of the primary tumour and the axilla, and may consist of a single sentinel lymph node biopsy, axillary node sampling (where 4 nodes are removed) or axillary clearance. It is important that an accurate assessment of the number of involved nodes is achieved, as this has prognostic implications (see Staging).

Post-operative radiotherapy to the chest wall or axilla is often also used to reduce the risk of recurrence.

Other treatment options include pre-operative adjuvant chemotherapy for advanced breast cancer, and primary hormonal therapy using tamoxifen or aromatase inhibitors, sometimes followed by surgery, for oestrogen receptor positive tumours in the elderly.

Table 3.8   TNM staging for breast cancer (American Joint Committee on Cancer 2010).

Tumour	T1	Tumour 2 cm or less, no fixation or nipple retraction. Includes pure DCIS and Paget's disease
	T2	Tumour 2–5 cm
	T3	Tumour >5 cm
	T4	Tumour of any size with direct extension into chest wall or skin
Nodes	N0	Node negative
	N1	1–3 lymph nodes positive
	N2	4–9 lymph nodes positive
		>10 axillary lymph nodes positive or metastasis in other lymph node groups
Metatasis	M0	No metastasis
	M1	Distant metastasis

Sentinel lymph node biopsy

Sentinel lymph node biopsy has recently been introduced in an attempt to reduce the morbidity associated with more extensive axillary node surgery. The first one or two lymph nodes draining a cancer are identified using a coloured dye, radioactive tracer or both, and removed for histological assessment. If negative, the chance of there being metastatic carcinoma in the remaining nodes is extremely small and further surgery can be avoided.

Prognosis and staging

The most important prognostic factors for all types of breast cancer are the size and grade of the primary tumour, the number of lymph nodes involved by metastatic tumour and the presence of distant metastases. These form the basis of the staging system, which is used to assess the extent of the disease and help to determine the most appropriate management for the individual patient. Other factors include hormone receptor status, Her2 status and lymphovascular invasion.

Table 3.9   The Nottingham Prognostic Index (NPI) gives an accurate prediction of survival for individual women with breast cancer. It relies on the measurement of three pathological factors.

Tumour size (cm)		
Lymph node involvement	Stage I	No nodes involved
	Stage II	1–3 nodes involved
	Stage III	4 or more nodes involved, or high node involved
Tumour grade	1	Well differentiated
	2	Moderately differentiated
	3	Poorly differentiated

The NPI is calculated as: size × 0.2 + stage + grade.

Table 3.10   Prediction of survival using the NPI.

Prognosis	NPI	15-year survival (%)	Adjuvant systemic therapy
Excellent	<3	90	Nil
Good	3.01–3.4	80	Nil
Moderate I	3.41–4.4	50	ER positive – endocrine therapy
			ER negative – advise chemotherapy depending on age, fitness and tumour size
Moderate II	4.41–5.3	30	As for Moderate I
Poor	>5.4	8	ER positive – endocrine therapy
			ER negative – chemotherapy if fit

Nottingham Prognostic Index

See Tables 3.9 and 3.10.

Tumour grade

The tumour grade refers to the degree of differentiation of the tumour – how well the tumour resembles the tissue of origin. Generally, patients with well differentiated tumours have a much better prognosis than those with poorly differentiated tumours.

Tumour size

Small tumours, less than 1 cm, have an excellent prognosis in the absence of lymph node metastases and may not require systemic therapy.

Lymph Node Involvement

The presence of metastatic breast carcinoma in the regional lymph nodes is a strong indicator of poor prognosis, particularly if four or more nodes are involved.

Hormone Receptor Status

Oestrogen receptor (ER) status of invasive tumours is routinely assessed by immunohistochemistry on the core biopsy in most laboratories. Progesterone receptor status is often only assessed in those cases where the ER is negative. The presence of hormone receptors does confer a slightly improved prognosis, but the main reason for determining their status is to predict response to antioestrogen endocrine therapy, such as tamoxifen.

Her2 Status

Her2 (also known as c-erbB2) is a gene on chromosome 17, which encodes for a membrane protein in normal cells. Approximately 30% of breast cancers exhibit amplification of this gene, and hence over-expression of the protein product, which can be detected by *in-situ* hybridisation or immunohistochemistry, respectively. Over-expression of the Her2 protein is associated with a poorer prognosis, but as with ER status, the importance of determining the Her2 status is to predict response to therapy with Herceptin, which is an antibody targeted against the Her2 gene.

Reflective points

- Consider a patient you have nursed with early stage disease and one with late stage disease. How did the treatment plans differ?
- How would you communicate staging to a patient?
- How does staging relate to curative or palliative options?

References

Cancer Research UK. *Cancer Incidence Statistics*. www.cancerresearchuk.org/cancerstats/type

Cibas, E.S. (2003) Peritoneal washings. In: E.S. Cibas and B.S. Ducatman (Eds) *Cytology, Diagnostic Principles and Clinical Correlates*, 2nd edn. Edinburgh: W.B. Saunders, pp. 151–6.

Crum, C.P. (2005) The female genital tract. In: V. Kumar, A. Abbas and N. Fausto (Eds) *Robbins and Cotan Pathologic Basis of Disease*, 7th edn. Philadelphia, PA: W.B. Saunders, pp. 1059–117.

Federation of Gynaecology and Obstetrics (2009) FIGO committee on Gynaecologic Oncology. *International Journal of Gynaecology and Obstetrics* **105**, 103–4.

Haybittle, J.L., Blamey, R.W., Erston, C.W. et al. (1982) A prognostic index in primary breast cancer. *British Journal of Cancer* **45(3)**, 361–6.

Pecorelli, S., Odicino, F., Maisonneuve, P. et al. (1998) FIGO annual report on the results of treatment in gynaecological cancer: carcinoma of the ovary. *Journal of Epidemiology Biostatistics* **3(1)**, 75–102.

Rosai, J. and Ackerman, L. (eds) (1996) Female reproductive system. In *Rosai and Ackerman's Surgical Pathology*, 9th edn, Vol. 2. Edinburgh: Mosby, pp. 1483–736.

Stevens, A. and Lowe, J. (2000) Female genital tract. In: Stevens and Lowe, *Pathology*, 2nd edn. Edinburgh: Mosby, pp. 395–420.

TNM Staging for Breast Cancer (2010) American Joint Committee on Cancer. In: S.B. Edge, D.R. Byrd, C.C. Compton, et al. (Eds) *Cancer Staging Manual*, 7th edn. New York: Springer, pp. 347–76.

Underwood, J.C.E. (1996) Female genital tract. In: J.C.E. Underwood (Ed.) *General and Systemic Pathology*, 2nd edn. New York: Churchill Livingstone, pp. 551–84.

Woolfe, N. (1998) The female reproductive system. In *Pathology Basic and Systemic*. London: W.B. Saunders, pp. 752–801.

Useful websites

http://en.wikipedia.org/wiki/

http://info.cancerresearchuk.org

http://www.trachelectomy.co.uk/Trachelectomy.htm

http://www.meb.uni-bonn.de/cancer.gov

http://www.cancerscreening.nhs.uk/cervical/index.html

http://hcd2.bupa.co.uk/fact_sheets/html/cervical_cancer.html

http://www.mayoclinic.com/health/ovarian-cancer/DS00293

http://www.cancer.net/patient/Learning+About+Cancer/Genetics/The+Genetics+of+Ovarian+Cancer

http://www.figo.org/content/PDF/staging-booklet.pdf

Chapter 4

Tumour Markers

Michelle L. Harrison, Ana Montes and Martin Gore

Learning points

At the end of this chapter the reader will have an understanding of:
- Significance of tumour markers in clinical practice
- The different tumours markers used in different womens cancers
- The influence of tumour markers on progression
- The use of tumour markers in monitoring progression

Introduction and clinical significance

Tumour markers are proteins or peptides produced or expressed by tumour or normal cells and measures by *in vitro* assays (Hayes et al. 1996). These proteins can be found in blood, urine, tumour or other tissues in malignant and benign conditions. Some markers are specific to a particular cancer, whereas others can be found in different tumour types: one tumour may express several different markers at the same time. Tumour markers are used for diagnosis and can aid in the monitoring of treatment.

There are different types of markers, depending on their clinical use (Hayes et al. 1996):

- *Risk markers* indicate that a person is more likely to develop a particular type of cancer. These are generally genetic markers or cancer susceptibility genes.
- *BRCA1 and 2* are good examples of useful risk markers (Thull and Vogel 1992).
- *Screening markers* are used to detect cancers before they are clinically evident. They provide early diagnosis and treatment and can thus reduce mortality.
- *Diagnostic markers* help in the differential diagnosis cancers as opposed to a benign condition. They can aid in the diagnosis of metastatic cancers from an apparently unknown primary site.

Women's Cancers, First Edition. Edited by Alison Keen and Elaine Lennan.
© 2011 Blackwell Publishing Ltd. Published 2011 by Blackwell Publishing Ltd.

- *Prognostic markers* enable the prediction of the clinical behaviour of a tumour, independent of the effects of subsequent treatment (McGuire and Clark 1992).
- *Predictive markers* predict response to a specific treatment (McGuire and Clark 1992). Some factors can be both prognostic and predictive.
- *Monitoring markers* are used during treatment, to evaluate response or to detect relapse/ progression after treatment during follow-up.

A tumour marker is clinically useful only if it results in a change of practice. To be clinically useful, a tumour marker needs to be sensitive and specific. Sensitivity measures the likelihood of a marker being elevated in someone who has the particular tumour that the marker is associated with. Specificity is the percentage of people with a particular tumour who express the marker. Unfortunately, no marker is 100% sensitive or specific. It is therefore important to assess and validate all candidate markers on strict criteria before integrating them into routine clinical practice (Hayes et al. 1996). This is the reason why, despite a plethora of candidate markers, only a very few are used in routine clinical practice. Guidelines are available for the correct use of tumour markers from the American Society of Clinical Oncology (ASCO) p. 4, the National Academy of Clinical Biochemistry (NACB) (Sturgeon 2006), and the European Group for Tumour Markers (EGTM) (EGTM 1999) (Table 4.1).

Breast cancer tumour markers

There is no single tumour marker that is clinically useful in patients with breast cancer. However, there are several that have utility in specific clinical circumstances. Some are serum-based and others are tissue-based. We will only discuss those markers where there is consensus regarding their clinical utility (Bassett et al. 2000; Fitzgibbons et al. 2000).

Table 4.1 Utility of breast and ovarian markers.

Markers	Risk	Diagnosis	Prognosis	Predictive	Monitoring
			ER (weak)	ER.PR (Hormone Treatment)	
CA Breast	BRCA1 BRCA2	None	HER2 (weak) uPA, PAII	HER2 (Trastuzumab)	CA 15.3
	BRCA1 BRCA2	Ca 125			Ca 125
Ca Ovary				Ca 125	

Screening and early detection

There are no proven serum markers for routine screening or early detection, and the recommendation for both these continues to be breast examination and mammography. For those families with a proven family history of breast and/or ovarian cancer, or with know mutations in the BRCA1 and 2 genes, genetic testing can be performed in specialist centres where patients can be appropriately counselled and monitored (Thull and Vogel 2004; ASCO 2003).

Diagnosis

There is no evidence base to recommend any tumour marker with this indication at present.

Prognostic and predictive markers

Hormone receptors: Estrogen and Progesterone Receptor (ER and PR)

ER is a weak prognostic factor that indicates a good prognosis. In combination with other established factors, it can be used to predict recurrence and assist in decision-making regarding the choice of adjuvant treatment for newly diagnosed breast cancer patients (Ravidin et al. 2001; EBCTCG 1998a,b).

In pre- and post-menopausal patients, ER and PR are predictive of response to hormonal treatments, both in early and advanced disease (McGuire and Clark 1992; Bassett et al. 2000; Colleoni et al. 2006). They are used to select those patients that are more likely to respond to hormone manipulation. Adjuvant hormone treatment has a significant impact on the overall survival of patients with early breast cancer, as demonstrated in several trials (EBCTCG 1998; Colleoni et al. 2006).

All current guidelines recommend that ER and PR should be assessed in all newly diagnosed patients with breast cancer (Bassett et al. 2000; Sturgeon 2006; EGTM 1999; Sturgeon 2002). They can be reliably measured by biochemical or immunohistochemical methods from tumour tissue (Golouh et al. 1997).

Her2

The use of Her2 as a prognostic factor is not clear, although many papers have addressed the issue. Overall, studies suggest that HER2 over expression is a poor prognostic factor, although its magnitude appears weak, as with hormone receptors. When used in addition to other factors, it is useful as an assessment of prognosis, mainly in node positive patients (Adjuvant online 2006).

Determination of the over expression of HER2 in the pathology samples of newly diagnosed breast cancer patients helps to select patients that will obtain a response from Trastuzumab treatment, both in early and advanced cancer.

Recent randomized trials have demonstrated that addition of Trastuzumab to conventional treatment improves survival for HER2 positive patients (Piccart-Gebhart et al. 2005; Romond et al. 2005; Slamon et al. 2001; Yamauchi et al. 2001a). There are some data suggesting that HER2 over expression might help the choice of type of hormone therapy or chemotherapy. However, the evidence for this is poor and it is not currently recommended that the choice of drugs is based on these results (Ellis et al. 2001; Yamauchi et al. 2001a,b).

It is important that HER2 status is determined by performing tests that use standardized approved assay methodology, either with immunohistochemistry or Fluorescence *in-situ* hybridisation (FISH) (Fitzgibbons et al. 2000).

Urokinase plasminogen activator (uPA) and Plasminogen activator inhibitor 1 (PAI 1)

These two markers, when used in conjunction, are strong independent prognostic factors of poor outcome in breast cancer, as determined in a study that included over 8000 patients. These data has been prospectively confirmed for axillary node negative-patients (Look et al. 2002; Janicke et al. 2001). Lymph node negative patients with low levels of either uPA or PAI 1 have a low risk of relapse and may not benefit from adjuvant chemotherapy (Harbeck et al. 2002). However, only a few centres in Europe perform these tests. The recommended assay for uPA and PAI 1 is validated ELISA performed in fresh frozen tumour biopsy (Sweet et al. 2009).

Monitoring recurrence

Monitoring the levels of Ca 15.3 (see below) may allow the detection of recurrence earlier than radiological or clinical examination in 7% of patients (Bassett et al. 2000). However, to date there is no indication that detecting recurrence and initiating therapy early has any impact on patient outcome. At present there are no markers that are of routine benefit when monitoring patients for recurrence.

Monitoring therapy

Ca 15.3 and CA 27.29

These serum assays detect the same antigen on the MUC protein, but Ca 15.3 has been more widely investigated. Their serum levels correlate well with the stage of disease and most guidelines recommend the use of one of these markers before the start of therapy for metastatic breast cancer and at every other cycle of chemotherapy (or every 3 months of hormone treatment) to evaluate response in cases where measurable disease is not present (Duffy 2006).

Carcinoembryonic antigen (CEA)

CEA is foetal glycoprotein found on cell surfaces and produced by foetal gastrointestinal tract, pancreas and liver. In adults it is found in small quantities in the blood and other normal tissues. Elevations of CEA are found in several tumours, generally those from gastrointestinal or hepato-biliary origin, making it unreliable for diagnosis. Its usefulness is limited to follow-up in patients with elevated pre-treatment levels. CEA can also be elevated in breast cancer and can be used to monitor response in cases with no measurable disease and normal pre-treatment Ca 15.3 (Molina et al. 1998).

Epithelial ovarian cancer tumour markers

Ca 125 is most commonly used in women with epithelial ovarian, fallopian tube and primary peritoneal cancer. Elevation in Ca 125 may be seen in a number of other malignancies, including endometrial breast, gastrointestinal tract and lung cancer. Benign conditions may also produce a raised serum Ca 125, including endometriosis, benign tumours of the ovary and uterus, pregnancy, menstruation, benign diseases of the liver and gastrointestinal tract, conditions causing inflammation of the peritoneum and pleura, and right heart failure (Meden et al. 1998).

Screening and early detection

Several studies of screening, which have enrolled women at moderate to high risk of ovarian cancer, have been reported. These have used Ca 125 and transvaginal ultrasound either alone or together. In a recent review, the difficulties of detecting early stage epithelial ovarian cancer were highlighted. Only 25% of ovarian cancers detected by screening were stage I, whilst the majority were stages IIC and III, and interval cancers accounted for almost 30% of reported cancers (Hogg and Friedlander 2004).

There is a high rate of false positives and negatives. In early-stage ovarian cancer, the Ca 125 is normal in approximately 40–50% of patients, and up to 20% of those with advanced disease (Bast 2003). In screening studies of women at high risk, a raised Ca 125 was documented in up to 25.5% and abnormal transvaginal ultrasound in up to 23% undergoing screening (Bast 2003; Laframboise et al. 2002; Dorum et al. 1996; Muto et al. 1993; Taylor et al. 2001; Bourne et al. 1991, 1993). As a result of an abnormal screen, 3–8.7% of high risk women had a surgical procedure performed, with the majority having benign lesions. In women with BRCA1 or 2 mutations, this increased to 16% (Vasen et al. 2005; Laframboise et al. 2002; Dorum et al. 1996; Muto et al. 1993; Taylor et al. 2001; Bourne et al. 1991, 1993; Liede et al. 2002; Scheuer et al. 2002). A model incorporating age, baseline Ca 125 level and rate of change of Ca 125, may improve the performance of Ca 125 as a screening tool (Skates 2003, Menon et al. 2005).

There is no role for screening women with no increased risk for ovarian cancer. Women with familial breast and ovarian cancer should be referred to a cancer genetics service for formal examination. Options for women who are at high risk include salpingo-oophorectomy or surveillance using regular Ca 125 estimations and transvaginal ultrasound acknowledging the limitations of such screening.

Diagnosis

The standard assessment for a patient with suspected ovarian cancer includes tumour marker measurement. A risk of malignancy index (RMI) was developed by Jacobs and colleagues. This is calculated by the product of menopausal status (1 pre-menopausal, 3 post-menopausal), suspicious ultrasound features (0 none, 1 one, 3 more than one) and the Ca 125 level. A threshold of 200 was used to discriminate between benign and malignant adnexal masses (Jacobs et al. 1990). This simple scoring system can facilitate the identification of patients who should be referred to gynaecological cancer centres for treatment (Bailey et al. 2006; Anderson et al. 2003; Tingulstad et al. 1999).

Once ovarian cancer is diagnosed, standard treatment includes surgery followed by chemotherapy. However, neo-adjuvant chemotherapy is often given in patients unfit for primary surgery or where it is anticipated from the pre-operative assessment that optimal debulking is unlikely to be achieved. Several retrospective studies have addressed the role of Ca 125 in predicting whether optimal debulking can be achieved. Patients with optimally debulked tumours had a lower median Ca 125 than those with sub-optimally debulked tumours. However, there is no agreement as to the precise level of Ca 125 above which optimal debulking is unlikely to be achieved. Amongst various studies, the suggested Ca 125 level has ranged from 400–912, with several proposing Ca 125 level of 500 (Gemer et al. 2005; Brockbank et al. 2004; Eltabbakh et al. 2004; Memarzadeh et al. 2003; Cooper et al. 2002; Chi et al. 2000). The Ca 125 forms part of the pre-operative assessments and although it has predictive value in this setting, it cannot be used in isolation.

Monitoring response

Patients receiving chemotherapy are primarily assessed for response using CT; however, in ovarian cancer, the Ca 125 is reflective of response if measured serially during chemotherapy. A 50% response is defined by a confirmed more than 50% decrease from the pre-treatment level and a 75% response was by a more than 75% decrease over three samples from the pre-treatment level (Rustin et al. 1996). The GCIG has a proposed definition based on a 50% reduction in Ca 125 that is confirmed and maintained for at least 28 days (Table 4.2).

There are several reports suggesting that the Ca 125 may overestimate response rate; however, the Ca 125 may be a better indicator of survival (Bridgewater et al. 1999; Grondlund et al. 2004). A possible explanation is that the pattern of disease in ovarian cancer usually involves small tumour deposits spread throughout the peritoneal cavity and these are not readily evaluated by CT. Thus target lesions seen on CT may not necessarily reflect the total tumour burden.

In patients who achieve a complete response after first-line chemotherapy with normalisation of the Ca 125 (below 35IU), the nadir value is predictive of serological progression-free survival and overall survival (Crawford and Pearce 2005).

Table 4. 2   GCG proposed Ca 125 response definition.

To be evaluated for response by Ca 125 requires 2 pre-treatment samples at least twice the upper limit or normal and at least 2 additional samples after the start of treatment.
A response to Ca 125 has occurred if after 2 elevated levels before therapy there is at least a 50% decrease that is confirmed by a 4th sample.

The 2 pre-treatment samples must both be at least twice the upper limit of normal and at least 1 day but not >3 months apart. At least 1 of the samples should be within 1 week of starting treatment.
The 3rd sample must be <50% of the second sample.
The confirmatory fourth sample must be >21 days after sample 3 and <110% of sample 3.

Any intervening samples between samples 2 and 3 and between samples 3 and 4 must be <110% of the previous sample, unless considered to be increasing because of tumour lysis.
Patients are not evaluated by Ca 125 if they have received mouse antibodies or if there has been medical or surgical interference with their peritoneum or pleura during the previous 28 days.

Timing of Ca 125 measures
Samples should be taken at the following time intervals:

2 samples prior to treatment
At intervals of 2–4 weeks during treatment
Once every 2 or 3 months during follow-up

For each patient the same assay method must be used. The assay must be tested in a quality control scheme.

Monitoring progression

Following primary treatment, patients are reviewed every three months and the serum Ca 125 is usually measured at these visits. Serum Ca 125 is a sensitive marker for relapse, with a rise typically preceding the development of symptoms or measurable disease on CT. In women with normal pre-operative Ca 125 levels, CTs are used, as Ca 125 levels are unreliable in identifying disease relapse.

Table 4.3   GCIG proposed Ca 125 progression definition.

Patients with elevated Ca 125 pre-treatment and normalisation of Ca 125 (Group A)
Ca 125 (2 × ULN documented on 2 occasions)
Date of progression: 1st date that Ca 125 (2 × ULN)
Patients with elevated Ca 125 pre-treatment that never normalises (Group B)
Ca 125 (2 × nadir documented on 2 occasions)
Date of progression: first date that Ca 125 (2 × nadir)
Patients with normal Ca 125 pre-treatment (Group C)
As per group A
ULN – upper limit of normal
Repeat Ca 125 at any time, but normally not less than after 1 week of the 1st elevated level

With the knowledge that the Ca 125 will generally increase before clinically apparent recurrences, criteria to define the changes in a Ca 125 that reliably predict recurrence have been sought. Several definitions have been suggested: serial Ca 125 levels with an increase of 25% over four occasions, 50% over three occasions or persistent elevation of 100 IU have all been used (Rustin et al. 1992). The CGIG has proposed a simplified definition: Ca 125 greater than twice the upper limit of normal, and in patients with a nadir Ca 125 above the normal range, and a doubling of the Ca 125 (Vergote et al. 2000) (Table 4.3).

Monitoring recurrence

In patients with a history of ovarian cancer, a rise in the Ca 125 within the normal range may be predictive of disease recurrence. In a small study with 39 patients, an absolute rise of 5 or 10 IU, or a relative rise of 100% above the nadir, was predictive with a sensitivity of 100% and a specificity of 94% (Santilan et al. 2005).

The practice of regularly measuring Ca 125 levels allows the identification of those patients who will develop clinical disease recurrence. A rise in the Ca 125 typically predicts recurrence 3–9 months prior to clinical and radiological recurrence. However, this frequent leads to great anxiety for patients and a syndrome of Ca 125 addiction has been described (Harries et al. 2002). Likewise, there is no evidence that early treatment of relapsed epithelial ovarian cancer (EOC) is associated with an increased survival and relapsed EOC is an incurable situation. Therefore it is our view that clinicians need to reserve the use of chemotherapy for patients with documented recurrence as dictated by symptoms or measurable disease on CT. Chemotherapy should not be commenced on the basis of an elevated Ca 125 alone (Gore 2006).

Tumour markers other than Ca 125 in epithelial ovarian cancer

Tumour markers other than Ca 125 may also be elevated in epithelial ovarian cancer. The common tumour markers routinely tested include CEA, Ca 19.9 and Ca 15.3, and these all may also be raised in EOC. If the CEA is significant, further investigations are required. A Ca 125 to CEA ratio of more than 25 was found to discriminate between ovarian and colorectal primaries (Yedema et al. 1992). An alternate approach is a relative rise in CEA greater than the relative rise in Ca 125. In addition, parenchymal liver or lung metastasis should be regarded as suspicious for a colorectal primary (Kolomainen et al. 2002). An elevated CEA may also be useful in the diagnosis and management of patients with an undifferential intra-abdominal cancer, where the primary is unknown.

Germ cell ovarian cancer tumour markers

Alpha-fetoprotein (AFP) and human chorionic gonadotrophin (hCG) are elevated in germ cell tumours and should be measured in all young women presenting with a complex ovarian mass. Lactate dehydrogenase (LDH) should also be measured routinely. The Ca 125 may also be elevated, but this rise is non-specific.

Amongst the different histological types, there is a variation in the pattern of tumour markers. Dysgerminomas typically exhibit a high LDH and a variable elevation of bhCG. Elevation in both AFP and bhCG may represent embryonal pathology or a mixed tumour (Talerman et al. 1980; Kawai et al. 1992).

Germ cell tumours are highly sensitive to chemotherapy and tumour markers should be serially measured weekly during chemotherapy. AAs with the Ca 125 in women with epithelial ovarian cancer, AFP and βhCG rise in those women who have had fertility sparing surgery (Mitchell et al. 1999)

Granulosa cell ovarian cancer tumour markers

Inhibin levels are used primary in the diagnosis and monitoring of granulose cell tumours (GCT) and other sex-cord stromal tumours. Inhibin levels are very low or undetectable in post-menopausal women; however, they fluctuate during the menstrual cycle and are therefore not reliable in pre-menopausal women at diagnosis. Serial inhibin measurements are useful in detecting relapse, and a rise should prompt appropriate imaging to be performed (Lappohn et al. 1989; Jobling et al. 1994).

Conclusion

Monitoring tumour markers is now well established in clinical practice and offers an easy way to establish responsiveness of the tumour to treatment. However, they are only a guide and must not be used in isolation. The clinical picture, the radiological tests and the tumour markers all provide information to guide the clinician to assess disease repose or disease relapse. They are a valuable addition to practice.

The meaning of Ca 125 for women

As the above chapter highlights, the clinical relevance of tumour markers indicates that there is often a dichotomy for patients – it has been described as a 'double edged sword' many times by women. On the one hand, each clinic appointment holds the promise that the Ca 125 has normalised after treatment and is staying stable or on the other, the it can inspire fear when it rises even within normal limits. Very few women opt not to have their Ca 125 results. One patient having her fifth line of chemotherapy tells any nurse or doctor looking after her that she never wants to hear her Ca 125 result; she is happy for the team to know and advise accordingly, but does not even want to know whether it is up or down. The following paragraph was written by a woman who has completed treatment. but it does reinforce the way many women feel about this test.

'Having ovarian cancer is rubbish'

A patient's story on the meaning of tumour markers

It's filled with uncertainty and it affects every part of your life, I mean I can't plan much or ... It took ages to get my diagnosis and eventually I had a Ca 125 test done. I know everyone's cancer is not sensitive to Ca 125, but mine was. It made me think, why didn't I have this test in the beginning ... it's just a blood test. At one point it was over 3000! My god! To be precise, my level was 3026. 3026 became a number I latched on to, to try to sort my head out. I have 3026 of the little buggers and I was determined to kill 'em off one by one if necessary! I know it's just a figure and not really little buggers as I describe, but 3026 became my symbol of cancer. This was as bad as it got and right now its only 24 last time we looked. Some of the doctors told me Ca 125 was only part of the picture but for me it became the centre of my cancer. The doctor said she could probably predict the Ca 125 level by examining me and listening to my symptoms but I wasn't convinced. I wanted to know the number. When it was down I was positive and it sort of helped energise me to face treatment. When it jumped slightly, which it did only once in my first lot of chemo, I was saying 'oh my god, the chemo's not working, I'm dying.' I was down and worried and I didn't have a good week. By the following time it was back going down and I felt a sense of relief and more ok that it was just a blip.

They say it can happen like that, it goes up and goes down, but in the beginning of course you don't know that. I have spoken to some women who just don't want to know and I do understand that, but for me it's become part of my life. I have had several relapses over the past 2 years and each time the Ca 125 has risen. Not to 3026, but up all the same. My head is not so down now if it does start to rise. I just think time to get back on treatment, which in a way is a positive thing. I have learned to live with the uncertainty of ovarian cancer and though it offers some restrictions I am trying to live my life. Thankfully I am currently off treatment and feeling good. I get it measured once every couple of months, but for me I would have it done weekly if I could.

Reflective points

- Think about a patient you have recently nursed with ovarian cancer. Map out the Ca 125 tumour marker and see how it corresponds to her clinical picture.
- Consider the psychological impact of the Ca 125 result. How could you support a lady with a rising Ca 125?

References

Adjuvant Online breast cancer help files (2006). Prognostic estimates.

American Society of Clinical Oncology (2003) Policy statement update; genetic testing for cancer susceptibility. *Journal of Clinical Oncology* **21(12)**, 2397–406.

Anderson, E.S., Knusden, A., Rix, P. and Johansen, B. (2003) Risk of malignancy index in the preoperative evaluation of patients with adnexal masses. *Gynecological Oncology* **90**, 109–112.

Bailey. J., Tailor, A., Naik, R. et al. (2006) Risk of malignancy index for referral of ovarian cancer cases to a tertiary centre: does it identify the correct cases? *International Journal of Gynecological Cancer* **16(Suppl 1)**, 30–4.

Bassett, R.C. et al. (2000) Update of recommendations for the use of tumour markers in breast and colorectal cancer; clinical practice guidelines of the American Society of Clinical Oncology. *Journal of Clinical Oncology* **19(6)**, 1865–78.

Bast, R.C. (2003) Status of tumour markers in ovarian cancer screening. *Journal of Clinical Oncology* **21(Suppl 10)**, 200–205.

Bourne, T.H., Campbell, S., Reynolds, K.M., et al. (1993) Screening for early familial ovarian cancer with transvaginal ultrasound and colour blood flow imaging. *British Medical Journal* **306(6884)**, 1025–9.

Bourne, T.H., Whitehead, M.I., Campbell, S. et al. (1991) Ultrasound screening for familial ovarian cancer. *Gynecological Oncology* **43**, 92–7.

Bridgewater, J.A., Nelstrop, A.E., Rustin, J.R. et al. (1999) Comparison of standard and Ca 125 response criteria in patients with epithelial ovarian cancer treated with platinum or paclitaxel. *Journal of Clinical Oncology*: **17**, 501–508.

Brockbank, E.C., Ind, T.E., Barton, D.P. et al. (2004) Preoperative predictors of suboptimal primary surgical cytoreduction in women with clinical evidence of advance primary epithelial ovarian cancer. *International Journal of Gynecological Oncology* **14**, 42–50.

Chi, D.S., Venkatraman, E.S., Masson, V. and Hoskins, W.J. (2000) The ability of preoperative serum Ca 125 to predict optimal primary tumour cytoreduction in stage III epithelial ovarian carcinoma. *Gynecological Oncology* **77**. 227–231.

Colleoni, M. et al. (2006) Tamoxifen after adjuvant chemotherapy for pre-menopausal women with lymph node-positive breast cancer. International Breast Cancer Study Group Trial 13–93. *Journal of Clinical Oncology* **24(9)**, 1332–41.

Cooper, B.C., Sook, A.K., Davis, C.S. et al. (2002) Preoperative Ca 125 levels: an independent prognostic factor for epithelian ovarian cancer. *Obstetrics and Gynaecology* **100**, 59–64.

Crawford, S.M. and Pearce, J. (2005) Does the nadir Ca 125 concentration predict a long-term outcome after chemotherapy for carcinoma of the ovary? *Annals of Oncology* **16**, 47–50.

Dorum, A., Kristensen, G.B., Abelere, V.M. et al. (1996) Early detection of ovarian cancer. *European Journal of Cancer* **32A(10)**, 1645–51.

Duffy, M.J. (2006) Serum tumour markers in breast cancer: are they of clinical value? *Clinical Chemotherapy* **52(2)**, 109–19.

Early Breast Cancer Trialists' Collaborative Group (1998a) Polychemotherapy for early breast cancer: an overview of the randomised trials. *Lancet* **352(9132)**, 930–42.

Early Breast Cancer Trialists' Collaborative Group (1998b) Tamoxifen for early breast cancer: an overview of the randomised Early Breast Cancer Trialists' Collaborative group. *Lancet* **352(9114)**, 1451–67.

Chia, S., Bryce, C. and Gelmon, K. (2005) Effects of chemotherapy and hormonal therapy for early breast cancer on recurrence and 15-year survival: an overview of the randomised trials. *Lancet* **365(9472)**, 1687–717.

Ellis, M.J. et al. (2001) Letrozole is more effective neoadjuvant endocrine receptor-positive primary breast cancer: evidence from a phase III randomized trial. *Journal of Clinical Oncology* **19(18)**, 3808–16.

Eltabbakh, G.H., Mount, S.L., Beatty, B. et al. (2004) Factors associated with cytoreducibility among women with ovarian carcinoma. *Gynecological Oncology* **95(3)**, 77–33.

European Group on Tumour Markers (1999) Quality requirements and control: EGTM recommendations. *Anticancer Research* **19(4A)**, 2791–4.

Fitzgibbons, P.L. et al. (2000) Prognostic factors in breast cancer. College of American Pathologists Consensus Statement 1999. *Archives of Pathology and Laboratory Medicine* **124(7)**, 966–78.

Gemer, O., Lurian, M., Gdalevich, M. et al. (2005) A multicenter study of Ca 125 level as a predictor of non-optimal primary cytoreduction of advanced epithelial ovarian cancer. *European Journal of Surgical Oncology* **31**, 1006–10.

Golouh, R. et al. (1997) Comparison of standardized immunohistochemical and biochemical assays for oestrogen and progesterone receptors in breast carcinoma. *Pathological Research Practice* **193(8)**, 543–9.

Gore M. (2006) Controversies in surveillance options for patients after initial treatment for ovarian cancer. *American Society of Clinical Oncology (ASCO) Education Book*, pp. 335–3338.

Grondlund, B., Hogdall, C., Hilden, J. et al. (2004) Should Ca 125 response criteria be preferred to response evaluation criteria in solid tumours (RECIST) for prognostication during second-line chemotherapy of ovarian carcinoma? *Journal of Clinical Oncology* **22**, 4051–8.

Harbeck, N., Kates, R.E. and Schmitt, M. (2002) Clinical relevance of invasion factors urokinase-type plasminogen activator and plasminogen activator inhibitor type 1 for individualized therapy decisions in primary breast cancer is greatest when used in combination. *Journal of Clinical Oncology*, **20(4)**, 1000–7.

Harries, M. and Gore, M. (2002) Chemotherapy for epithelial ovarian cancer-treatment of recurrent disease: Part II. *Lancet Oncology* **9**, 537–45

Hayes, D.F. et al. (1996) Tumour marker utility grading system: a framework to evaluate clinical utility of tumour markers. *Journal of National Cancer Institute* **88(20)**, 1456–66.

Hogg, R. and Friedlander, M. (2004) Biology of epithelial ovarian cancer: implications for screening women at high genetic risk. *Journal of Clinical Oncology* **4(22)**, 1315–27.

Jacobs, I., Oram, D., Fairbanks, J. et al. (1990) A risk of malignancy index incorporating Ca 125, ultrasound and menopausal status for the accurate preoperative diagnosis of ovarian cancer. *British Journal of Obstetrics and Gynaecology* **97**, 922–9.

Janicke, F. et al. (2001) Randomised adjuvant chemotherapy trial in high-risk lymph node-negative breast cancer patients identified by urokinase-type plasminogen activator and plasminogen activator inhibitor type 1. *Journal of the National Cancer Institute* **93(12)**, 913–20.

Jobling, T., Marmers, P., MacLachlan, V. et al. (1994) A prospective study of inhibin in granulosa cell tumours of the ovary. *Gynecological Oncology* **55**, 285–9.

Kawai, M., Kano, T., Kikkawa, F. et al. (1992) Seven tumour markers in benign and malignant germ cell tumours of the ovary. *Gynecological Oncology* **45**, 248–53.

Kolomainen, D.F., Ross, P.J., Webb, A.R. et al. (2002) Is there a role for measuring serum CEA in patients with a diagnosis of 'ovarian cancer'. *Gynecological Oncology* **68**, 5.

Laframboise, S., Nedlcu, R., Murphy, J. et al. (2002) Use of Ca 125 and ultrasound in high-risk women. *International Journal of Gynecological Cancer* **12**, 86–91.

Lappohn, R.E., Burger, H.G., Bouma, J. et al. (1989) Inhibin as a marker for granulosa cell tumours. *New England Journal of Medicine* **321,** 790–3.

Liede, B., Karlan, B.Y., Baldwin, R.L. et al. (2002) Cancer incidence in a population of Jewish women at risk of ovarian cancer. *Journal of Clinical Oncology* **20(6)**, 1570–7.

Look, M.P. et al. (2002) Pooled analysis of prognostic impact of urokinase-type plasminogen activator and its inhibitor PAI-1 in 8377 breast cancer patients. *Journal of the National Cancer Institute* **94(2)**, 116–28.

McGuire, W.L. and G.M. Clark (1992) Prognostic factors and treatment decisions in axillary-node-negative breast cancer. *New England Journal of Medicine* **326(26)**, 1756–61.

Meden, H. and Fattahi-Meibodi, A. (1998) Ca 125 in benign gynaecological conditions. *International Journal of Biological Markers* **13**, 231–7.

Memarzadeh, S., Lee, S.B., Berek, J.S. and Farias-Eisner, R. (2003) Ca 125 levels are a weak predictor of optimal cytroeductive surgery in patients with advanced epithelial ovarian cancer. *International Journal of Gynecological Cancer* **13**, 120–4.

Menon, U., Kates, S.J., Lewis, S. et al. (2005) Prospective study using the risk of ovarian cancer algorithm to screen for ovarian cancer. *Journal of Clinical Oncology* **23**, 7919–26.

Mitchell, P.L., Al-Naisiri, N., A'Hern, R. et al. (1999) Treatment of non-dysgerminomatous ovarian germ cell tumours: an analysis of 69 cases. *Cancer* **85**, 2232–44.

Molina, R. et al. (1998) c-erbB-2 oncoprotein, CEA and CA 15.3 in patients with breast cancer: prognostic value. *Breast Cancer Research and Treatment* **51(2)**, 109–19.

Muto, M.G., Cramer, D.W., Brown, D.L. et al. (1993) Screening for ovarian cancer: the preliminary experience of a familial cancer centre. *Gynecological Oncology* **51(1)**, 12–20.

Piccart-Gebhart, M.J. et al. (2005) Trastuzumab after adjuvant chemotherapy in HER2-positive breast cancer. *New England Journal of Medicine* **353(16)**, 1659–72.

Ravidin, P.M. et al. (2001). Computer program to assist in making decisions about adjuvant therapy for women with early breast cancer. *Journal of Clinical Oncology* **19(4)**, 980–91.

Romond, E.H. et al. (2005) Trastuzumab plus adjuvant chemotherapy for operable HER2-positive breast cancer. *New England Journal of Medicine* **353(16)**, 1673–84.

Rustin, G.J., Nelstrop, A.E., McClean, P. et al. (1996) Defining response of ovarian carcinoma to initial chemotherapy according to serum Ca 125. *Journal of Clinical Oncology* **14**, 1545–51.

Rustin, G.J., Nelstrop, A., Stilwell, J. et al. (1992) Savings obtained by Ca 125 measurements during therapy for ovarian carcinoma: The North Thames Ovary Group. *European Journal of Cancer* **28,** 9–82.

Santilan, A., Garg, R., Zahurak, M.L. et al. (2005) Risk of epithelial ovarian cancer recurrence in patients with rising serum Ca-125 levels within the normal range. *Journal of Clinical Oncology* **23**, 9388–43.

Scheuer, L., Kauff, N., Robson, M. et al. (2002) Outcome of preventive surgery and screening for breast and ovarian cancer in BRCA mutation carriers. *Journal of Clinical Oncology* **20(5)**, 1260–8.

Skates, S.J., Menon, U., MacDonald, N. et al. (2003) Calculation of the risk of ovarian cancer from serial Ca 125 values for preclinical detection in postmenopausal women. *Journal of Clinical Oncology* **21(10s)**, 206–10s.

Slamon, D.J. et al. (2001) Use of chemotherapy plus a monoclonal antibody against HER2 for metastatic breast cancer that over expresses HER2. *New England Journal of Medicine* **344(11)**, 783–92.

Sturgeon, C. (2006) *Practice Guidelines and Recommendations for the Use of Tumour Markers in the Clinic.* www.nacb.org/lmpg/tumor [cited.

Sturgeon, C. (2002) Practice guidelines for tumour marker use in the clinic. *Clinical Chemotherapy* **48(8)**, 1151–9.

Sweet, C.G. et al. (2009) External quality assessment of trans-European multicentre antigen determinations (enzyme-linked immunosorbent assay) or urokinase-type plasminogen activator (uPA) and its type 1 inhibitor. (PAi-1) in human breast cancer tissue extracts. *British Journal of Cancer* **78(11)**, 14,324–41.

Talerman, A., Jaije, W.G., Baggerman, L. et al. (1980) Serum alphafetoprotein (AFP) in patients with germ cell tumours of the gonads and extragonal sites: correlation between endomermal sinus (yolk sac) tumour and raised serum AFP. *Cancer* **46**, 380–5.

Taylor, K.J. and Schwartz, P.E. (2001) Cancer screening in high risk populations: clinical trial. *Ultrasound Medical Biology* **27**, 461–6.

Thull, D.L. and Vogel, V.G. (2004) Recognition and management of hereditary breast cancer symptoms. *Oncologist* **9(1)**, 13–24.

Tingulstad, S., Hagen, B., Skjeldestad, F.E. et al. (1999) The risk of malignancy index to evaluate potential ovarian cancers in local hospitals. *Obstetrics and Gynaecology* **93**, 448–52.

Vasen, H.F.A., Tesfay, E., Boonstra, H. et al. (2005) Early detection of breast cancer and ovarian cancer in families with BRCA mutations. *European Journal of Cancer* **41**, 549–54.

Vergote, I., Rustin, J.S., Eisenahue, E.A. et al. (2000) New guidelines to evaluate the response to treatment in solid tumours (ovarian cancer). *Journal of National Cancer Institute* **92**, 1534–5

Yamauchi, H., Stearns, V. and Hayes, D.F. (2001a) The role of c-erb B-2 as a predictive factor in breast cancer. *Breast Cancer* **8(3)**, 171–83.

Yamauchi, H., Stearns, V. and Hayes, D.F. (2001b) When is a tumour marker ready for prime time? A case study of c-erbB-2 as a predictive factor in breast cancer. *Journal of Clinical Oncology* **19(8)**, 2334–56.

Yedema, C., Kenemans, P., Wobbes, T. et al. (1992) Use of serum tumour markers in the differential diagnosis between ovarian and colorectal adenocarcinomas. *Tumour Biology* **13**, 18–26.

Chapter 5

Genetic Susceptibility to Female Cancers

Gillian Crawford

Learning points

By the end of this chapter, the reader will have an understanding of:
- Genetics susceptibility to female cancers
- Genetics including basic cancer genetics
- Process of genetic testing
- Inherited predisposition
- Strategies to manage an increased risk of malignancy
- Psychological impact of genetic testing

Introduction

In an ageing population, cancer incidence, including female cancers, is increasing. More than one in three people will develop some form of cancer during their lifetime. The majority of diagnoses are in the last few decades of life; only 1 in 27 are diagnosed with cancer below the age of 50 (Toms 2004). The most common cancer that affects women is breast cancer (around 30% of all cancers diagnosed in women). Uterine and ovarian cancers each account for 5% of all cancers affecting women, with other gynaecological cancers (e.g. cervix and vulva) occurring less commonly (Toms 2004).

This chapter will discuss inherited cancer predisposition, exploring in detail genetic conditions where female cancers occur with increased frequency. The inheritance, associated cancer risks and available management strategies for these cancers will be explored. Prior to discussing these specific cancers, information about cancer genetics, how to identify 'at risk' families and genetic testing will be presented. These details will equip nurses caring for female cancer patients to have the necessary information to be able to make an initial risk assessment for their patients, referring on to specialist services as indicated. In addition, there will be an understanding of risk assessment and options available to women (e.g. screening, surgery and other medical options).

Women's Cancers, First Edition. Edited by Alison Keen and Elaine Lennan.

Basic cancer genetics

The vast majority of cancers occur as a result of somatic (acquired) mutations in genes that control cell proliferation. The biggest risk factor for the development of these tumours is age, with other environmental factors also playing a part (e.g. smoking, hormonal exposure, diet, alcohol intake), as well as yet unknown factors. In a small proportion (in the region of 5%) of women affected by cancer, an inherited predisposition constitutes the bulk of cancer risk. This inherited or germline mutation is present in almost every cell of the body, and the amount of somatic damage that is required before a cancer is initiated is much less on this background. Consequently, cancers arising from an inherited germline mutation tend to arise at younger ages. A germline mutation is not sufficient to cause cancer (Figure 5.1 illustrates this), but it significantly increases the chances in an individual's lifetime.

The vast majority of women seen in clinical practice will not have a strongly inherited predisposition to cancer; their cancers will have developed as a sporadic or 'one-off' event or a combination of weaker gene effects and environmental factors. It is important to be able to recognise which individuals and families may have an inherited predisposition to developing cancer, so they can access information about the risks of specific cancers developing and the possibility of genetic testing, screening programmes and possible surgical and other preventive options. In addition, even in families where there is a confirmed high risk gene alteration, cancers can still occur in individuals who are non-carriers, because they continue to have a population risk of developing cancer. These cancers are called phenocopies, which are the same cancers but with a different aetiology. This can have implications in the genetic counselling of families, as these individuals may be incorrectly identified as being at a significantly increased risk and make inappropriate management decisions on this basis.

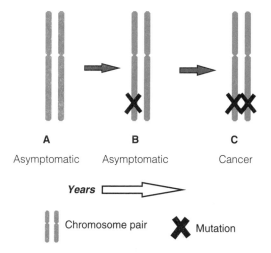

Figure 5.1   Genetic mutations and cancer. In a sporadic cancer, a person is born without any mutations in the particular genes concerned (A). The chances of acquiring one mutation (B) are quite high, but a second mutation needs to be acquired in exactly the same chromosomal location in the same cell (C) before cancer can develop. In a hereditary cancer, a person is born with situation B. The probability of having just one mutation in a lifetime is quite high and cancer therefore usually arises many years earlier than in sporadic cancers. Used with permission from Professor Anneke Lucassen.

Female cancers can be seen in a range of inherited cancer predisposition syndromes. Features in a family, which may indicate an inherited predisposition, will now be discussed. The process of genetic testing will then be explored. The rest of the chapter will discuss the female cancers and the inherited cancer syndromes they present in. Breast and ovarian cancer will be discussed in the conditions BRCA1 and 2, and endometrial and ovarian cancer within Lynch syndrome. The less common conditions of Peutz-Jeghers, Cowden's and Li Fraumeni will also be discussed. The genetic basis of the other female cancers will then be explored. The chapter will finish with an overview of some of the psychosocial issues that face these families.

Features which may indicate an inherited predisposition to cancer in a family

There are a range of features that may indicate that there is an inherited cancer predisposition syndrome present within a family. For example, the following may indicate that a family should be investigated further and a referral to clinical genetics considered:

(1) Young age at onset of a cancer, for example, a breast cancer diagnosed below the age of 50 or an ovarian cancer diagnosed below the age of 60. The more cases that are diagnosed at a young age in a family, the more likely there is an inherited predisposition.
(2) Multiple tumours seen in one individual. This can be either multiple primary cancers of the same site, for example, bi-lateral breast cancer or of different sites.
(3) The occurrence of recognised associated cancers in the same family (e.g. breast and ovarian cancer or bowel and endometrial cancer). These diagnoses, when seen together, may indicate a specific cancer predisposition.
(4) Suggestion of a characteristic inheritance pattern in the family. Most strongly inherited cancer predisposition shows autosomal dominant inheritance. One copy of a pair of genes is mutated and so with each generation the mutated gene is passed on to an average half the offspring, the other half receiving the normal copy. A family where approximately half the 'at risk' individuals are affected, through successive generations, is therefore suggestive of this inheritance pattern. Dominant inheritance is shown in Figure 5.2.

Recessive inheritance (where both parents are carriers of the genetic condition, i.e. have one mutated and one normal copy of the gene) (Figure 5.3) can also be seen in a small number of cancer genetic syndromes. To be affected, a child needs to receive a faulty copy from both parents. In these families, the disease will not be apparent in parents or previous generations. Recessive inheritance is shown in Figure 5.3.

(5) Histological features of the cancers can make an inherited cancer predisposition more or less likely. For example, mucinous ovarian cancers are more commonly seen in high risk bowel cancer predisposition syndromes, whilst medullary breast cancers are suggestive of a mutation in the high risk breast cancer gene, BRCA1. Whilst a medullary breast cancer is unusual, more common features, such as a grade 3 invasive ductal breast carcinoma that is oestrogen receptor negative, may also be suggestive of a BRCA1 mutation in the context of a strong family history.

Patients with a malignancy will often be concerned about their family history and seek advice on risk and management options (such as surveillance) for their children. In order

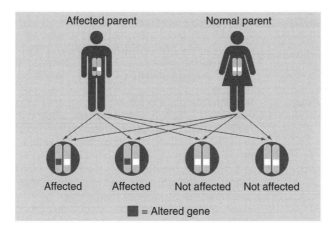

Figure 5.2   Dominant inheritance. Used with permission from Wessex Clinical Genetics
Service.

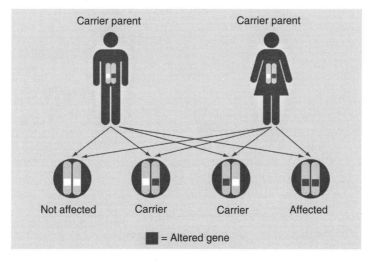

Figure 5.3   Recessive inheritance. Used with permission from Wessex Clinical Genetics
Service.

to address these questions, it is important to take a family history, asking about three
generations where possible, about the types of cancers that have occurred in the family
and the ages of diagnosis. There are many facilities available to assess a family history of
cancer. These include computer programs, such as Boadicea (Antoniou et al. 2004) and
Cyrillic (www.cyrillicsoftware.com), which assess breast cancer risk, manual assessment
methods, for example, the Manchester scoring system for family history of breast cancer
(Evans et al. 2004) and International criteria, for example, the Amsterdam criteria (see
Table 5.1), which assesses the likelihood of Lynch syndrome in a family (Vasen et al.
1999). Risk assessment is usually completed within a clinical genetics service that has the
appropriate expertise to interpret the findings. Family pedigrees showing both a moderate
and high risk breast cancer family history are illustrated in Figures 5.4 and 5.5.

Table 5.1   Amsterdam/Modified Amsterdam criteria.

Amsterdam	Three relatives with colorectal cancer, one of whom is a 1st degree relative of the other two; CRC involving at least two generations; one or more CRC cases diagnosed before the age of 50.
Modified Amsterdam (1)	Very small families, which cannot be further expanded, can be considered as Lynch, even if only two CRCs in 1st degree relatives; CRC must involve at least two generations, and one or more CRC cases must be diagnosed under age 55.
	or
Modified Amsterdam (2)	In families with two 1st degree relatives affected by colorectal cancer, the presence of a third relative with an unusual early onset neoplasm or endometrial cancer is sufficient.
Amsterdam 2	Three relatives with an Lynch associated tumour (CRC, endometrial, small bowel, ureter, or renal pelvis), one of whom must be a first degree relative of the other two; involving at least two generations; one or more cases being diagnosed before the age of 50.

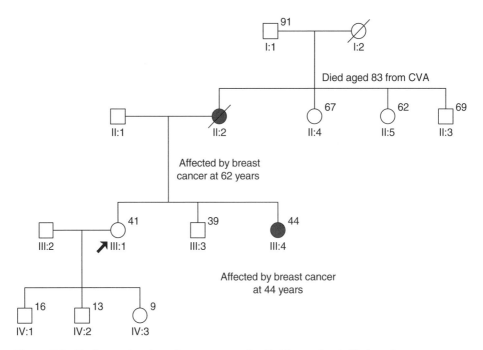

Figure 5.4   Pedigree showing a breast cancer family history that is likely to be moderate risk.

Twenty-three regional cancer genetic services cover the UK and accept referrals from primary and secondary care. National, and where not yet available, local referral criteria exist for individuals with a personal and/or family history of cancer. Referral to a regional genetics service may be helpful for advice on genetic testing and surveillance. An example

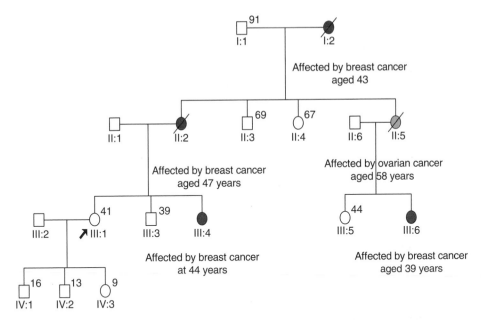

Figure 5.5 Pedigree showing a breast cancer family history that is likely to be high risk.

of cancer referral criteria for a regional genetics service is outlined in Figure 5.6. Some hospitals may also have secondary care family history clinics in breast or gynaecology services. These are often nurse led and appropriate for patients who have a 'moderate' family history, are eligible for additional screening but unlikely to have a high risk cancer predisposition syndrome (see *NICE Guidelines on the Familial Breast Cancer 2004*).

Genetic testing

If there is a clear suggestion of an inherited cancer predisposition in a family, then genetic testing may be offered. If a causative mutation is identified, then genetic testing should be made available to family members who wish to know their genetic status. However, family members may differ in their desire to avail themselves of the options of genetic testing or risk reduction/screening strategies. It is important to involve the regional genetics service to ensure appropriate access to mutation testing and interpretation of results. Genetic testing is a multistage process; it involves mutation searching in an affected family member first and where a mutation is identified, predictive genetic testing is then offered to 'at risk' relatives.

Mutation searching (the diagnostic test)

This involves obtaining a DNA sample (through a blood test) from an affected family member (preferably the person who was diagnosed at the youngest age). Techniques for

These guidelines are to help health care professionals decide when to refer a patient to clinical genetics. If your patient's family history fulfils one of the following categories, then genetic assessment may be appropriate.

To meet the following criteria for referral, your patient is required to have at least one affected 1st degree relative. The only exceptions are:

1) In a breast/ovarian family where the risk is coming down through the paternal line. In this situation, the father may be unaffected and therefore a referral would be accepted with 2nd degree affected relatives.
2) Where there is a known gene mutation within the family, e.g. Familial Adenomatous Polyposis, MYH, Juvenile Polyposis, Peutz Jegher Syndrome, HNPCC, BRCA1, BRCA2.

For GPs, please refer using the referral form and questionnaire found at www.wcgs.nhs.uk. Please ask your patient to complete the questionnaire and then send the referral form and completed questionnaire, as referrals will not be accepted without the questionnaire.

FAMILY HISTORY OF BREAST AND/OR OVARIAN CANCER:

- **Two** close* relatives with breast cancer with average age at diagnosis **under 50** from same side of family
- **Three** close* relatives with **breast** cancer with average age at diagnosis **under 60** from same side of family
- **Four** close *relatives diagnosed at **any age** from same side of family
- One **male** breast cancer at any age **plus** 1 close* relative with breast cancer diagnosed before age 50 from same side of family
- One **male** breast cancer at any age **plus** 2 close* relatives with breast cancer diagnosed before average age 60 from same side of family
- A parent, sibling or child diagnosed with **bilateral** breast cancer before average age 50
- One close* relative diagnosed with bilateral breast cancer **plus** one close relative* diagnosed with **breast** cancer before average age 60 from same side of family
- One relative diagnosed with **ovarian** cancer at **any age plus** one close* relative with breast cancer before **age 50** from same side of family
- **Two** close* relatives with **ovarian** cancer at any age from same side of family
- One relative with **ovarian** cancer at any age **plus** two close* relatives with **breast cancer** before average age 60 from same side of family

Please ring for advice for any other cancer family history that you may be concerned about.

*For the purpose of these guidelines the definition of a 'close' relative is a 1st or 2nd degree relative.
1st degree relative, i.e. child, sibling, parent.
2nd degree relative, i.e. grandparent, aunt or uncle, niece, nephew.

Figure 5.6   Wessex Clinical Genetics Service: *Referral Guidelines to Genetics Service (Tertiary Care)* – Family History of Breast/Ovarian.

finding mutations are continually improving and most laboratories now offer a high throughput service with results available in 2–3 months (in comparison to 1–2 years only a short time ago). This is likely to improve further with results being available within 4 weeks. Because of the implications of a positive gene test result, informed consent prior to blood sampling is essential. The possible outcomes following completion of mutation analysis are listed in Table 5.2.

Table 5.2　Possible outcomes from diagnostic genetic testing.

Positive result	Negative result	Uninformative result
Mutation identified that is pathogenic (disease causing)	Mutation not identified	Mutation identified that has uncertain significance. Not clear if pathogenic (disease causing)
Predictive genetic test available to family members	Mutation not ruled out as testing not yet 100% sensitive	Further testing may clarify significance in due course
	Further testing may be available in the future No predictive genetic test available to family members	No predictive test available to family members until significance is clarified

Testing 'at risk' relatives (the predictive test)

Once a mutation considered to be pathogenic has been identified in a family, predictive testing can be offered to 'at risk' relatives. These individuals need to be carefully counselled to explore motivations for testing and expectations from results. Throughout the UK, predictive testing for cancer predisposition tends to follow the protocol for Huntingdon's disease, where individuals have an initial appointment to explore all relevant issues, followed by a 'cooling off' period of at least 1 month and then a second appointment where blood is usually drawn. Results are usually available within 1 month. A follow-up programme is negotiated between the individual and the genetics team, which may include an invitation to an annual appointment within a specialist multidisciplinary carrier clinic.

Inherited cancer predisposition

Breast and ovarian cancer predisposition (BRCA1 and BRCA2)

Approximately 5% of all breast cancers are due to an inherited dominant cancer predisposition gene, which results in a lifetime risk of breast cancer of approximately 80%. The lifetime risk for women in the general population is around 10%. The two most common genes that cause a strong predisposition to breast cancer are the BReast CAncer1 (Miki et al. 1994) and BReast CAncer2 (Wooster et al. 1995) genes (BRCA1 and 2). Both conditions are dominantly inherited. As well as increasing the risk of breast cancer, mutations in the BRCA1 or 2 genes also cause an increased risk of ovarian cancer. This is a lifetime risk of up to 50%, compared with a 2% general population risk.

It has become apparent that these genes also confer an increased risk of other cancers (e.g. male breast cancer, prostate cancer and pancreatic cancer in BRCA2 and prostate cancer in BRCA1). Specific data on the risk of developing these cancers is not available to families; these cancers are not seen in all BRCA1 and 2 families, and relative risks often demonstrate wide confidence intervals. The relative risks for prostate cancer presented by the Breast Cancer Linkage Consortium range from 3.48–6.22 in BRCA2 male carriers (Thompson and Easton 2001). Other cancers have also been reported in BRCA1/2 families, for example, cervical, laryngeal and colorectal cancer, but there is insufficient evidence that these do actually occur with an increased frequency. There may be other factors, for example, environmental (smoking) or the fact that these are common cancers that explain why these appear in BRCA pedigrees. Some of the uncertainties regarding risk may have arisen from the misreporting of certain cancers within families; it is not unusual for ovarian cancers, for example, to be reported as an abdominal cancer. These additional cancer risks may therefore be clarified over time, as family follow-up continues over many years.

Despite the high risks that an inherited BRCA1/2 mutation confers, it is clear that not all women who inherit a BRCA1/2 mutation go on to develop a breast or ovarian cancer. This reduced penetrance (the chance of a cancer manifesting itself in a gene carrier) may be the effect of protective genes or protective environment in that particular individual. Different mutations within these genes may also confer slightly different risks, the figures given are for all mutations and for any one individual family their own risk figures may fall at either end of the spectrum. Such genotype/phenotype correlations (where specific mutations in a gene result in different features or cancer risks) are emerging as more families are studied. The risk of ovarian cancer particularly seems to vary with different BRCA1/2 mutations; in some families there is preponderance to ovarian cancer rather than breast, and in other families there is no ovarian cancer seen in a number of females with the mutation.

Women who have been affected by breast cancer are also at a significant risk of a further breast cancer primary; around 4% of BRCA1/2 mutation carriers will develop a contra lateral breast cancer per year compared with 1% per year in age matched non-familial cases. In addition, BRCA1 associated breast cancers are often high grade and triple negative tumours (ER/PR/HER2 negative), so fall into a poorer prognosis group. The breast cancers will often occur pre-menopausally and women will be at significant risk from their 40s onwards.

The risk of an ovarian cancer in BRCA1/2 carriers starts to increase in the 40s but is generally at a later onset than the breast cancers (23% by 50 years and 63% by age 70 (Ford et al. 1994; Easton et al. 1995). It is rare to see an ovarian cancer occurring before the early 40s, even in these high risk families. The typical histology features of the ovarian cancers seen within BRCA1/2 are serous papillary cystadenocarcinomas.

Fallopian tube cancer is a rare cancer but occurs with an increased frequency in BRCA1 and 2 carriers. Indeed, BRCA1/2 carriers probably account for a significant proportion of all cases of fallopian tube cancers.

Management of women with a BRCA1/2 mutation

Breast cancer

Surveillance

High risk women are offered strategies to manage their increased risk of malignancy. There are a variety of different methods for the early detection of breast cancer, including mammography, Magnetic Resonance Imaging (MRI) and ultrasonography. *NICE Guidelines for the Management of Familial Breast Cancer* were published in 2004 (NICE 2004) and provide algorithms for which interventions are indicated in different circumstances. Guidelines for mammography examinations in BRCA carriers suggest that there is an individualised surveillance strategy for these women. Many centres offer annual mammography to 'at risk' women from the age of 35 (although in some centres this may start at 40). This will be reviewed at 50 when the National Breast Screening Programme starts, where it may be reduced to 18 monthly. Whilst mammography has been shown to reduce breast cancer mortality in the general population aged 50–64 years (normal screening range), a reduction in mortality in younger women who are screened because of a family history is of unproven benefit. Further research is required to try to establish the effects of mammography on mortality in this patient group. It also needs to consider the limitations of this type of surveillance, for example, false negative results, the efficacy of this test in pre-menopausal dense breast tissue and concerns about the exposure of breast tissue to radiation in women with a germline DNA mutation. This remains an area of debate.

Ultrasonography is not routinely offered to women at high risk of breast cancer, because there is little evidence of its effectiveness of reducing mortality. A study by Berg et al. (2008) suggested that adding ultrasound to mammography increases the number of breast cancers diagnosed, but with additional numbers of false positive results. It may be offered in rare circumstances, such as in women who will not tolerate mammography or have been advised to avoid radiation, but this should only be done with a careful explanation of its limitations.

The efficacy of MRI screening of the breasts has been assessed in younger women in several international research studies (Kriege et al. 2004; Warner et al. 2004; MARIBS Study Group 2005). All of these studies have indicated an increased sensitivity compared with mammography screening, and a combination of the two modalities gives the highest detection rate. NICE updated their 2004 guidelines in 2006 (NICE update 2006), to include the findings of these studies and recommended annual MRI surveillance from 30–49 years in BRCA carriers. Women at 50% risk of a mutation, or those who come from a high risk family where no mutation has been identified, are also offered this screening modality. The delivery of MRI is still rather patchy across the country, as funding and appropriate technology is established.

Despite these surveillance measures, women with a familial predisposition will still present with interval cancers. High risk women should be investigated promptly and thoroughly if they present with breast symptoms or non-specific changes in their breasts. Breast awareness is also discussed with these women routinely.

Chemoprevention

Research exploring the role of hormonal therapy as chemoprevention (e.g. Tamoxifen) has shown a reduction in risk of oestrogen receptor positive breast cancer (Cuzick et al. 2003). However, the increased risks of endometrial cancer associated with Tamoxifen usage has meant that such chemoprevention is not licensed for this use in the UK. Further trials of new agents and their role in reducing breast cancer risk in women at increased risk are therefore awaited.

Recruitment into such projects may be difficult for a variety of reasons. Potential participants are well so may not wish to take interventions that can give them side effects, do not want to enter a randomisation process or have already had preventive surgery, which will make them ineligible to take part. In addition, family members may make different decisions about taking part in research studies, which can lead to conflict and coercion in the family. However, research in these high risk families is very informative. The cancer risks for individuals in these families are greatly increased above the general population and therefore a smaller cohort of participants is required to obtain sufficient information and power to achieve a result.

Surgical options

Prophylactic bi-lateral mastectomy reduces the risk of breast cancer in high risk gene carriers, leading to an approximate 90% reduction in breast cancer diagnoses (Rebbeck et al. 2004; Hartmann et al. 2004). Women who carry a deleterious BRCA mutation should be offered appointments with a specialist breast surgeon and/or plastic surgeon to discuss prophylactic surgery. This is major surgery with significant associated morbidity and careful discussion is required before women proceed. Although the risks of breast cancer are significantly reduced, women should be told that cancers have been reported following prophylactic mastectomy. This is because neither subcutaneous nor total mastectomy by current standard techniques removes all 'at risk' breast tissue, for example, where the nipple areola complex has been preserved, cancers may arise there (Evans et al. 2001). The uptake of prophylactic surgery is more common in younger women and those with young children, with some centres reporting an uptake of 50% in their BRCA carriers. It can be helpful to have a care pathway for women contemplating such surgery, so that a range of specialities are involved; for example, psychological assessment and support for the woman and her partner (Figure 5.7). Complications post-operatively can occur, for example, infection, problems with implants and difficulties in adjusting to the surgery. Positive outcomes of this procedure have been described as a decreased concern about developing breast cancer and in addition, favourable psychological and social outcomes (Frost et al. 2000).

High risk women, who have already undergone mastectomy as part of their breast cancer treatment, may wish to consider a contra-lateral prophylactic mastectomy once their cancer treatment is complete. Following diagnosis, their greatest risk in the short term is a recurrence of their original breast cancer, but as time passes this risk will diminish and the risk of a contra lateral cancer will increase. It is important therefore to have a careful discussion around this question, as women may make different choices at different times.

All the interventions discussed above are based on varying degrees of evidence and patient acceptability. Women therefore have difficult choices to make and these may differ from other family members. This can lead to conflict and possible isolation and these women will need support and careful counselling to support them through decision-making.

Ovarian cancer

Surveillance

There is no evidence that ultrasound (± Ca 125) screening is effective in reducing the mortality from ovarian cancer in the general population. Whether these modalities are

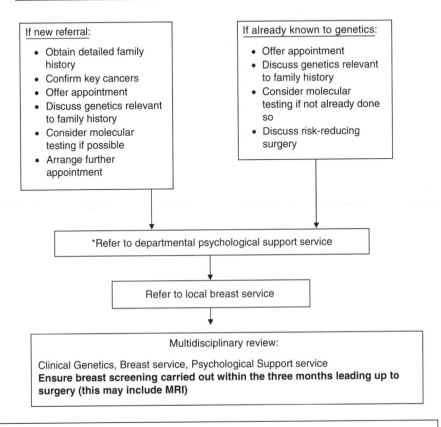

Figure 5.7   Wessex Clinical Genetics Service: Risk-Reducing Mastectomy Pathway.

more effective in a high risk population is being researched in a UK-wide Familial Ovarian Cancer Screening Study (UKFOCSS) (ukfocss@ucl.ac.uk). Women with a BRCA1/2 mutation are eligible to join and undergo an annual ultrasound examination and serial Ca 125 measurements. The primary aim of the project is to develop an optimised screening strategy for ovarian cancer in women at high risk because of a strong family history or inherited genetic predisposition.

Surgery

Because of the limitations of ovarian screening as highlighted above, women may also consider a prophylactic bi-lateral salpingo-oophorectomy. This has been shown to significantly reduce ovarian cancer by up to 90% (Rebbeck et al. 2009; Kauff et al. 2002; Finch et al. 2006). As for prophylactic mastectomy, not all the risk is removed by surgery and peritoneal cancers have been reported in women who have undergone prophylactic oophorectomy. It is important that women undergo a pre-operative assessment to check for occult disease and that post-operatively specimens are carefully analysed for malignancy. Removal of the ovaries pre-menopausally also results in a reduction in breast cancer risk. The earlier this surgery is completed, the greater the reduction in risk. If prophylactic oophorectomy is completed at 40 years, there is a 50% reduction in breast cancer risk (Rebbeck et al. 2005; Eisen et al. 2005). This is thought to be due to the reduction in circulating oestrogen following surgery. However, the breast cancer risk reduction is seen in BRCA1 and BRCA2 carriers, even though the breast cancers seen with BRCA1 mutations are likely to be oestrogen negative.

Because of the risk of fallopian tube cancer, women with BRCA1/2 mutations should also have their fallopian tubes removed, and subsequently analysed for occult mali, at the time of their prophylactic oophorectomy.

Hormone Replacement Therapy (HRT) in a surgical menopause

There has been much media coverage of several high profile trials in the general population, which have fuelled debate that long-term use of HRT increases the risk of developing breast cancer. This has raised anxiety in women who have undergone a prophylactic oophorectomy procedure and are taking or wish to take HRT for menopausal symptoms. It is difficult to interpret these results in women with a family history of breast cancer, because their circumstances are different. Although these women are at an increased risk of breast cancer because of a family history, they will have had surgery completed prior to their natural menopause, and will be replacing hormones they would normally be producing. They are therefore not extending the numbers of years that they are exposed to these hormones. Recent studies have suggested that HRT for this group of women is safe to use, especially in the short term (3–5 years) and does not negate the effect of prophylactic oophorectomy on reducing breast cancer risk (Rebbeck et al. 2005).

Case report from woman after prophylactic oophorectomy with BRCA1 or 2 mutations

Endometrial and Ovarian cancer predisposition (Lynch syndrome or Hereditary Non-Polyposis Colorectal Cancer HNPCC)

Lynch syndrome or Hereditary Non-Polyposis Colorectal Cancer (HNPCC) is an autosomal dominantly inherited cancer predisposition syndrome. The common genes associated with Lynch syndrome are the hMLH1, hMSH2, hMSH6 and PMS2 genes.

A pathogenic mutation in one of these genes results in an increased risk of both colorectal and endometrial cancer for women. The lifetime risk of colorectal cancer is in the region of 28–75% in males (6% in the general population) and 24–52% in females (5% in the general population). These risk figures are broad, because HNPCC mutations demonstrate reduced penetrance and other factors (i.e. environmental) will affect cancer risk. There is a lifetime risk of up to 70% for women of endometrial cancer (Vasen et al. 2007) compared to a risk of 1% in the general population. One in five (20%) women with HNPCC will present with endometrial cancer before they reach the menopause. Ovarian cancer has a lifetime risk of around 7–13% in HNPCC carriers (Vasen et al. 2007; Watson et al. 2008) compared to a 2% population risk and adenocarcinoma of the endocervix also occurs at an increased frequency.

The so-called Amsterdam criteria (Vasen et al. 1999), and subsequently modified Amsterdam criteria, have been devised to identify families who may have a diagnosis of HNPCC (Table 5.1). It is important to note that these are highly specific criteria; this means that those who meet the criteria are very likely to have HNPCC, but does not exclude those who do not, especially if they come from a small family or there is minimal family history information available. Genetic testing can then be offered to confirm the diagnosis and help in the management of family members. If women decide that they do not wish to pursue a genetic test, then they will still be offered screening as per the protocol for confirmed carriers.

Management of women from HNPCC families

This next section will discuss management options for 'at risk' women from HNPCC families. It will focus on the female cancers that present in HNPCC carriers. However, as there is a significant risk of colorectal cancer in HNPCC, 2-yearly colonoscopy surveillance will be recommended for women from 25 years of age. This will usually continue until at least 70, and the decision to stop these examinations is guided by the individual's health status. If polyps are found on examination, the 2-yearly screening intervals may be amended, depending on histology results. Where possible, polyps will be removed at the time of colonoscopy and undergo detailed histological examination. Further surgery may then be required.

Endometrial cancer

Surveillance

There is insufficient evidence available on the efficacy of different surveillance modalities for endometrial cancer. Because of this, there are no widely accepted surveillance guidelines available. Further clarification is needed on the usefulness of screening and there is data suggesting that there may be value in further assessing approaches to endometrial screening using endoscopic biopsy (Renkonen-Sinisalo et al. 2007).

Chemoprevention

Research to assess endometrial screening modalities and possible chemoprevention agents is ongoing. An example of this is the Prevention of Endometrial Tumour (POET) project www.poet-trials.co.uk, where women with Lynch syndrome are randomised to endometrial screening (annual trans-vaginal ultrasound or hysteroscopy with endometrial biopsy or pipelle) and the Mirena (progesterone) intrauterine device vs screening only. Women remain on the study for 5 years, with the primary aim of the project being to determine if treatment with an intrauterine progestogen reduces the incidence of atypical endometrial hyperplasia and endometrial cancer. Again, recruitment to these studies is problematic, as women often do not want to undergo the randomisation process.

Surgical options

Because of the high risk of developing endometrial cancer in HNPCC, women may wish to consider a prophylactic hysterectomy. This may include bi-lateral salpingo-oophorectomy, because of an increased risk of ovarian cancer in female carriers. The decision to undergo prophylactic surgery may be easier if women have concurrent benign gynaecological pathology and are already considering surgery.

HRT following surgery

HRT should be considered following surgery, including prophylactic oophorectomy, particularly if the surgery is completed pre-menopausally. The use of HRT is not contra-indicated for female HNPCC carriers and there is no significantly increased risk of breast cancer in female carriers. One consideration pre-surgery is the associated risk of post-operative adhesions, which can make the colonoscopy required for colorectal cancer risk technically difficult and painful for the woman. This may result in an incomplete examination, and thus subsequent further examinations under general anaesthetic or other investigations such as barium enema.

Ovarian cancer

Because of the increased risk of ovarian cancer in HNPCC, management options, as described in the section on BRCA genes, will be available to women. This includes prophylactic surgery and eligibility for the UKFOCSS study.

Cowden syndrome

This is a hamartoma tumour syndrome caused by mutations on the PTEN gene. Prevalence is likely to be more than 1/200,000. It presents with an array of features, with the major diagnostic criteria including breast, thyroid and endometrial cancer with macrocephaly (>95th centile). Minor criteria include benign thyroid disease, developmental delay, fibrocystic breast disease, lipomas and fibromas. There are also pathognomonic criteria with muco-cutaneous lesions, facial trichilemmomas and papillomatous papules. Genetic testing is possible in this syndrome and screening of the breast and thyroid recommended if the diagnosis is confirmed either clinically or through a genetic test. This will include annual mammography (usually from 40 years), annual thyroid examination and consideration of endometrial screening.

Peutz-Jeghers syndrome (PJS)

This syndrome is characterised by gastro-intestinal hamartomas, mucocutaneous pigmentation (freckling of lips and oral mucosa) and a predisposition to gastrointestinal tumours, breast and other cancers. Women either diagnosed with the condition or 'at risk', should be offered 3-yearly cervical smears (ecto- and endo-cervical) and annual breast screening from 35 years, until they enter the National Breast Screening Programme at 50.

Li-Fraumeni syndrome (LFS)

This is a rare cancer syndrome characterised by a clustering of childhood and adult cancers. The condition is caused by mutations in the TP53 gene. The common cancers seen within LFS are breast cancer, soft tissue sarcomas, osteosarcomas, brain tumours and adrenocortical tumours. Cancer of other sites has also been reported and the lifetime cancer risk is practically 100% in females. There is concern about the effects of radiation in this condition and therefore women are offered annual breast MRI screening from their early 20s. Screening for the other cancers commonly seen in LFS is not routinely offered, but women are carefully counselled about having a low threshold for having symptoms promptly investigated because of the high malignancy risk.

Other gynaecological cancers

Cervical cancer

An inherited predisposition to this cancer is rare and there is now clear evidence of the role of environmental factors in its development (e.g. exposure to the Human Papilloma Virus (HPV) and smoking). An increased risk of cervical cancer has been proposed in BRCA1 and 2 female carriers, but this has not been robustly supported in the literature and there is an increased incidence in PJS. There is a national cervical screening programme and no additional screening is recommended to women from BRCA families. When women with a BRCA1/2 or HNPCC mutation are considering prophylactic surgery to remove their ovaries and/or uterus, a full hysterectomy procedure may be discussed by their surgeon. This may be because of other gynaecological problems that would make this a reasonable option or because of concerns about malignancy risk of other reproductive organs, which are not yet clearly established.

Vulval cancer

This cancer is rarely considered to be 'genetic', but may be associated with HPV and smoking. Vulval cancer has been reported to occur with increased frequency in some rare genetic conditions, for example, Fanconi's anaemia and Morris' syndrome.

Psychosocial issues in genetic assessment and testing

Cancer risk assessment and genetic testing is not an easy process for families. It does not only have implications for the person being assessed/tested, but also for other family members both current and future. Some individuals would prefer not to know this information, which can become difficult if family members want different things from a genetics referral. Other issues that may be important during the genetic counselling process are insurance and financial concerns, family dynamics, coercion, non-disclosure of results in a family, testing of identical twins and non-paternity. These factors will all need to be considered when counselling families. Access to specialist psychotherapeutic counselling may be available in genetic services, if indicated.

This chapter has outlined the importance of identifying women with a possible genetic predisposition to cancer. This includes both women affected by cancer and those at an increased risk of developing it. These women can then avail themselves of specialist advice and make decisions about the benefits and limitations of genetic testing, surveillance possibilities and other options such as prophylactic surgery and chemoprevention. In addition, information from one person may reveal other family members who are at increased risk (including male relatives). This chapter has discussed the information that needs to be gathered to be able to identify families who may be at an increased risk of cancer and might benefit from referral to specialist services for further assessment.

The author would like to acknowledge Professor Anneke Lucassen for her very helpful comments on this chapter.

Genetic appointment: a patient's story

I first learnt that I may have a gene mutation 3 years after the death of my younger sister.

There was no clear history breast cancer in our family and my sister was diagnosed with breast cancer at the age of 34, 4 months after the birth of her second child. She had advanced breast cancer and was told her disease was terminal within 1 month of diagnosis. She survived a further two and a half years, but was confined to a wheelchair after a spinal cord compression and died having experienced much aggressive oncology treatment and leaving behind young children and a family who were shocked and devastated by the trauma of her death.

As you might imagine, the thought of receiving a letter out of the blue from the genetic service via my brother-in-law was at least alarming. I opened a letter from an anonymous doctor suggesting I might wish to discuss with my local genetic team the possibility of my carrying similar DNA as my sister. I was aware my sister had asked for a test, as her son had a cancerous tumour in his kidney at the same time as she was being treated, but also that they had been told their cancers were unrelated and just one of those unfortunate tragic events.

I work professionally in the NHS, so attending an outpatient appointment was both familiar and yet I felt very detached. I knew the purpose of the first meeting in the genetic department would be to discuss whether to take a blood test and to discuss what to do if I carried a familiar gene. What I didn't expect was the way in which the two people who met with me were able to adapt to exactly what I needed. We were able to make a decision to take the test and I was initially surprised about how long it might take to get the results.

I went back for the results 2 months later, meeting again with the same two members of the genetic team. I had convinced myself that I did not have the mutated gene and that everything would be ok. It came as an overwhelming shock to find I did carry the gene. I was able to get all the information I needed to make a decision, but my immediate feeling was 'I can't go through what my sister did – I can't risk not seeing my children grow up', and if there was a way for me to not to be in that place then, I would take it.

I was able to get all the information about surgery, insurance and also about the next steps; it felt like I was being guided through the process and I left the appointment knowing I needed time to digest the information but also with lots of things to think about. I was relieved to hear that something could be done; but had not realised that if I did take the surgical option it would be so radical.

I was able to think about less invasive options over the next couple of days; but really what informed me most were my feelings of never wanting to be in my sister's position. My friends who spoke with me reacted differently; what was most helpful were those who listened to me and said we will support you whatever. Some friends felt surgery was too drastic, even though they understood my motives and some worried about my emotional well-being after having such major surgery. For me, I knew I would struggle emotionally but knew also I was strong enough to manage the surgery and recovery period. I felt if I could recover physically, I would then allow myself the longer period of emotional healing. I knew that the loss of my breasts and womb would back the loss of my sister amongst other things, but felt I was taking action to make sure this was not going to have the same outcome as my sister. I was taking my life back, getting away from the uncertainty and fragility of feeling out of control.

What I appreciated from the specialist staff at the genetics service was the regularity of being able to meet the same person and being able to discuss the different options. There was an open honesty to our conversations and I was still able to ask for information as needed. What I had not appreciated was that as I carried this gene, it wasn't just about me but had more far reaching consequences. I watched my husband and children adjust to my decisions and support me through the surgery, even though they were worried for me. My own mother was so terrified, she had lost one daughter and wanted to do all she could to help me. My mum took the blood test herself as she wanted to know if she carried the gene and had passed it on. It was a huge relief to know she did not carry the same mutation, which had been passed to me from my father, who had since died. At every stage I would get a phone call saying 'how are you?' and 'is the path your taking going ok?' The approach the staff took was to be guided by my questions and in time we spoke about how to talk to my own family and children about how I could not feel 'guilty' that I carried a genetic mutation. What surprised me was how it was important to keep building up my family tree and how it is important to communicate information so others could have the opportunity to make their minds up. Two of my extended family took opposing views, one cousin went though the same process of testing that I had done and decided to have the same extensive surgery. Another cousin decided she did not want to get tested and took the view if she developed cancer it would be fate and she would deal with if it occurred.

It was a long and complicated process to discover I had the genetic mutation and then to make a decision about what I might do. Looking back, I felt much supported along this journey and am completely happy with the decisions I have made. I have been able to speak with my own children and family and know now that the door is open to have further conversations as time moves on.

Reflective points

- Using symbols provided, outline your own family tree.
- Consider the issues that women have, knowing that they have an increased risk of malignancy.

References

Antoniou, A.C., Pharoah, P.P.D., Smith, P. et al. (2004) The BOADICEA model of genetic susceptibility to breast and ovarian cancer. *British Journal of Cancer* **91**, 1580–90.

Berg, W.A., Blume, J.D., Cormack, J.B. et al. ACRIN 6666 Investigators (2008) Combined screening with ultrasound and mammography vs mammography alone in women at elevated risk of breast cancer. *JAMA* **299(18)**, 2151–63.

Cuzick, J., Powles, T., Veronesi, U. et al. (2003) Overview of the main outcomes in breast-cancer prevention trials. *Lancet* **361**, 296–300.

Easton, D.F., Ford, D. and Bishop, D.T. (1995) Breast and ovarian cancer incidence in BRCA1 mutation carriers. Breast Cancer Linkage Consortium. *American Journal of Human Genetics* **56(1)**, 265–71.

Eisen, A., Lubinski, J., Klijn, J. et al. (2005) Breast cancer risk following bi-lateral oophorectomy in BRCA1 and BRCA2 mutation carriers: an international case-control study. *Journal of Clinical Oncology* **23(30)**, 7491–6.

Evans, D.G., Eccles, D.M., Rahman, N. et al. (2004) A new scoring system for the chances of identifying a BRCA1/2 mutation outperforms existing models including BRCAPRO. *Journal of Medical Genetics* **41(6)**, 474–80.

Evans, D.G., Lalloo, F., Shenton, A. et al. (2001) Uptake of screening and prevention in women at very high risk of breast cancer. *Lancet* **358(9285)**, 889–90.

Finch, A., Beiner, M., Lubinski, J. et al. (2006) Salpingo-oophorectomy and the risk of ovarian, fallopian tube, and peritoneal cancers in women with a BRCA1 or BRCA2 mutation. *JAMA* **296(2)**, 185–92.

Ford, D., Easton, D.F., Bishop, D.T. et al. (1994) Risks of cancer in BRCA1 mutation carriers. Breast Cancer Linkage Consortium. *Lancet* **343(8899)**, 692–5.

Frost, M.H., Schaid, D.J., Sellers, T.A. et al. (2000) Long-term satisfaction and psychological and social function following bilateral prophylactic mastectomy. *JAMA* **284(3)**, 19–24.

Hartmann, L.C., Degnim, A. and Schaid, D.J. (2004) Prophylactic mastectomy for BRCA1/2 carriers: progress and more questions. *Journal of Clinical Oncology* **22(6)**, 981–3.

Kauff, N.D., Satagopan, J.M., Robson, M.E. et al. (2002) Risk-reducing salpingo-oophorectomy in women with a BRCA1 or BRCA2 mutation. *New England Journal of Medicine* **346(21)**, 1609–15.

Kriege, M., Brekelmans, C.T., Boetes, C. et al. Magnetic Resonance Imaging Screening Study Group (2004) Efficacy of MRI and mammography for breast cancer screening in women with a familial or genetic predisposition. *New England Journal of Medicine* **351(5)**, 427–37.

MARIBS Study Group (2005) Screening with magnetic resonance imaging and mammography of a UK population at high familial risk of breast cancer: a prospective multicentre cohort study (MARIBS). *Lancet* **365(9473)**, 1769–78.

Miki, Y., Swensen, J., Shattuck-Eidens, D. et al. (1994) A strong candidate for the breast and ovarian cancer susceptibility gene BRCA1. *Science* **266(5182)**, 66–71.

National Institute for Clinical Excellence (2004) Familial breast cancer. The classification and care of women at risk of familial breast cancer in primary, secondary and tertiary care (www.nice.org. uk/CG041NICEguideline)

National Institute for Clinical Excellence (2006) Familial breast cancer. The classification and care of women at risk of familial breast cancer in primary, secondary and tertiary care. Update (www. nice.org.uk/CG041NICEguideline)

Rebbeck, T.R., Friebel, T., Lynch, H.T. et al. (2004) Bilateral prophylactic mastectomy reduces breast cancer risk in BRCA1 and BRCA2 mutation carriers: the PROSE study group. *Journal of Clinical Oncology* **22(6)**, 1055–62.

Rebbeck. T.R., Friebl, T., Wagner, T. et al. (2005) Effect of short-term hormone replacement therapy on breast cancer risk reduction after bi-lateral prophylactic oophorectomy in BRCA1 and BRCA2 mutation carriers: The Prose Study Group. *Journal of Clinical Oncology* **23(31)**, 7804–10.

Rebbeck, T.R., Kauff, N.D. and Domchek, S.M. (2009) Meta-analysis of risk reduction estimates associated with risk-reducing salpingo-oophorectomy in BRCA1 or BRCA2 mutation carriers. *Journal of the National Cancer Institute* **101(2)**, 80–7.

Renkonen-Sinisalo, L., Butzow, R., Leminen, A. et al. (2007).Surveillance for endometrial cancer in hereditary nonpolyposis colorectal cancer syndrome. *Inernational Journal of Cancer* **120**, 353–62.

Thompson, D. and Easton, D., Breast Cancer Linkage Consortium (2001) Variation in cancer risks, by mutation positive, in BRCA2 carriers. *American Journal of Human Genetics* **68(2)**, 410–9.

Toms, J.R. (Ed.) (2004) *CancerStats monograph (2004)*. London: Cancer Research UK.

Vasen, H.F., Watson, P., Mecklin, J.P. et al. (1999) New clinical criteria for hereditary nonpolyposis colorectal cancer (HNPCC, Lynch syndrome) proposed by the International Collaborative group on HNPCC. *Gastroenterology* **116**, 1453–6.

Vasen, H.F., Moslein, G., Alonso, A. et al. (2007) Guidelines for the clinical management of Lynch syndrome (hereditary non-polyposis cancer). *Journal of Medical Genetics* **44(6)**, 353–62.

Warner, E., Plewes, D.B., Hill, K.A. et al. (2004) Surveillance of BRCA1 and BRCA2 mutation carriers with magnetic resonance imaging, ultrasound, mammography and clinical breast examination. *JAMA* **292(11)**, 1317–25.

Watson, P., Vasen, H.F., Mecklin, J.P. et al. (2008) The risk of extra-colonic, extra-endometrial cancer in the Lynch syndrome. *International Journal of Cancer* **123**, 444–9.

Wooster, R., Bignell, G., Lancaster, J. et al. (1995) Identification of the breast cancer susceptibility gene BRCA2. *Nature* **378(6559)**, 789–92.

www.cyrillicsoftware.com

Chapter 6

Lifestyle and Prevention

Elaine Lennan

Learning points

At the end of this chapter, the reader will have an understanding of:
- Cancers potentially caused by lifestyle choices
- The public health strategies aimed at reducing the risk of developing cancer

Introduction

Currently over 1 million women are living with cancer in the UK. One in three people will develop cancer at some point in their lives and it is estimated that over 285,000 people are diagnosed with the disease every year (DH 2000).

Although many cancers tend to be put down to bad luck or fate, or in some cases faulty genes, the environment and lifestyle choices also pay a significant part of cancer incidence. Cancer Research UK state that half of all cancers could be prevented by lifestyle changes (CRUK 2009). Commonly cited lifestyle changes include:

- not smoking
- cutting back on alcohol
- keeping a healthy body weight
- eating a healthy, balanced diet
- keeping active
- staying safe in the sun
- staying sexually healthy.

This chapter aims to discuss the role of lifestyle in developing cancer and looks at strategies to adopt a healthier approach. The latter part of the chapter will look at specific screening programmes.

Women's Cancers, First Edition. Edited by Alison Keen and Elaine Lennan.
© 2011 Blackwell Publishing Ltd. Published 2011 by Blackwell Publishing Ltd.

Prevention

Adopting a healthy lifestyle free from high risk behaviour does of course not guarantee cancer will be prevented. In practice, everyone can cite many patients who have never been ill, never visited the GP, never drunk to excess, maintained a healthy diet and body weight, exercised regularly and then have been struck by a cancer diagnosis. However, there is evidence that avoiding certain risks can significantly reduce the risk of developing cancers. Indeed, the World Cancer Research Fund Report (2007) estimates that cancers could be prevented in the UK by the following:

- 42% breast cancer
- 56% endometrial cancer
- 26% all cancers

This chapter will discuss lifestyle issues and outline preventative measures.

Smoking

Smoking is the single biggest cause of cancer in the world (DH 2009). Half of all smokers eventually die from cancer, or other smoking-related illnesses, and a quarter of smokers die between 35 and 69 years of age.

Whilst the epidemic of women smoking has passed in the later quarter of the twentieth century, 20% of all women actively smoke on average 13 cigarettes per day (Office for National Statistics 2009). The age range for the peak prevalence is 25–34. This prevalence is predicted to fall further following intense campaigning and health awareness benefits. In addition, the world has now begun smoking bans in public places. Cancer of the cervix is known to be linked to smoking (Berrington de Gonzalez et al. 2004). Benzyrene in cigarettes is thought to change the potential of the lining of the cervix to fight infection. It is also known that once smoking ceases, these cells return to normal. The risk of cervical cancer further increases if you smoke and also have Human Papilloma Virus (HPV).

Smoking cessation

The overall health benefits of smoking cessation cannot be underestimated. Studies have shown that stopping smoking can greatly reduce the risk of smoking-related cancers (Doll 2003). The earlier you stop, the better, but it is never too late. However, this is well recognised as a difficult task (IARC 2004). The American Cancer Society state that 70% of smokers want to quit, 40% try, but only 4–7% succeed. Reasons for this are the powerful physical and emotional aspects of nicotine addiction. Certainly trying to quit smoking alone is associated with high failure rates and there is now evidence to show that providing help to stop smoking is the most clinically proven cost-effective prevention action that health care professionals can undertake (West et al. 2000). Indeed, the DH (2009) advocates the need for 'referral to quit' services to become embedded in everyday practice, and Perceival (2009) suggests that helping individuals to quit smoking is an extremely productive use of nurses' time.

So just how can nurses help others to stop smoking? Experts suggest it is a combination of good communication skills, motivational support and pharmacological treatment that generate high success rates. Nurses involved with cancer patients can begin the process by firstly taking a smoking history, and acknowledging quitting smoking following a cancer diagnosis may not be the immediate best approach. Indeed, many smokers describe a smoking habit that relates to stress or a coping mechanism. Obviously being told you have a cancer diagnosis is extremely stressful and may well be associated with a sense of guilt because they have smoked. Nurses need to look for opportunities to raise the benefits of quitting smoking at any time and can extend this to family members, as those that do quit often do so in response to a health crisis (Perceival 2009). Once an initial assessment has been made, nurses should refer to specialist advice and support services. Evidence suggests that whilst awareness of smoking cessation services is high, this does not necessarily relate to high referrals to such services (Elsheikh et al. 2006; West et al. 2000). Nurses are well placed to bridge this gap.

There are now many resources to help an individual quit smoking, which include:

- NHS Smoking Helpline
- www.quit.org
- www.nhsdirect.nhs.uk
- Quitters

In addition, ongoing support from the primary care team cannot be underestimated:

I always smoked right from school days, I guess it just built up over time, everyone did it … it's one of those things, it's never gonna happen to me but here I am. I was confused at first, once I was diagnosed I smoked more, it was my way of getting through. I would have a smoke before I came through the doors of the hospital and if there were delays. Of course there were delays. I would nip out and have another, it kind of prepared me for what I was going to hear and what I had to face. Even after I used to say to Charley, 'don't talk till we get outside', he knew really but I still said it. I'd light up and then I'd say, 'ok what do you think?' I have thought about quitting and tried a couple of times, once went 6 weeks but then started again, can't remember why now. But I like I said, I was confused, I thought people got lung cancer, no one told me smoking can cause my cervix cancer, no one even mentioned it to me, when I started treatment, but when I was getting over the shock I was looking on the internet and I read smokers can get cervix cancer. I felt oh my god I did this to myself whereas before that I kind of thought I was just unlucky. I loaded myself again with a smoke before I made the phone call to ask whether my smoking had caused my cancer. From then on I decided to quit. I was over the initial shock of being told I had cancer and I was now looking for ways to help myself. I was referred to a quitters programme at my GPs and they have been great. I guess its early days but I feel stronger than before to do this. Even Charley is giving it a go. I am now 11 weeks without a cigarette and it's still hard, but I am going to beat it and am going to beat my cancer. I have put 2 and 2 together.

Alcohol

Alcohol is a well established cause of cancer, accounting for about 6% of cancer deaths. Of particular note is the increased risk of breast cancer in women who regularly drink alcohol, i.e. 3 units a day to about 7% (Doll 2003). If the woman is also smoking, this increases the risk further.

Even small amounts of alcohol can increase your risk of breast cancer. Several studies have found that every alcohol unit drunk a day increases the risk of breast cancer risk by about 7–11% (Key et al. 2006; Allen et al. 2009a).

A recent very large study, known as "The Million Women Study", tracked cancer incidence and alcohol use in nearly 1,300,000 middle-aged women in the UK. Women in the study had an average age of 55, and 3 out of 4 identified themselves as 'drinkers'. Of these 'drinkers', the average alcohol intake was about one drink per day (Allen et al. 2009b).

Follow-up was for 7 years and during this time approximately 69,000 women were diagnosed with cancer. 'Drinkers' were found to be at increased risk of cancers of the oral cavity, pharynx (throat), oesophagus, rectum, liver and breast. The risk for these cancers increased with the number of drinks a woman consumed, regardless of the type of alcohol.

These findings raised interesting points; the researchers estimated that in the UK, alcohol accounts annually for about 11% of all breast cancers, 22% of liver cancers, 9% of rectal cancers and 25% of cancers of the oral cavity, pharynx, oesophagus and larynx (Allen et al. 2009b). This research then questions the confusing public health message. On the one hand, the public is told of the favourable cardiovascular benefits of small alcohol consumption and yet it is unlikely there will be a safe level of alcohol consumption that does not increase the risk of breast cancer.

Whilst it is known that alcohol does cause cancer, it remains unclear how it does and it is likely to be multi-factorial. These are listed below:

- *Acetaldehyde*. This is the hangover chemical thought to distort DNA and encourage liver cells to grow more rapidly
- *Hormones*. Alcohol is known to increase oestrogen, testosterone and insulin
- *Alcohol* makes it easier for smoking chemicals to enter the blood stream, therefore increasing the risk of cancer if you smoke and drink

Help in cutting down on alcohol consumption

The current advice to individuals through a public health message is that women should not consume more than 2–3 units regularly per day (DH 1995). For most, understanding the links between alcohol with the development of cancer will be enough to encourage a immediate cutting down in alcohol consumption. However, for many it might be a surprise to realise just how much they do intake per week. A helpful leaflet is available called *Units and You*, for those who might not be aware of just how much alcohol they consume. This leaflet offers awareness advice and tips for when to recognise that drinking patterns are becoming more dependent (www.dh.gov.co.uk). For individuals who do develop a dependence, referral to an alcohol dependency service will be necessary through their GP:

I really didn't realise how much alcohol I was drinking. I would always have a glass of wine at night and sometimes 2, but I would never open a second bottle . . . but sometimes one bottle rolled into the next. It was a habit I guess, I would too have a few at the weekend, not every weekend and I guess when you think about it I would binge drink. I never get into trouble of anything or fall over but I was always merry. Even now as I'm talking it seems so normal. I was asked about drinking as I suppose a routine question and I said you know one a day and I was told to cut back. I thought, 'O oh heck I probably take in more than that!' I thought about it and sure enough I had myself down as a raging alcohol but I wasn't it was just normal, everyone was doing it. I still like my wine but not every night.

Body weight

Maintaining a healthy body weight is an important step in reducing the risk of developing a cancer. Being overweight increases the risk of developing cancer, due to the increase in production of hormones particularly insulin and oestrogen. Ideal body weight is calculated using the body mass index (BMI). It is thought to reduce the risk of cancer, your BMI needs to be less than 25 (Renehan et al. 2008).

Preventing weight gain can reduce the risk of many cancers. Establishing habits of healthy eating and physical activity early in life to prevent obesity are current public health messages. Weight loss strategies are appropriate at any time of life and avoiding additional weight gain is important. A small weight loss of only 5–10% of total weight can provide health benefits (Cui et al. 2002; Huang et al. 1997).

The cancer burden through obesity is important and when taken in the context of other health concerns related to obesity, is significant to the health economy. Several studies in the US suggest the direct link between obesity and cancer is in the range of 3–20% (Calle et al. 2003; Polednak 2003). There is sufficient evidence to establish a link between obesity and two women's cancers, breast and endometrium (Weiderpass et al. 2000). In addition, there is a probable link between obesity and ovarian cancer (CRUK 2009) (Figure 6.1).

Breast cancer and obesity

The link between breast cancer and obesity only becomes important when considering post-menopausal breast cancer. It is thought that heavier women are at a lower risk of developing breast cancer than lighter women, but after menopause this reverses (van den Brandt et al. 2000; Trentham-Dietz et al. 1997).

Both the increased risk of developing breast cancer and dying from it after menopause are believed to be due to increased levels of oestrogen in obese women. In pre-menopausal women, circulating oestrogen comes primarily from the ovary with little from fat tissues.

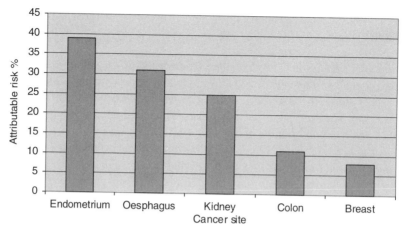

Figure 6.1   Proportion of selected cancers caused by overweight and obesity.

However, after the menopause, the fat tissue becomes the primary source of oestrogen and consequently obese women can double their circulating oestrogen when compared to thinner women. Exposure to oestrogen sensitive cells can become overwhelming and a tumour develops (Cui et al. 2002).

Distribution of fat or body shapes have also been found to play a significant role. Those with abdominal fat (apples) are thought to be at greater risk than those with thigh fat (pears). Finally, any cancer in an obese person is often diagnosed late due to difficulties in detection.

Endometrial cancer and obesity

It is unclear why obesity is a risk factor for developing endometrial cancer, but a link has been established. It is again thought to be due to increased circulating oestrogens and insulin. Unlike breast cancer, menopause status does not appear to play a part (Salazar-Martínez et al. 2000; Shoff et al. 1998; Goodman et al. 1997; Bergstrom et al. 2001).

The benefits of maintaining a healthy BMI cannot be underestimated in reducing the risk of cancer. Health education messages are important in this regard and should continue once a diagnosis of cancer has been made. However, in a similar way to smoking cessation programmes, often a cancer diagnosis creates a stress response and entering into talks about losing weight may not be appropriate. Health professionals need to look for opportunities to engage in positive health messages and offer support when required. Referrals to dieticians may be appropriate.

Eating well and keeping active

A healthy eating plan and maintenance of a BMI of more than 25 of course go hand in hand. According to CRUK and the American Cancer Society, there are no associations between diet and the women's cancer described in this book, with the exception of a potential link between saturated fats and breast cancer (Thiebaut et al. 2007; Boyd et al. 2003).

The WCRF (2007) looking at preventable cancer has recommended 10 simple messages, mostly dietary. They are:

- Stay lean throughout adult life
- Limit food and drinks that promote weight gain
- Be physically active
- Limit red meat consumption
- Avoid processed meat
- Eat non-starchy vegetables
- Eat non-starchy fruit
- Limit alcohol consumption
- Limit salt intake
- Breastfeed children

These are clear messages that have filtered into public health services, but it has been recognised that individuals alone find it difficult to make lifestyle shifts. To this end, a subsequent report from WCRF (2009) urged governments, schools and industry to accept responsibility for presenting and encouraging positive lifestyle changes. Examples include promoting healthy eating in schools, introducing cycle routes, nutrient messages on food packs, and legislation to ensure women can breastfeed, to name a few.

Diet is extremely important to a cancer patient. It is something they can take control of and use to help themselves. It is also particularly important to relatives, as it is something they can do or help with. Unfortunately, despite the rhetoric, there are no magic dietary answers in either prevention or treating cancer. The message remains consistent with general public health messages – eat healthily and avoid extremes of weight.

Keeping active helps control weight and therefore has a positive benefit in preventing cancers. It is also known that activity helps to promote positive hormone levels and boosting immune systems. However, there is no robust evidence to suggest exercise decreases a risk of developing cancer. Despite this, CRUK (2009) have recently suggested there is probable evidence for the positive benefits of reducing the risk of breast cancer for those who are physical active. The public health message currently recommends at least 30 minutes vigorous exercise 5 times a week:.

When I was diagnosed I wanted to help myself as much as possible. I had spent years in and out of weight watchers – life long member. In one way you've got a cancer diagnosis, you think what the hell and then another you want to give yourself the best possible chance. That's quite a dilemma! I decided I would like this experience to once and all fix my weight. I asked about diet, you know read a bit and they said do this, don't eat this. I read I was to stop all diary products and to be honest I felt gutted. I was, am never a chocolate person but cheese, can't get enough and really it's really hard to cut out all diary, so I decided just to be healthy. I know all the rules anyway and I put on about a stone through treatment, stress I guess but I've now lost that stone and another half a stone. I don't think I'll manage much more but the cancer definitely kick started me.

Staying safe in the sun

Whilst preventing skin cancer may seem out of place in a book on women's cancer, it is relevant as a lifestyle message to women in general, as the image of the modern women is with a tan. Indeed, skin cancer rates have soared over the past few years. Over the past 30 years, the incidence of malignant melanoma has tripled in women in the UK CRUK (2005). This is a worldwide trend (de Veries et al. 2005).

There are many causes but there is a clear correlation between sun damage, prolonged exposure to UV light and skin cancer. Exposure to UV light has increased due to increased holidays abroad, which involves short intense exposure, reduction in ozone layer and the use of sun beds.

All people are affected by sunlight but some populations are more at risk than others. Light coloured people are more susceptible than darker, but this does not exclude darker skins from sun damage. In addition to skin tone, there are further risk factors associated with developing skin cancer as follows:

- Those with lots of moles or freckles
- Fair skin, blonds and red heads
- Previous history of skin cancer
- Family history
- High altitude living
- Intense sun exposure
- Outdoor working
- Underlying immune diseases
- Previous organ transplant
- Regularly taking certain medications (American Cancer Society 2009).

Skin cancer prevention campaigns aim to increase sun damage awareness. Avoidance of midday sun, use of high factor sun cream and covering up are the three key messages. Some campaigns also add in the need to wear sunglasses to protect the eyes.

Health professionals have the opportunity to promote positive lifestyle messages whenever possible, and skin cancer prevention is no exception:

I obviously don't have skin cancer but just having a cancer makes you more health aware. I am your typical 'lie out in the sun till I'm pink person' but then I go nicely brown. I do like the look of a tan but I'm not so bothered that I would go on a sunbed, I do think that's extreme. My worry is I live in the north, you know the old saying,' its grim up north' and we head to the sun for our holidays twice' sometimes 3 times a year and it's a real boost. I couldn't give it up. I think I will be more aware of sun damage and the need to wear lotion' etc. and I guess for my daughter and son for that matter I need to be making them really aware before they develop my bad habits.

Sexual health

Sexual health is important, particularly in the prevention of cervix cancer. Screening programmes are crucial in detecting pre-cancerous states and offering treatment before a cancer develops. It is known that 99% of cervical cancers occur as a result of sexually transmitted virus HPV. This is a very common virus, with over 100 different strains, but only 13 cause cancer (Women's Health Concern 2007). Most people will have the virus at some point in their lives and be asymptomatic (Health Promotion Agency 2008). The recent introduction of immunisation for girls aged 12–14 is aimed at reducing the incidence of cervix cancer by 70%, by developing immunity before sexual activity begins. This is a major medical advance but importantly it should be remembered that the vaccine does not protect against all HPV or other sexually transmitted diseases, and therefore good sexual health practices and continued cervical smears are important throughout life (Women's Health Concern 2007).

The link between promiscuity and cancer of the cervix is now thought to be a misguided. It is possible to have only one partner throughout life and still develop cervical cancer if your one partner has HPV. The promiscuity link is more likely to be exposure to the virus the more partners you have, than actually amount of partners.

Sexual health education can help women reduce their risk of cervical cancer. Several approaches to sexual health are needed, including practical advice and behavioural strategies. Shepperd et al. (1999) recommend the following:

- How to use a condom
- To avoid sex when they are young
- To reduce their number of sexual partners
- How to negotiate safe sex

In addition, some researchers have found that the risk of cancer was almost half in women who bathed more often than compared to women who bathed less. Others have shown this poor hygiene link and summarized the increased risk due to a lasting HPV infection if they are exposed to the virus (CRUK 2009).

Conclusion

Clearly lifestyle has a bearing on health and well-being in general. However, it is clear that lifestyle choices have the potential to increase a risk of developing cancer. Adopting a healthy lifestyle free from high risk behaviour does of course not guarantee cancer will be prevented. However, there is evidence that avoiding certain risks can significantly reduce the risk of developing cancers. Education via public health messages is ongoing and will continue.

Reflective points

- What lifestyle advice would you give a lady diagnosed with breast cancer when she asks if she can have a drink?
- Why does obesity have an increased risk of developing endometrial cancer?
- Think about a patient with cervix cancer. How might you coach them to stop smoking?

References

Allen, N.E., Beral, V., Casabonne, D. et al. (2009a) Moderate alcohol intake and cancer incidence in women. *Journal of National Cancer Institute* **20**, 514.

Allen, A., Beral, V., Casabonne, D. et al. Million Women Study Collaborators (2009b) Moderate alcohol intake and cancer incidence in women. *Journal of National Cancer Institute* **101**, 296–305.

Bergstrom, A., Pisani, P.M., Tenet, V., Wolk, A. and Adami, H.O. (2001) Overweight as an avoidable cause of cancer in Europe. *International Journal of Cancer* **91(3)**, 421–30.

Berrington de Gonzalez, A. et al. (2004) Comparison of risk factors for squamous cell and adenocarcinomas of the cervix: a meta-analysis. *British Journal of Cancer* **90(9)**, 1787–91.

Boyd, N.F., Stone, J., Vogt, K.N., Connelly, B.S., Martin, L.J. and Minkin, S. (2003) Dietary fat and breast cancer risk revisited: a meta-analysis of the published literature. *British Journal of Cancer* **89**, 1672–85.

Calle, E.E., Rodriguez, C., Walker-Thurmond, K. and Thun, M.J. (2003) Overweight, obesity, and mortality from cancer in a prospectively studied cohort of US adults. *New England Journal of Medicine* **348(17)**, 1625–38.

CRUK (2005) *Cancer Statistics – Malignant melanoma*. London: CRUK.

CRUK (2009) *Cancer Statistics – Breast Cancer*. London: CRUK.

Cui, Y., Whiteman, M.K., Flaws, J.A. et al. (2002) Body mass and stage of breast cancer at diagnosis. *International Journal of Cancer* **98(2)**, 279–83.

de Veries, E. and Coebergh, J. (2005) Cutaneous malignant melanoma in Europe. *European Journal of Cancer* **40(16)**, 2355–66.

Doll, R. et al. (2003) Mortality in relation to smoking: 50 years' observations on male British doctors. *British Medical Journal* **328**, 1519.

Department of Health (1995) Sensible drinking: the report of an interdepartmental working group In: S.E. Vollset, et al. Smoking and Deaths between 40 and 70 Years of Age in Women and Men. *Annals International Medicine*, 2006. **144(6)**, 381–9.

Department of Health (2000) *The NHS Cancer Plan*. London: HMSO.

Department of Health (2009) *NHS Stop Smoking Services-Service and Monitoring Guidance 2009/10*. London: HMSO.Elsheikh, A. et al. (2006) The NHS stop smoking services: hospital staff awareness and the pattern of referral to local services. *Thorax* **61(Suppl. 2)**, 23.

Goodman, M.T., Hankin, J.H., Wilkensm L.R. et al. (1997) Diet, body size, physical activity, and the risk of endometrial cancer. *Cancer Research* **57(22)**, 5077–85.

Health Promotion Agency (2008) *Beating Cervical Cancer*. Scotland: HMSO.

Huang, Z., Hankinson, S.E., Cloditz, G.A. et al. (1997) Dual effects of weight and weight gain on breast cancer risk. *Journal of the American Medical Association* **278(17)**, 1407–11.

IARC (2004) *Monographs on the Evaluation of Carcinogenic Risks to Humans: Tobacco Smoke and Involuntary Smoking*, Vol. 83. Lyon: IARC Press.

Key, J., Hodgson, S., Omar, R.Z. et al. (2006) Meta-analysis of studies of alcohol and breast cancer with consideration of the methodological issues. *Cancer Causes Control* **17**, 759–70.

Office for National Statistics (2009) *Living in Britain: General Household Survey 2007*. London: TSO.

Perceival, J. (2009) Smoking cessation 2: targeting, engaging and supporting hard to reach groups. *Nursing Times 6* **105(39)**, 28–29.

Polednak, A.P. (2003) Trends in incidence rates for obesity-associated cancers in the US. *Cancer Detection and Prevention* **27(6)**, 415–421.

Renehan, A.G., Tyson, M., Egger, M. et al. (2008) Body-mass index and incidence of cancer: a systematic review and meta-analysis of prospective observational studies. *Lancet* **371**, 569–578.

Salazar-Martínez, E., Lazcano-Ponce, E.C., Lira-Lira, G.G. et al. (2000). What biological mechanisms are thought to be involved in explaining the link between obesity Case-control study of diabetes, obesity, physical activity and risk of endometrial cancer among Mexican women. *Cancer Causes and Control* **11(8)**, 707–11.

Shepherd, J.J., Peersman, G. and Napuli, I. (1999). Interventions for encouraging sexual lifestyles and behaviours intended to prevent cervical cancer. *Cochrane Database of Systematic Reviews* **4(CD001035)**. DOI: 10.1002/14651858.CD001035.

Shoff, S.M. and Newcomb, P.A. (1998) Diabetes, body size, and risk of endometrial cancer. *American Journal of Epidemiology* **148(3)**, 234–240.

Thiebaut, A.C., Kipnis, V., Chang, S.C. et al. (2007) Dietary fat and post-menopausal invasive breast cancer in the National Institutes of Health-AARP Diet and Health Study cohort. *Journal of National Cancer Institute* **99**, 451–62.

Trentham-Dietz, A., Newcomb, P.A., Storer, B.E. et al. (1997) Body size and risk of breast cancer. *American Journal of Epidemiology* **145(11)**, 1011–19.

van den Brandt, P.A., Spiegelman, D., Yuan, S.S. et al. (2000) Pooled analysis of prospective cohort studies on height, weight, and breast cancer risk. *American Journal of Epidemiology* **152(6)**, 514–27.

Weiderpass, E., Persson, I., Adami, H.O. et al. (2000) Body size in different periods of life, diabetes mellitus, hypertension, and risk of post-menopausal endometrial cancer (Sweden). *Cancer Causes and Control* **11(2)**, 185–92.

West, R. et al. (2000) Smoking cessation guidelines for health professionals: an update. *Thorax* **55(12)**, 987–99.

Women's Health Concern (2007) *Cervical Screening.* www.womens-health-concern.org (accessed 6 February 6 2009).

World Cancer Research Fund (2007) *Food, Nutrition, Physical Activity, and the Prevention of Cancer: A Global Perspective.* www.diet and cancer report.org (accessed 6 July 2009).

World Cancer Research Fund (2009) *Policy and Action for Cancer Prevention.* www.diet and cancer.org (accessed 6 July 2009).

Useful websites

NHS Smoking Helpline
www.quit.org
www.nhsdirect.nhs.uk

Chapter 7

Cancer of the Breast

Alison Farmer

Learning points

At the end of this chapter the reader will have an understanding of:
- The incidence and mortality of breast cancer
- The pathology and staging of breast cancer
- The differences between the management of adjuvant and metastatic disease
- The psychological impact of breast cancer

Introduction

Almost all women share a mythology of breast cancer. It's as if a stream of ideas and images circling this topic moves continuously from woman to woman. We lean towards each other, share information in low, confiding voices. 'It happened to me once. The doctor said we should watch it.' There are questions: Is the lump very hard? Can you move it with your fingers? Where is it in your breast? Questions, observations, intimacies, everything rushes towards a final, deeply drawn breath of relief. 'Oh in that case – because it's hard, soft, movable, immovable, in the inner quadrant, out towards your armpit – it can't be cancer.

Juliet Whitman (1993)

Mention you have discovered a lump in your breast to a room full of people and there will be few, if any, who are unaware of the significance of the statement. Our cultural model of breast cancer is deeply ingrained and is one of advanced disease, mutilating surgery, unpleasant treatments and ultimately death. It goes without saying that a diagnosis of any cancer is distressing, but breast cancer is compounded by the significance of the breasts as nurturing and sexual organs. They are intrinsically linked with a sense of attractiveness, femininity and motherhood. Newspapers, magazines, soap

Women's Cancers, First Edition. Edited by Alison Keen and Elaine Lennan.
© 2011 Blackwell Publishing Ltd. Published 2011 by Blackwell Publishing Ltd.

operas and celebrities have gone some way to dispel some of the fear and myths and ensure a more open dialogue, but the diagnosis and treatment can still have a signifi-cant physical and psychological impact.

The topic of breast cancer is vast and some might say deserves a book of its own. Whilst making no claims to cover all aspects of breast cancer, this chapter will endeavour to provide an overview of the main topics. These will include epidemiology, modes of detection, diagnosis, pathology, adjuvant therapy, survivorship, recurrence and the psy-chological impact. This chapter will only address female disease, although approximately 300 cases of breast cancer are found in men annually.

Incidence and mortality

Approximately 44,500 women are diagnosed with breast cancer in the UK each year. One in nine women will develop breast cancer in their lifetime (Cancer Research UK). Although the majority of women are post-menopausal, 8000 women under the age of 50 are also diagnosed annually. Since the 1970s, advances in detection and treatment have reduced the mortality from breast cancer, possibly by as much as 30% (Peto 2000). In 2006 there were 12,319 female breast cancer deaths compared to 15,625 deaths in 1989 (Cancer Research UK). The multidisciplinary approach to treating breast cancer, which is now common practice, appears to have been largely responsible for the reduction in mortality we are now seeing. The multidisciplinary approach includes diagnostic imaging, breast screen-ing, surgery, radiotherapy and chemotherapy. Identification of high-risk women who may benefit from surveillance, prophylactic drug treatment and/or surgery has also contributed to the recent reduction in mortality (Moulder and Hortobagyi 2008).

Risk factors

Although the cause of breast cancer is uncertain, there are a number of risk factors associ-ated with the disease (Breakthrough Breast Cancer 2009) (Table 7.1). More recently, *in utero* and early life factors are also being considered, with some studies showing a link between the development of breast cancer in later life and above average birth weight, twin-ship and rapid childhood growth (dos Santos Silva 2005).

Detection

Breast cancer may be symptomatic or asymptomatic and can occasionally present as wide-spread metastasis with no obvious primary in the breast. Symptomatic breast cancer usually presents as a lump, change in size or shape of the breast, indrawn nipple, puckering of the skin (peau d'orange), nipple discharge or swelling in the axilla. Whilst symptomatic breast cancer is usually detected by the patient, her partner or a health professional, asymptomatic breast cancer is often found following routine mammographic breast screening by the NHS Breast Screening Programme (NHSBSP).

Table 7.1   Risk factors for developing breast cancer.

Known risk factors
Increasing age
Ethnicity
Genetic predisposition
Gender – women > men
Height
Early menarche
Benign disease
Alcohol consumption
HRT
Contraceptive pill
Later pregnancy
Increasing weight post menopause
Exposure to radiation
Possible risk factors
Diet
IVF treatment
NSAIDs
Shift-work
Stress
Doubtful risk factors
Abortion
Implants
Chemicals
Deodorants
Non-ionizing radiation
Under wire bras

The NHSBSP was introduced in England and Wales in 1988, following the success of large randomised, controlled trials of mammographic breast screening in New York and Sweden (Shapiro 1977; Tabar et al. 1985). These showed a reduction in mortality of up to 30% in women invited to attend. Currently all women in the UK between the ages of 50 and 64 are invited to attend every 3 years. Despite some high profile criticism (Baum 1995), the programme continues and is considered a success by most, as it saves approximately 1400 lives per year (NHSBSP 2006). Further reductions in mortality are anticipated and we are not expected to see the full effect of screening until 2010 (Blanks et al. 2000).

Pathology

Amongst the various procedures employed to reach a diagnosis of breast cancer, perhaps the most important is the histological examination of the tumour. The histopathologist will want to know the cell type and whether the cells are confined within the ducts or lobules, *'non-invasive'*, or have spread beyond the basement membrane into neighbouring breast tissue and perhaps elsewhere, *'invasive'*.

Non-invasive breast cancer

The two main types of non-invasive breast cancer are ductal carcinoma *in situ* (DCIS) and lobular carcinoma *in situ* (LCIS). DCIS is a proliferation of malignant duct epithelial cells, which are confined to the breast ducts and show no evidence of spread and LCIS is confined within the lobules of the breast. These conditions, often described as 'pre-cancerous', if left untreated may spread beyond the ducts and lobules, becoming invasive. The introduction of the National Breast Screening Programme has not only contributed to the reduction in mortality, but has had an impact on the number of non-invasive breast cancers, such as (DCIS), that are detected. Numbers have risen from a pre-screening level of 5% of breast cancer cases to a post-screening level of approximately 20% (Morrow and O'Sullivan 2007).

Invasive breast cancer

Invasive breast cancer has spread beyond the basement membrane. There are a number of different types of invasive breast cancer that are differentiated by their growth and cellular morphology. Tumours with specific features are known as invasive cancers of 'special type', whereas those that have no specific features are known as invasive cancers of 'no special type'. Those tumours of special type tend to have a better prognosis than those of no special type (Sainsbury et al. 2000). There are a number of subtypes of breast cancer, the most common being adenocarcinoma of the breast, which arises from the epithelial lining of the terminal duct lobular unit and accounts for 75% of all breast cancers.

Staging

An important part of breast cancer treatment is staging of the disease. Staging relates to the patient's prognosis and has implications for treatment. Staging can only be done after the lesion is excised and the axilla has been dissected. Patients with stage I disease currently have approximately an 84% chance of surviving 5 years, whereas those with a stage IV cancer have approximately an 18% chance of surviving 5 years (Cancer Research UK). The most common method for staging breast cancers is the TNM classification (Appendix X). The American Joint Committee of Cancer modified the TNM classification of staging in 2002, to include assessment by a pathologist (Singletary et al. 2002).

Diagnosis

Patients who are suspected of having breast cancer are referred for further procedures and investigations. These include clinical breast examination, ultrasound, mammography and fine needle aspiration (FNA). Ideally the patient is examined and given the diagnosis on the same day to avoid the distress of waiting for test results. If the mammogram or FNA prove conclusive, then an excision biopsy may be performed under anaesthetic. All patients also have liver function tests, full blood count and a chest X-ray to assist with the diagnosis of metastatic disease. Patients with early stage disease require no further investigations, but those with evidence of more extensive disease might also be offered bone and liver scans.

Treatment

Surgical options for invasive breast cancer are removal of the breast tissue, usually along with the nipple (mastectomy), removal of the tumour, together with a 1 cm margin of healthy tissue (wide excision) or removal of a quadrant (quadrantectomy). The most common form of mastectomy performed today is the simple mastectomy. This does not necessitate removal of the underlying muscles as was the case with the more radical Halstead mastectomy. If wide excision is the treatment of choice, then healthy margins are crucial as any remaining disease significantly increases the likelihood of recurrence (Sainsbury et al. 2000). As the cosmetic result will be very important for some women, wide local excision is discouraged if the tumour is over 4 cm or too close to the nipple. A wide excision is almost always followed by radiotherapy. Treatment of the disease not only depends on stage but the patient's wishes, age, health, hormone receptor status and human epidermal growth factor 2 (HER2) status. Irrespective of whether mastectomy or wide excision is chosen, the procedure is usually accompanied by some form of axillary dissection.

Axillary dissection

Establishing whether the cancer has spread from the breast to the axillary lymph nodes is an essential part of breast cancer staging. Assessing the axilla may take the form of node sampling. Sampling involves the removal of a few of the lymph nodes and only if cancer is found, will the axilla be completely cleared. Complete axillary clearance, removal of all the lymph nodes, carries the risk of lymphoedema but is favoured by some surgeons. More commonly, the sentinel node or nodes are taken. A sentinel node biopsy involves the injection of a dye and a radioactive material into the area of the breast close to the tumour. The dye and radioactive tracer then drain away to the first group of lymph nodes, which are removed and examined for any traces of cancer. This procedure results in less arm stiffness or swelling than complete axillary lymph node dissection, and further surgery is only required should cancer be detected (Samphao et al. 2008).

  Consensus has still to be reached regarding the best way to manage the axilla in women with breast cancer. Whether a woman is offered axillary sampling, clearance or sentinel node biopsy, may be simply down to the preference of the surgeon. The results of long-term follow-up and randomised controlled trials should help determine the optimum treatment (Samphao et al. 2008).

Non-invasive breast cancer

Non-invasive breast cancer or ductal carcinoma *in situ* (DCIS) is, according to Morrow and O'Sullivan (2007), notoriously difficult to treat due to the natural history of the disease being poorly understood. Little is known about which cases of DCIS will become invasive and what the time interval is between recurrence of DCIS and/or development of invasive disease. Treatment varies from centre to centre and women may be offered local excision or, if the disease is widespread, i.e. affects multiple ducts, mastectomy or simply a diagnostic biopsy, hormones and observation. Although there is some evidence that radiotherapy reduces the incidence of local recurrence, the absolute benefit is small and there is a lack of survival difference between all forms of treatment (Morrow and O'Sullivan 2007). Until more is known about which lesions will become invasive on a molecular level, women will continue to be offered a range of treatments. This can lead to some confusion and distress (De Morgan et al. 2002).

Choice of treatment

The lack of survival difference between mastectomy and wide excision has not only led to more conservative surgery but has enabled more women to have a role in choosing their treatment. Early research showed that women who were offered a choice of treatment had less psychological morbidity (Morris and Royal 1988). However, a review of studies by Fallowfield (1997) failed to find a psychological benefit and in some cases there appears to be an increase in psychological morbidity. Choosing treatment may burden a woman with responsibility, especially if the disease recurs. This is an instance in which it is essential to take account of the woman's individual coping style and preferences. It should also be borne in mind that a woman who declines the chance to take part in treatment decisions at one point may well want to be more involved at another. It should certainly not be assumed that all women would prefer to keep their breasts.

Adjuvant therapy

For the majority of women, surgical excision is followed by some form of adjuvant therapy. The choice of adjuvant therapy is dictated by a woman's age, hormone receptor status and stage of disease.

Chemotherapy

Adjuvant chemotherapy is an important part of the treatment for breast cancer and is particularly beneficial for women up to the age of 70 with moderate- to high-risk breast cancer (Smith and Chua 2006b). Traditionally, the drugs cyclophosphomide, methotrexate and fluououracil (CMF) were the treatment of choice, but there is now evidence that anthracycline regimens with doxorubicin or epirubicin can achieve a significant further improvement in survival of 4–5% (Smith and Chua 2006b). Indeed, anthracyclines followed by CMF are frequently used in the UK. Trials of the drug docetaxel, a taxane, are also complete and NICE guidelines recommend its use after surgery in women with early stage breast cancer with positive nodes.

The physical impact on the patient of several months of chemotherapy should not be underestimated and many women find the treatment gruelling. Fatigue, hair loss, nausea, cognitive impairment, lowered resistance to infection, anaemia, peripheral neuropathy, bruising and sore mouth can all occur to a lesser or greater degree.

Chemotherapy can also lead to a premature menopause. Attempts are being made to establish the efficacy of shorter courses. The CALBG 9741 trial randomised women to receive conventional treatment, every 3 weeks, or 'dose dense' treatment, every 3 weeks. Results showed a survival advantage and a reduction in neutropenic sepsis (Smith and Chua 2006b). Shorter duration of treatment is likely to be an attractive option for many women, as this will mean less time spent visiting the hospital and shorter duration of side effects such as alopecia. However, it is important that women get the planned dose at the correct time, as the proportion of the prescribed dose that is given can have a significant impact on overall and relapse-free survival (Bonadonna et al. 1995).

Chemotherapy may also be given prior to surgery, known as neo-adjuvant, to reduce the size of the tumour or as a palliative treatment in advanced breast cancer.

Adjuvant online

A fairly recent addition to the breast cancer armory is the decision-making tool 'Adjuvant! Online'. This tool enables patients with early breast cancer and their oncologists to assess the risks/benefits of adding additional therapy such as chemotherapy and/or hormone therapy after surgery. The information provides an estimate of the risk of negative outcome should further treatment not be used. The patient is usually given a print-out as an aid to decision-making. Due to the complexity of the input information, it must be entered by a health professional with a knowledge of cancer.

Radiotherapy

Patients who have a wide excision are highly likely to be offered adjuvant radiotherapy to the remaining breast tissue and any remaining axillary lymph nodes if they have not been surgically removed. Irradiating the axilla does increase the risk of the patient developing lymphoedema of the arm on the affected side (Cancer Research UK). Radiotherapy is not usually offered to women after mastectomy, unless they are at high risk of local recurrence, such as those with involvement of pectoralis major (Sainsbury et al. 2000). Treatment is usually given daily over 3 or 5 weeks. Side effects can include fatigue, nausea and soreness of the skin. Higher doses of radiation used formerly often led to cardiac damage and pneumonistis, but these side effects are now seen much less commonly since the adoption of lower dose regimens.

Although radiotherapy has been in use for many years, there remains a high level of ignorance amongst the general public surrounding the treatment. In a qualitative study by Halkett et al. (2008), women reported a great deal of fear of radiotherapy prior to commencing treatment and were particularly scared of being burnt or having their internal organs damaged. Most women found that their fears were much worse than the actual experience and the authors urge health professionals to listen to patients' fears and provide reassurance during the planning stage.

As with chemotherapy, radiotherapy may be given prior to surgery to reduce the size of the tumour.

Endocrine therapy

In 1896, Sir George Beatson performed oophorectomies on two women with advanced breast cancer. The first patient's response was dramatic; however, the second patient failed to respond (Cheung 2007). It was not until 70 years later, when oestrogen receptors were discovered, that the difference in response was explained.

It is Beatson's early work that forms the basis of the use of hormones in the treatment of breast cancer (Cheung 2007), as it is the oestrogen receptor (ER) status of the patient's cancer that dictates whether or not endocrine therapy is used. Historically, surgical techniques were used to achieve oestrogen ablation such as oophorectomy, adrenalectomy and hypophysectomy. These operations were risky and irreversible and it is now more common to achieve the same results with the use of drugs, luteinizing hormone-releasing hormone (LHRH) agonists. The advantage of LHRH agonists is that the treatment is reversible, unlike surgical or radiotherapy procedures. The benefits of endocrine therapy alone have been shown to be either equivalent, or greater than, those of chemotherapy in ER positive women (Cheung 2007). Ovarian ablation, tamoxifen and chemotherapy have all shown survival advantages in randomised controlled trials. Ovarian ablation has been shown to provide a survival advantage in pre-menopausal women with ER positive tumours. The absolute gain in survival after 15 years was 6.3 and 12.5% for all patients and node positive patients, respectively (Cheung 2007).

Tamoxifen

Tamoxifen, a partial oestrogen agonist, was introduced in 1971 and for years was the single most important addition to breast cancer treatments. Recently, however, third generation selective aromatase inhibitors are frequently the drug of choice. It is effective in all age groups, and in pre-menopausal and post-menopausal women. Tamoxifen is used in a number of different circumstances. It is used as a sole treatment in the elderly who are unfit for surgery and, as the tumour is still present, it can be observed for response. It is used as an adjuvant therapy following surgery for operable breast cancer and in this situation, as there is no visible tumour present, response cannot be assessed. Adjuvant treatment currently lasts for 5 years, but there is no evidence that continuing treatment for more than 5 years is of benefit (Smith and Chua 2006a). Trials have shown that tamoxifen given after chemotherapy is more effective than if it is given at the same time (Smith and Chua 2006a). Tamoxifen is also being evaluated as a pre-operative/neo-adjuvant therapy and a preventative treatment in women at risk of developing breast cancer (Cheung 2007).

The side effects of tamoxifen can be particularly distressing for some women. These include vaginal dryness, venous thromboembolism, hot flushes, altered libido, gastrointestinal symptoms, weight gain, menstrual disturbance and endometrial cancer. Endometrial cancer risk is increased three or four times with prolonged use, but absolute risk of serious side effects remains low and can be balanced by a decreased risk of bone loss and osteoporosis (Smith and Chua 2006a).

Aromatase inhibitors

Post-menopausal women with ER positive tumours may be offered aromatase inhibitors. These have been shown to be more effective than tamoxifen (Cheung 2007). Aromatase inhibitors inhibit oestrogen synthesis, are effective only in post-menopausal women and improve both disease-free and metastatic-free survival (Smith and Chua 2006a). The aromatase inhibitors that may be offered are Anastrazole, Exemestane and Letrozole.

Trastuzumab

One drug that has made significant headlines in the last 5 years is Trastuzumab (Herceptin). Trastuzumab has been shown to be very effective in women with breast tumours that over express HER2 and has greatly improved remission rates (Smith and Chua 2006c). Herceptin is an expensive drug which, until recently, was not funded by all Primary Care Trusts in the UK. This lead to several high profile court cases, where women attempted to force their health authorities to allow prescription of the drug for them. Trastuzumab is now a recommended and funded treatment for all HER2 positive women.

Survivors

Once surgery and adjuvant therapy are completed, women have to adjust to their status as a breast cancer survivor. Breast cancer survivors are the largest group of cancer survivors. The quality of life of this large, and growing, group is of great importance and the aim of any physical and psychological treatment should be to return the patient to pre-morbid functioning.

As the risk of recurrence is highest in the first 3 years, the breast cancer survivor will be followed up regularly. The aim of breast cancer follow-up is to detect recurrence and assess the patient for physical and psychological side effects of diagnosis and treatment. How often, and by whom, the follow-up should be administered is an ongoing debate. The European Society of Medical Oncology (ESMO 2005) recommends history taking, eliciting of symptoms and physical examination every 3–6 months for 3 years, every 6–12 months for 3 years, and then annually. They also recommend mammography every 1–2 years and, if the patient is symptomatic, blood tests, chest X-ray, bone scans, liver ultrasound, CT scans and tumour markers such as CE 15-3 and CEA.

Transferring follow-up to the patient's GP has been considered and has been found to be an effective way of detecting recurrence. In a study by Grunfield et al. (2006), no significant differences in outcome were found between the group who had regular cancer centre follow-up and those that were followed up by their GP. Patient initiated follow-up has also been considered. Brown et al. (2002) randomised two groups of women with stage 1 breast cancer to either routine clinic follow-up or self-referral after instruction on what signs and symptoms to look for. There were no major differences in quality of life or psychological morbidity between the two groups, although the routine clinic group did report more reassurance.

Lymphoedema

Lymph is a straw coloured fluid, which is formed in the body. This fluid drains back into the circulatory system through a network of vessels and lymph nodes. The lymph nodes form a filtering system, helping to remove excess protein, dead and abnormal cells and bacteria.

Lymphoedema occurs when the drainage routes through the lymphatic system become blocked or damaged. For women having removal of axillary lymph nodes or receiving radiotherapy, there is significant risk of the development of lymphoedema of the arm. Women who are at risk should have instruction on preventative measures, and if lymphoedema occurs should be referred to a lymphoedema clinic.

Reconstruction

For many survivors who have had a mastectomy, breast reconstruction is an attractive prospect. Reconstruction can either be in the form of breast implants, pedicled flaps or free flaps.

Breast implants

Breast implants may be made of silicone gel or saline and are placed beneath the skin either with or without prior tissue expansion. Tissue expansion gives a more natural look than the insertion of silicone implants without it.

Pedicled Flaps

Pedicled flap reconstruction involves taking either the latismus dorsi or the rectus abdominis muscle, along with its skin and blood supply, and tunnelling it under the skin before stitching it in place. This type of surgery occasionally requires an implant as well and also a breast reduction or lift for the uninvolved breast.

Free flap

Free flap reconstruction uses skin and fat from the abdomen or buttock, but rather than use existing blood supply, a new blood supply is established using microsurgery.

The surgeon will discuss the most suitable method of reconstruction with the patient and will take into account her age, breast size and preference. Reconstruction can either be performed at the time of the initial cancer surgery (immediate) or some years later (delayed). Research has shown that breast reconstruction post-mastectomy has a positive effect on body image and confers a psychosocial benefit long term. Satisfaction does not appear to be related to the type of procedure used (Atisha et al. 2008).

Recurrence

Recurrent breast cancer is devastating for the patient, their family and friends. The disease is no longer curable and although women with recurrent disease are likely to die from it, advances in treatment means that it is possible for some women to live for many years, managing their breast cancer more as a chronic condition than an acute one. If breast cancer spreads, then the most likely places for it to metastasise to are the bones, brain, liver and lungs.

Spread to the bones

Patients whose breast cancer has metastasised to the bones may experience pain and weakness. They are also at risk from pathological fractures, spinal cord compression and hypercalaemia. The metastatic bone cancer stimulates osteoclast mediated bone resorption. The broken down bone then provides nutrients for the cancer, accelerating tumour growth. A recent advance in the treatment of bone metastases has been the use of Bisphosphonates. Bisphosphonates act by inhibiting osteoclastic bone resorption and, although there is currently no evidence that they prolong survival, they can reduce the incidence of pathological fracture, spinal cord compression, hypercalaemia and pain. Further research is needed to assess the role of Bisphosphonates in the development of bone metastasis and survival (Gralow 2002).

Spread to the liver

Spread to the liver is often characterised by discomfort, nausea, loss of appetite and ascites (swelling of the abdomen due to fluid build up). Occasionally the skin and whites of the eyes become yellow (jaundice). This is due to the presence of bile salts in the blood, which along with making the eyes and skin yellow, can lead to itching of the skin. The nature of the liver means that it can still function if some of it is removed or is out of action due to secondary disease (Cancer Research UK).

Spread to the lungs

If breast cancer spreads to the lungs, women may experience a persistent cough or become short of breath. If the cancer has spread to the pleura (the lining of the lungs) fluid may build up, which then presses on the lung and may make it difficult to breathe. This fluid can be drained off by a doctor, which will relieve the symptoms; however, the procedure may need repeating if the fluid builds up again (Cancer Research UK).

Spread to the brain

If the breast cancer has spread to the brain, women may experience headaches, nausea, arm or leg weakness or memory loss. As the brain is large it can, like the liver, continue to function quite well despite secondary spread.

Treatment for secondary breast cancer

The treatment for secondary breast cancer may involve hormone therapy, chemotherapy and or radiotherapy. Hormone therapy has the advantage of being easy to administer and relatively safe; however, the side effects can impact of the patient's quality of life (Smith and Chua 2006a). Another advantage of hormone therapy is that there are many different types of hormone treatment available and if the cancer is not responding to one then it may respond to another. Those women with oestrogen receptor positive tumours are more likely to respond favourably to hormone therapy for secondary breast cancer (Cancer Research UK).

Although the chemotherapy drugs used for advanced breast cancer may, in some cases, be the same as those used for primary breast cancer, there are a number of new drugs available specifically for advanced disease. NICE (2009) recommends first line docetaxel, second-line single agent Vinorelbine or Capecitabine and third-line single agent Vinorelbine or Capecitabine (whichever was not used as a second-line treatment). It is recommended that Capecitabine and Gemcitabine are given in combination with docetaxel (Cancer Research UK).

In the palliative setting, chemotherapy may be given to women with inoperable fungating tumours, to reduce their size and dry them out.

A good quality of life up until death should be the aim and involving the palliative care team sooner rather than later will help ensure that all that is possible is done to manage the psychological as well as the physical effects of recurrence.

Psychological aspects of diagnosis and treatment

The relatively recent discipline of 'Psycho-social Oncology' has led to a more thorough empirical understanding of the psychological and social aspects of the diagnosis and treatment of cancer (Greer 1994). Initially derided by the medical profession, psychological care is now considered to be an essential part of the cancer care package although, sadly, the service remains patchy, with only a few dedicated psycho-oncology units around the country.

All cancers have been studied, but the emotive nature of breast cancer has meant that this particular disease has received a great deal of attention from psycho-oncologists. Early research identified a number of common psychological reactions following mastectomy, with as many as 25–30% of women reporting significant long-term distress, including anxiety, depression, anger, lack of concentration and inability to cope with breast loss (Morris et al. 1977; Maguire et al. 1978; Meyerowitz 1980). The revelation that wide excision and radiotherapy offered the same survival advantage for women as mastectomy (Fisher et al. 1985) was greeted by many with relief, as it was anticipated that psychological morbidity would disappear along with mastectomy (Lasry et al. 1987). Unfortunately, this was not found to be the case, with similar levels of psychological morbidity found in women undergoing both mastectomy and wide excision (Fallowfield et al. 1990).

Women appear to be more concerned about losing the cancer than the extent of the surgery:

> *Sometimes I think that doctors don't really believe you when you say 'I'm not bothered by how much you take, just as long as you take it all' and I wonder whether the doctors believe you, because so many women are worried about losing their breasts, but me, I'd rather lose the cancer.* (Farmer 2000)

One would expect women to be distressed on learning they have breast cancer and then having to cope with the unpleasant side effects of treatment. Of importance is how long the distress lasts. Looking at prevalence of anxiety and depression in the 5 years after diagnosis, Burgess et al. (2005) found that 50% of women had anxiety and depression in the first year after diagnosis, 25% in the second, third and fourth years and 15% in the fifth year. There appears to be little evidence of long-term serious psychological morbidity in breast cancer survivors (Kornblith 2007; Burgess et al. 2005; Helgeson and Tomich 2005), and some studies have found that psychological morbidity in stable cancer survivors is similar to that found in the general population (Hanson-Frost et al. 2000).

The early breast cancer studies used participants with symptomatic disease, so when breast screening was introduced, there was considerable debate as to whether the diagnosis of screen detected disease would lead to an increase or a decrease in breast cancer related psychological morbidity. Maguire (1983) suggested that it might cause significant psychological morbidity and 'cancerphobia' due to apparently well women being invited to attend, and subsequently being given a diagnosis of breast cancer.

Some studies did report an increase in breast cancer worry (Dean 1986, Marteau 1994) and breast self examination (Dean et al. 1986; Bull and Campbell 1991; Farmer et al. 1995) following breast screening. Also women who perceive themselves to be susceptible to breast cancer, or have a false positive result, do appear to be most at risk of psychological distress (Ellman et al. 1989; Absetz et al. 2003). However, several studies have failed to find high levels of long-term clinical anxiety and depression in women with a diagnosis of screen detected breast cancer (Farmer 2000; Absetz et al. 2003).

A more recent systematic review of 54 papers (Brett et al. 2005) found that although women who receive an invitation to screening and subsequently have a clear result do not appear to suffer from psychological distress, those that have a false positive result and undergo further investigations have reported significant anxiety in the short term. Brett identified a number of characteristics of women most likely to experience distress and they include younger age, lower education, dissatisfaction with information and communication, fear of cancer and greater perceived risk.

Although the incidence of clinical anxiety and depression may be low in both screen detected and symptomatic women, a significant proportion of patients report cancer related worries many years after diagnosis (Deimling et al. 2006). These 'cancer related worries' include fear of recurrence, fear of new cancers and fear that any symptoms they experience might be cancer. Cancer related worries have been linked with anxiety and depression (Deimling et al. 2006). According to Kornblith et al. (2007), younger survivors report greater fear of recurrence, distress about long-term treatment related problems and sexual dysfunction. This is thought to be due to the added stress of being primary carers for their children, parents and sometimes partner, and having financial and work commitments (Kornblith et al. 2007).

It is hardly surprising that research has shown a sharp increase in anxiety and depression associated with recurrence (Burgess et al. 2005). Hanson-Frost et al. (2000) also looked at the psychological and social well-being of women in different disease phases. The recurrent group experienced more difficulties in terms of health perception, physical functioning, impact on life and medical interactions, than the newly diagnosed, adjuvant and stable groups.

Perhaps the most important finding is that it is factors relating to the patient rather than the disease or treatment that increase the risk of anxiety and depression. Previous psychiatric history, the presence of an affective disorder, lack of confiding relationship or social support, lack of optimism, being under the age of 50, unemployment and being emotionally labile, have all been linked with poor adjustment (Watson 1983; Burgess et al. 2005). Ideally psychological resources should be channelled towards these vulnerable women.

All health professionals should be alert for both physical and psychological problems and although some survivors have reported that their need for information and emotional support are often not met by their oncology team (Vivar and McQueen 2005; Turner et al. 2005), improvements do continue to be made. Many health professionals have the opportunity to attend communication workshops and the introduction of the role of Breast Care Nurse (BCN) has been a welcome addition to the multidisciplinary team (McArdle et al. 1996).

Conclusion

Receiving a diagnosis of breast cancer can be devastating, and sadly in some cases fatal, but thanks to advances in treatment, there has been a significant reduction in the mortality rate and more and more women are surviving breast cancer and returning to pre-morbid functioning. Even women with metastatic disease are surviving long periods. We have also seen a significant reduction in long-term psychological morbidity. The media, celebrities and voluntary sector have all contributed to making breast cancer less of a taboo subject. Greater awareness of the importance of psychological support and the appointment of specialist nurses have all helped reduce psychological distress (McArdle et al. 1996).

Although long-term psychological distress is less common there, continues to be significant anxiety and depression at the time of diagnosis and recurrence and we should also acknowledge the importance of more existential concerns such as fear and vulnerability. An awareness of potential periods of heightened distress, and of the characteristics of women less likely to adjust, will hopefully mean that psychological resources can be concentrated where they are needed most.

Breast cancer: a patient's perspective

I have breast cancer for 10 years now. When I was first diagnosed, I was menopausal and I thought I was just going through the dreaded change. I felt this lump but I always felt lumpy, and so let it go. Eventually I decided to get my menopause symptoms sorted and I just sort of mentioned it in passing to the GP, but she was straight to it and got me in for a mammogram. I was sent a letter saying I needed to come back and it might or might not be a cancer. I wasn't even worried then, just thought they'd got it wrong, it's been there ages. Then I had an ultrasound and was told I needed a biopsy. Mammograms are painful enough but that first core biopsy was awful. I don't know if it was the doctor or not enough anaesthetic or what, but it hurt like hell at the time and for ages after. Anyway, it came back as cancer. Again I thought, 'No you've got it wrong'. It took a while to sink in. I was told I needed a mastectomy and that it needed to be done soon. I asked if it was necessary and they said 'yes'. I've heard since some people only have the lump out but that wasn't offered to me and I never asked. Once it sank in, I knew surgery was the right thing for me. I just wanted it out and the operation couldn't come quick enough. I think I waited about 5 weeks in the end and I would probably say even now that was the most difficult time. I built up in my head that this cancer was growing and spreading. The surgery was ok, not nice but exactly as I'd expected. I was in for five days and to be honest I made some good friends there, people who I've kept in touch with. One of my friends died actually and that was difficult to deal with, as I couldn't help but think about it could be me. Anyway, I had to come back to the hospital after 3 weeks and was told that my cancer was removed but I had positive nodes. Because of this I had to go for further tests to see if it had spread; this was a terrible because the doctor told me if it had spread it wasn't curable. I started to think every ache and pain was cancer and it took about 2 more weeks to get all the tests done and I was given the 'all clear'. Next step was chemotherapy and radiotherapy. I had my chemo first and I think I would say I was ok through this, just tired mainly. I mean you don't expect to get through scot free, do you? It took 6 months and then you think what now. I mean I hated going for chemo but when it came to the end I was thinking what next, will it start to grow. I also had to have radiotherapy and this was unpleasant. Mainly because I had to strip off every day with a stranger and it's not right to be half naked in a big room with a stranger, especially as I was disfigured and not normal. I got used to my flat chest very quickly. My husband too was ok with it. We just took it gently in getting used to it. It was harder though to lose my hair. This was a very public event and I could hide the mastectomy but there was no avoiding the image of the bald head that must be cancer! I didn't get on well with the wig, too hot, too conscious, so I just wore the scarf. As soon as I'd finished radiotherapy I went back to work. I was knackered but I just needed to be normal so I pushed myself through it and before too long I was ok. I still went for a check-up every now and then but I was fine. I needed to take Tamoxifen as I was ER+ but that wasn't a problem. I was clear for about 4½ years when I started to get a niggle in my side. I thought I had twisted myself and so ignored it for a couple of weeks, but it didn't seem to get any better. Eventually I called my GP but then I called my breast nurse and she got me in to see the specialist. I was due in a couple of months anyway. He did an X-ray and sure enough they suspected a cancer. I went for a bone scan and I had 3 hot spots. It was back! At first I thought that's ok, some more treatment and I'll be back to normal again. It took a little while to realise I now was living with this cancer and it was going to get me in the end. I felt cheated as people had told me usually at 5 years you get discharged. I was so nearly there. I was told I needed more treatment and this time they also tested me for HER2, which came back positive. Suddenly I was back on the treadmill of fitting life around treatment. I was started on Herceptin, more chemo and some bone strengtheners. Treatment made work more and more difficult. Not necessarily the side effects, though I did get a lot of muscle aches, this time but it was more the frequency. After a little while I decided to go off sick. This was diffi-cult because I was unoccupied and it made me think, it made me put things in order and decide what I wanted to do. That was 5 years ago now and I've had several set backs, different treatments but I've always come through. I've made friends, lost friends and made some new ones. It's been up and down and hard going at times but I'm still here. I only have Herceptin at the moment and I take tablets for my bones. More treatment will come and I do know eventually it will beat me but I have learned to live for the moment. The worst thing now is living with the uncertainty. Twice we have cancelled holidays because it came back and I needed more treatment; you just never know when it's going to hit you again. It affects the whole family, not just me. I don't work now so it's just my husband's wage. He works so hard and he needs a holiday, he says he'd just rather be sure I'm ok but I feel bad, then as he and we need a break sometimes. It's lovely to have him there always by my side in sickness and health and I guess we have rewritten our path.

It's never going to go away, we have learned to just live whilst we can. My only plan at the moment is to see my first grandchild due in 3 months time. After that we'll see...

Reflective points

- Discuss with your team how you provide tailored information at the appropriate time for women with breast cancer.
- Consider how you would provide support and the resources necessary for a woman with recurrent metastatic breast cancer.

References

Absetz, P., Aro, A.R and Sutton, S.R. (2003) Experience with breast cancer, pre-screening per-ceived susceptibility and the psychological impact of screening. *Psychooncology* **12**, 305–18.

Atisha, D., Alderman, A.K., Lowery, J.C., Kuhn, L.E., Davis, J. and Wilkins, E.G. (2008) Prospective Analysis of long-term psychosocial outcomes in breast reconstruction: Two-year post-operative results from the Michgan breast reconstruction outcomes study. *Annals of Surgery* **247(6)**, 1019–28.

Baum, M. (1995) Screening for breast cancer, time to think and stop? *Lancet* **346**, 436.

Blanks, R.G., Moss, S.M., McGahan, C.E., Quinn, M.J. and Babb, P.J. (2000) Effect of NHS breast screening programme on mortality from breast cancer in England and Wales, 1990–1998: com-parison of observed with predicted mortality. *British Medical Journal* **321**, 665–9.

Bonadonna, G. et al. (1995) Cyclophosphamide, methotrexate, and fluorouracil in node-positive breast cancer. The results of 20 years of follow-up. *New England Journal of Medicine* **332**, 901–6.

Breakthrough breast Cancer (2009). *Breast Cancer Risk Factors. The Facts*. London: Breakthrough Breast Cancer.

Brett, J. et al. (2005) The psychological impact of mammographic screening: a systematic review. *Psychooncology* **14**, 917–38.

Brown, L., Payne, S. and Royle, G. (2002) Patient-initiated follow-up of breast cancer. *Psychooncology* **11**, 346–55.

Bull, A.R. and Campbell, M.J. (1991) Assessment of the psychological impact of a breast screening programme. *The British Journal of Radiology*, **64**, 510–15.

Burgess, C., Cornelius, V., Love, S., Graham, J., Richards, M. and Ramirez, A. (2005) Depression and anxiety in women with early breast cancer: five year observational cohort study; doi:10.1136/bmj.38343.670868.D3 (published 4 February 2005).

Cheung, K.L. (2007) Endocrine therapy for breast cancer: an overview. *The Breast* **4**, 327–43.

Dean, C., Roberts, M.M., French, K. and Robinson, S. (1986) Psychiatric morbidity after screening for breast cancer. *Journal of Epidemiology Community Health* **40(1)**, 71–5.

De Morgan, S., Redman, S., White, K.J., Cakir, B. and Boyages, J. (2002) 'Well, have I got cancer or haven't I?' The Psycho-social issues for women diagnosed with ductal carcinoma *in situ*. *Health Expectations* 5(4), 310–18.

Deimling, G.T., Bowman, K.F., Sterns, S., Wagner, L.J. and Kahana, B. (2006) Cancer-related health worries and psychological distress among older adult, long-term cancer survivors. *Psychooncology* **15(4)**, 306–20.

Dos Santos Silva, I. (2005) Breast cancer aetiology: shifting the emphasis from adult to early life risk factors. In: R. Leonard, A. Polychronis and A. Miles (Eds) *The Effective Management of Breast Cancer*, 2nd edn. London: Aesculapius Medical Press.

Ellman, R., Angeli, N., Christians, A., Moss, S., Chamberlain, J. and Maguire, P. (1989) Psychiatric morbidity associated with screening for breast cancer. *British Journal of Cancer*, **60(5)**, 781–4.

ESMO (2005) Minimum clinical recommendations for diagnosis, adjuvant treatment and follow-up of primary breast cancer. *Annals of Oncology* **16((Suppl 1)**, i7–i9.

Fallowfield, L., Hall, A., Maguire, G.P. and Baum, M. (1990) Psychological Outcomes of Different treatment policies in women with early breast cancer outside a clinical trial. *British Medical Journal* **301**, 575–80.

Fallowfield, L. (1997) Offering choice of surgical treatment to women with breast cancer. *Patient Education and Counseling* **30(3)**, 209–14.

Farmer, A.J., Payne, S. and Royle, G. (1995) A comparative study of psychological morbidity in women with screen detected and symptomatic breast cancer. In: A. Richardson and J. Macleod Clrke (Eds) *Nursing Research in Cancer*. London: Scutari Press, pp. 189–204.

Farmer, A.J. (2000) The minimization to clients of screen-detected breast cancer: a qualitative analysis. *Journal of Advanced Nursing* **31(2)**, 306–13.

Fisher, B. et al. (1985) Five year results of a randomized trial comparing total mastectomy with or without radiation in the treatment of breast cancer. *New England Journal of Medicine* **312(11)**, 665–73.

Gralow, J.R. (2002) Biophosphonates as adjuvant treatment for breast cancer. *British Medical Journal* **325**, 1051–2.

Greer, S. (1994) Psycho-oncology: Its aims, achievements and future tasks. *Psychooncology* **3**, 87–101.

Grunfield, E., Levine, N.M., Julian, J.A. et al. (2006) randomized trial of long-term follow-up for early-stage breast cancer: a comparison of family physician vs specialist care. *Journal of Clinical Oncology* **24**, 848–55.

Halkett, G.K.B., Kristjanson, L.J. and Lobb, E.A. (2008) 'If we get too close to your bones they'll go brittle': women's initial fears about radiotherapy for early breast cancer. *Psychooncology* **17**, 877–84.

Hanson-Frost, M., Suman, V.J., Rummans, T.A. et al. (2000) Physical, psychological and social well-being of women with breast cancer: the influence of disease phase. *Psychooncology* **9**, 221–31.

Helgeson, V.S. and Tomich, P.L. (2005) Surviving cancer: a comparison of 5-year disease-free breast cancer survivors with healthy women. *Psychooncology* **14(4)**, 307–17.

Kornblith, A.B., Powell, M., Regan, M.M. et al. (2007) Long-term psychosocial adjustment of older vs younger survivors of breast and endometrial cancer. *Psychooncology* **16(10)**, 895–903.

Lasry, J.M., Margolese, R.G., Poisson, H.S. et al. (1987) Depression and body image following mastectomy and lumpectomy. *Journal of Chronic Diseases* **40(6)**, 529–34.

Maguire, G.P., Lee, E., Bevington, D., Kuchemann, C., Crabtree, R. and Cornell, C. (1978) Psychiatric problems in the first year after mastectomy. *British Medical Journal* **1**, 963–5.

Maguire, G.P. (1983) Possible psychiatric complications of screening for breast cancer. *British Journal of Radiology* **56**, 284 (abstract).

Marteau, T.M. (1994) Psychology and screening: Narrowing the gap between efficacy and effectiveness. *British Journal of Clinical Psychology* **33**, 1–10.

McArdle, J., George, W.D., McArdle, C.S. et al. (1996) Psychological support for patients undergoing breast surgery: a randomised study. *British Medical Journal* **312**, 813–16.

Meyerowitz, B.E. (1980) Psychosocial correlates of breast cancer and its treatment. *Psychological Bulletin* **87(1)**, 108–31.

Morris, J. and Royle, G. (1988) Offering patients a choice of surgery for early breast cancer: A reduction in anxiety and depression in patients and their husbands. *Social Science and Medicine* **26(6)**, 583–5.

Morris, T., Greer, S. and White, P. (1977) Psychological and Social adjustment to mastectomy: A two year follow-up study. *Cancer* **40**, 2381–7.

Morrow, M and O'Sullivan, M.J. (2007) The dilemma of DCIS. *The Breast* **16(Suppl 2)**, 59–62.

Moulder, S. and Hortobagyi, G.N. (2008) Advances in the treatment of breast cancer. *Pharmacology and Therapeutics* **83(1)**, 26–36.

National Institute for Health and Clinical Excellence (2009) *Advanced Breast Cancer: Diagnosis and Treatment. NICE Clinical Guideline*. London: National Collaborating Centre for Cancer.

NHSBSP (2006) *Screening for Breast Cancer in England: Past and Future*. Advisory Committee on Breast Cancer Screening, 2006 (NHSBSP Publication no 61).

Peto, R., Boreham, J., Clarke, M., Davies, C. and Beral, V. (2000) UK and USA breast cancer deaths down 25% in year 2000 at ages 20–69 years. *Lancet* **355**, 1822–3.

Sainsbury, J.R.C., Anderson, T.J. and Morgan, D.A.L. (2000) ABC of breast diseases. Breast Cancer. *British Medical Journal* **321**, 745–50.

Samphao, S., Eremin, J.M., El-Sheemy, M. and Eremin, O. (2008) Management of the axilla in women with breast cancer: Current clinical practice and a new selective targeted approach. *Annals of Surgical Oncology* **15**, 1282–96.

Shapiro, S. (1977) Evidence on screening for breast cancer from a randomized trial. *Cancer* **39**, 2772–82.

Singletary, S.E., Allred, C., Ashley, P. et al. (2002) Revision of the American Joint Committee on Cancer Staging System for Breast Cancer. *Journal of Clinical Oncology* **20(17)**, 3628–36.

Smith, I.E and Chua, S. (2006a) ABC of breast diseases. Medical treatment of early breast cancer. I: adjuvant treatment. *British Medical Journal* **332**, 34–6.

Smith, I.E and Chua, S. (2006b) ABC of breast diseases. Medical Treatment of early breast cancer. III: Chemotherapy. *British Medical Journal* **332**, 161–2.

Smith, I.E and Chua, S. (2006c) ABC of breast diseases. Medical treatment of early breast cancer. IV: Neoadjuvant treatment. *British Medical Journal* **332**, 223–4, 162.

Tabar, L. et al. (1985) Reduction in breast cancer mortality by mass screening with mammography: First results of a randomized trial in two Swedish counties. *Lancet* **1**, 829.

Turner, J., Kelly, B., Swanson, C., Allison, R. and Wetzig, N. (2005) Psycho-social impact of newly diagnosed advanced breast cancer. *Psychooncology* **14**, 396–407.

Vivar, C.G. and McQueen, A. (2005) Information and emotional needs of long-term survivors of breast cancer. *Journal of Advanced Nursing* **51(5)**, 520–8.

Watson, M. (1983) Psychosocial intervention with cancer patients: a review. *Psychological Medicine* **13**, 839–46.

Whitman, J. (1993) *Breast Cancer Journal*: a century of petals. Colorado: Fulcrum Publishing.

www.CancerResearchUK.org

Appendix

TNM Classification of breast tumours

Tx	Primary tumour cannot be assessed To: no evidence of primary tumour. Tis: Cancer *in situ* or Paget's disease of the nipple with no associated tumour
T1	≤2 cm (T1a ≤0.5 cm, T1b >0.5–1, T1c >1–2 cm)
T2	>2 cm–5cm
T3	>5 cm
T4a	Involvement in chest wall
T4b	Involvement of skin (includes ulceration, direct infiltration, peau d'orange, and satellite nodules)
T4c	T4a and T4b together
T4d	Inflammatory cancer
No	No regional node metastases
N1	Palpable mobile involved ipsilateral axillary nodes
N2	Fixed involved ipsilateral axillary nodes
N3	Ipsilateral internal mammary node involvement (rarely clinically detectable)
pNx	Regional lymph nodes cannot be assessed
pNo	No regional lymph node metastasis
pN1	Metastasis to movable ipsilateral axillary lymph node(s)
pN1a	Only micro metastasis (none >0.2 cm)
pN1bi	Metastasis in 1 to 3 lymph nodes, any >0.2 cm and all <2.0 cm in greatest dimension
pN1bii	Metastasis to 4 or more lymph nodes, any >0.2 cm and all <2.0 cm in greatest dimension
pNn1biii	Extension of tumour beyond the capsule of a lymph node metastasis <2.0 cm in greatest dimension
pN1biv	Metastasis to a lymph node 2.0 cm or more in greatest dimension
pN2	Metastasis to ipsilateral axillary lymph node(s) fixed to each other or to other structures
pN3	Metastasis to ipsilateral internal mammary lymph node
Mx	Presence of distant metastasis cannot be assessed
Mo	No evidence of metastasis
M1	Distant metastasis (includes ipsilateral supraclavicular nodes)

Chapter 8

Cancer of the Ovary

Kate Gregory

Learning points

At the end of this chapter, the reader will have an understanding of:
- The factors involved in the development of ovarian cancer
- The difficulties that can be involved in diagnosing cancer of the ovary and to understand the staging process
- The multi-disciplinary approach to the primary treatment of ovarian cancer
- The options for the treatment of relapsed disease

Introduction

The normal ovary is approximately the size of a walnut. The ovaries are filled with follicles, which are fluid filled structures in which the oocyte grows to maturity. Females are born with their lifetime supply of gametes (~1–2 million). These gametes undergo growth and maturation each month, which usually takes 14 days. In order to grow and fully develop, the oocytes rely on pituitary-derived gonadal hormone stimulation. When the egg is fully developed, the follicle bursts and the mature egg is released into the fallopian tube towards the uterus. The egg is capable of being fertilised for a short period. If this does not occur, then the egg dies and 7–10 days later a new egg begins the cycle of maturation. Normal ovulation can be affected by the oral contraceptive pill, illness, malnutrition and endocrine imbalances.

Epidemiology and aetiology

Ovarian cancer is the commonest gynaecological cancer in the UK. There were 6615 new cases in 2004 and 4447 deaths from ovarian cancer in 2005 in the UK (CRUK website). Ovarian cancer is predominantly a disease of post-menopausal women, with over 85% of

Women's Cancers, First Edition. Edited by Alison Keen and Elaine Lennan.
© 2011 Blackwell Publishing Ltd. Published 2011 by Blackwell Publishing Ltd.

cases being diagnosed in the over 50 age-group. The incidence of ovarian cancer has risen over the last decades from an incidence of 15/100,000 in 1978 to 17/100,000 in 2004 (Cancer Research UK). The rise has been predominantly in the post-menopausal group, with rates being stable in younger women, potentially due to increased use of the oral contraceptive pill over this time.

Genetic factors

Carriers of the BRCA1 and BRCA2 genes are at an increased risk of developing breast and ovarian cancer. These genes are both tumour suppressor genes and can be passed through either the maternal or paternal line. The BRCA1 gene confers a 65% lifetime risk for breast cancer and a 39% risk of developing ovarian cancer (Thompson et al. 2002). The BRCA2 gene confers a 45% lifetime risk of breast cancer and an 11% lifetime risk of ovarian cancer (The Breast Cancer Linkage Consortium 1999).

A detailed family history is important for any patient diagnosed with ovarian cancer and those with first-degree relatives affected with either breast or ovarian cancer should be referred in to the local genetic service for consideration of testing. In non-affected carriers, once child-bearing is completed, consideration should be given to prophylactic surgery, which has been shown to reduce the risk of developing ovarian or primary peritoneal cancer to less than 1% (Rebbeck et al. 2002). This is particularly important, as screening for ovarian cancer is so unreliable.

Protective factors

It is well documented that there is a decreased incidence of ovarian cancer in users of the oral contraceptive pill (Franceschi et al. 1991). It is postulated that this is due to the ovary being 'rested' as one of the modes of action of the pill is to suppress ovulation. Conversely there is concern that the use of fertility drugs for assisted reproduction techniques may increase the risk or ovarian cancer as the ovary is hyper-stimulated, although this is not proven.

Screening for ovarian cancer

Screening programmes for ovarian cancer have proved to be disappointing and cannot be routinely recommended. To be successful, a screening test has to be able to identify patients with early stage, operable and hence curable disease. Ca 125 testing would seem a promising candidate, but it is only elevated in approximately 50% of patients with stage I ovarian cancer. The other test used is trans-vaginal ultrasound, but this has limited specificity and is operator dependent. Many centres offer a combination of ultrasound and serial Ca 125 testing in patients with an increased risk of the disease. The search for a more reliable way of screening these women is the ongoing subject of much research (see also Chapter 4 'Tumour Markers').

Pre-diagnosis

Ovarian cancer is often referred to as the silent killer, due to the non-specific and insidious symptoms that patients commonly present with. This frequently leads to delay in diagnosis and referral to inappropriate specialists. The commonly presenting symptoms are summarised in Table 8.1. The most common presentation is of non-specific abdominal pain, bloating and alteration in bowel habit. Some of these patients are falsely diagnosed as having irritable bowel syndrome or in some cases the symptoms are put down to the menopause. These are the patients who typically have a long path to diagnosis and many are angry and confused at the time taken. Less commonly, patients present with ascites, vaginal bleeding, a pelvic mass or a unilateral deep vein thrombosis. Very occasionally patients will present acutely with bowel obstruction to the general surgeons.

Many gynae-oncology clinics have special rapid referral proformas for patients with suspected ovarian cancer. In some instances, this requests that GPs do a blood test for Ca 125 (a glycoprotein antigen elevated in approximately 80% of women presenting with advanced ovarian cancer, and in 50% of women presenting with stage I disease) prior to the patients being seen in clinic and in some cases a pelvic ultra sound scan (USS) is also requested. The risk of malignancy index can be used to predict whether or not the patient has malignancy (Jacobs et al. 1990). This is a scoring system based on the patients age, menopausal status, Ca 125 reading and USS findings (detailed in Table 8.2). All patients in

Table 8.1 Symptoms and signs of ovarian cancer.

Abdominal pain
Bloating and abdominal distension
Change in bowel habit
Increased frequency of micturition
Nausea and vomiting
Vaginal bleeding
Swelling of the legs
Pelvic mass
Deep vein thrombosis
Bowel obstruction
Pleural effusion
Supra clavicular lymphadenopathy

Table 8.2 The risk of malignancy (RMI) scoring system.

Feature	RMI Score
Ultrasound features	no abnormality = 0,
Multilocular cyst	single abnormality = 1
Solid areas	multiple abnormalities = 4
Ascites	
Intraabdominal metastases	
Premenopausal	1
Postmenopausal	4
Ca 125 result	[]

RMI score = ultrasound score × menopausal score × Ca 125 result.

whom there is suspicion of malignancy should have a staging CT scan of abdomen and pelvis – this allows for the extent and operability of the disease to be assessed. If patients have ascites, then a diagnostic tap should be taken and sent for cytological investigation. In patients who are deemed to have inoperable disease and are to be considered for primary chemotherapy and in whom cytological diagnosis from ascitic tap is not obtained, it is imperative that a biopsy is obtained to confirm a malignant diagnosis – this can be done under radiological guidance or at laparoscopy.

Once all these investigations have been performed and a diagnosis made, the case should be presented at a multi-disciplinary meeting to formulate a treatment plan. This should involve discussion between radiologists, pathologists, medical and surgical oncologists and clinical nurse specialists.

Giving the diagnosis

By the time it comes to receiving a definitive diagnosis, many women with ovarian cancer will already have been symptomatic for some time. They will have had several investigations and some will be frustrated by the time the whole process has taken. Ideally, the patient should be seen with a support person and a specialist nurse, as they will be given a lot of information at this time when they will be understandably anxious and upset. If possible, a treatment plan should be available to be outlined to the patient, so they are aware of the next step. If at this point they are to be passed on to another specialist, then an appointment date should be given to them on that visit. Written information should be offered to the patient and a phone number given to them, so that they are able to reach the specialist nurse with any questions that may arise following the consultation. It is important that the patient's GP is kept fully informed of the diagnosis and treatment plan – this is best achieved with a fax to the surgery within 24 hours of the patient being informed of the diagnosis. This is particularly important when the patient's specialist may not be in the local hospital.

Infertility issues

In younger women, the diagnosis and treatment plan may bring with it the secondary devastating blow of infertility. It is essential that these issues are explored and referral to an infertility specialist offered – new developments in technology offer the possibility of preserving fertility with tissue or egg freezing, but at present this is essentially experimental. Women may benefit from information on future options, such as egg donation, if they are able to keep their uterus. For some women their grief at this loss is very hard to cope with and persists long after the treatment for cancer is complete – specialists caring for these women need to be aware of this and specialist counselling may be appropriate.

Classification and staging

Histological types of ovarian cancer

Ovarian cancer is a general term to cover malignant tumours of the ovary. The majority are epithelial (~60%) and these can further be divided into serous, mucinous, endometriod, carcinosarcoma (mixed Mullerian) clear cell and transitional cell. The other major groups are sex-cord stromal tumours, germ cell tumours and metastatic tumours. Borderline tumours of the ovary have low malignant potential and no evidence of invasion, but abnormal cytological and atypical features. Most borderline tumours present as stage I lesions and are cured by surgery. Primary peritoneal carcinoma is a tumour that shows similar histological features to ovarian cancer, but in which there is minimal ovarian involvement – the treatment is the same as for ovarian carcinoma. Pseudomyxoma peritonei is a clinical condition in which there is mucinous material within the peritoneal cavity. This can be of either ovarian or gastro-intestinal origin. The staging system for ovarian cancer does not take into account the grade of the tumour, but commonly pathologists will refer to the grade or differentiation of the cancer.

Staging of ovarian cancer

The most commonly used staging for ovarian cancer is the FIGO system (Table 8.3). Ovarian cancer is only accurately stage by a formal surgical procedure, but some idea can be obtained from CT scanning. Staging is important, both to give guidance on adjuvant therapy and to give prognostic information. One study looking at FIGO stage and survival demonstrated 5-year survival rates of 91.1%, 75.2%, 46.4% and 21.2% for stage I, II, III and IV, respectively (Chung et al. 2007).

Treatment

Primary Surgery

For the majority of patients, their treatment begins with surgery. This provides both definitive staging of their disease and de-bulking or complete removal of the tumour. There is

Table 8.3 FIGO staging of ovarian cancer (Pecorelli et al. 1998).

Stage I – Limited to the ovaries
        1a One ovary, capsule intact
        1b Both ovaries, capsule intact
        1c Capsule ruptured, tumour on surface, malignant cells in ascites or peritoneal washings

Stage II – Pelvic extension
        2a pelvic extension into uterus and fallopian tubes
        2b extension to other pelvic tissues
        2c pelvic extension and malignant cells in ascites or peritoneal washings

Stage III – Peritoneal metastasis beyond pelvis and or regional lymph node
        3a microscopic peritoneal metastasis
        3b macroscopic peritoneal metastasis <2 cm
        3c peritoneal metastasis >2 cm and/or regional lymph node metastasis

Stage IV – Distant metastasis

convincing evidence that patients do better if they are operated on in specialist centres by gynaecological oncologists. A Scottish retrospective review looked at the outcome of 1866 women – of those with stage III disease, those operated on by gynaecological oncologists had a 25% reduction in the risk of death compared to those operated on by general gynaecologists (Junor et al. 1999). It is now written into the COG guidelines in the UK that patients suspected of having an ovarian malignancy should be operated on by specialised surgeons. This can be difficult for patients who face being treated at a distance from their home and this is where the clinical nurse specialist is particularly important in guiding the patient through their journey. There has also been concern expressed that this may lead to the deskilling of experienced general gynaecologists.

Optimal surgery in early stage disease should be through a mid-line incision, to allow palpation of all peritoneal surfaces, bilateral oophorectomy, total abdominal hysterectomy, para-aortic node sampling, omentectomy and peritoneal washings. In patients of child-bearing age with early stage disease, then fertility preserving surgery may be considered. In patients with advanced disease, the aim of surgery is to achieve maximal cytoreduction. Several studies have shown that optimal cytoreduction correlates with survival (Hunter et al. 1992; Voest et al. 1989).

Adjuvant chemotherapy

As most patients present with advanced stage disease, the majority with ovarian cancer are referred for adjuvant chemotherapy. At the present time it is recommended that all patients of stage Ic and above should receive adjuvant chemotherapy. In addition, those with high risk histology (e.g. clear cell, grade 3) with lower stage disease should also be considered for adjuvant chemotherapy. The ICON-1 study looked at the role of adjuvant chemotherapy in patients with stages Ia and Ib disease – this showed a 9% reduction in the odds of death and an 11% improvement in recurrence free survival (Colombo et al. 2003). However, in this study, the majority of patients were not optimally staged and so it is speculated that many of them had in fact higher stage disease.

Historically, the treatment of choice in these patients was single agent carboplatin or cisplatin-cyclophosphamide and in some patients single agent carboplatin may still be acceptable, but the treatment of ovarian cancer changed with the results of the GOG1-11 study (Muggia et al. 2000), which showed improved survival with the combination of cisplatin-paclitaxel over the standard cisplatin-cyclophosphamide. Around the same time, the ICON-3 study reported (this used single agent carboplatin as the control arm and many centres dose-escalated and significant patients crossed over to receive a taxane) in this study that there was no survival advantage seen with the addition of the taxane (International Collaborative Ovarian Neoplasm Group 2002). The platinum-taxane regime is recommended by NICE for the adjuvant treatment of advanced ovarian cancer (National Institute of Clinical Excellence 2003).

A further UK study compared carboplatin-paclitaxel to carboplatin docetaxel – the regimes showed equivalent response rates and survival rates (Vasey 2001). However, Docetaxel is not approved by NICE in this setting and so is seldom used in the UK, despite the fact that its administration is more convenient being given over 1 rather than 3 hours.

More recent studies have looked at the inclusion of newer agents – the ICON5 study was a 5-arm study comparing the standard carboplatin paclitaxel to regimes containing in addition gemcitabine, liposomal doxorubicin and topotecan – none of these new regimes was found to be superior to the standard (Bookman et al. 2006).

There is no evidence to support the use of high dose chemotherapy with stem cell rescue in patients with ovarian cancer (Ozols 2007). However, there is interest in dose escalation of carboplatin and this is currently being investigated in the SCOTROC IV study.

Typically, patients receive 6 cycles of chemotherapy given at 3-week intervals, giving a total length of treatment in the order of 4 ½ months (see Table 8.4 on side effects of chemotherpy).

Interval de-bulking surgery

In patients in whom optimal cytoreduction is not achieved, consideration should be given to interval debulking surgery after three cycles of adjuvant chemotherapy. Ideally this should be discussed by the multi-disciplinary team (MDT) following the first operation and a provisional date for second laparotomy is made once chemotherapy commences to avoid delays in treatment down the line. A final decision regarding second surgery should be made with the help of a CT scan and Ca 125 estimation after three cycles of chemotherapy. The role for interval debulking surgery was established by a Dutch study, in which a 6-month extension in survival was seen in patients who had interval debulking (van de Berg et al. 1995). However, subsequent studies suggest no role for interval debulking surgery, if the initial operation is performed by a specialist surgeon (Rose et al. 2002).

Primary Chemotherapy

Some patients present with disease that is deemed inoperable on CT scanning at the outset of treatment, and the surgeons feel that they have little chance of achieving reasonable debulking. These are the patients who may have had 'open and close' laparotomies in the past. Also some patients are physically very unwell at presentation and there would be concerns about their ability to withstand a general anaesthetic and a major surgical procedure. Primary or neoadjuvant may be considered in these patients. The drug regimes are the same and the patients should be re-assessed and considered for surgery after three

Table 8.4 Side-effects of chemotherapy.

Nausea and vomiting
Hair loss (paclitaxel, docetaxel, topotecan, etoposide)
Fatigue
Myelosuppression
Hand and foot syndrome (liposomal doxorubicin)
Peripheral neuropathy (taxanes, platinum agents)
Joint and bone pain (taxanes)
Pulmonary fibrosis (bleomycin)
Mouth ulcers
Hypersensitivity reactions (taxanes)

cycles. To date, no randomised trials of neoadjuvant chemotherapy have been reported, but the CHORUS study (OVO6) is currently recruiting and will provide information of the impact of neoadjuvant chemotherapy on survival rates.

Intra-peritoneal chemotherapy

Ovarian cancer is intrinsically a chemo-sensitive disease and the fact that it tends to be confined in the peritoneal cavity for much of its course has led to interest in the use of intra-peritoneal (IP) therapy. A Cochrane review on the use of IP chemotherapy examined 8 randomised trials in which over 1800 women had been treated and found prolongation of both the disease-free interval and overall survival if IP therapy had been a component of treatment. However, they also noted the potential for catheter complications and toxicity (Cochrane Review abstract 2007). IP therapy would now be considered standard of care in the USA, but less so in Europe. A commentary on the meta-analysis stated that IP therapy could not yet be considered standard of care, as none of the trials used a control arm that would be deemed to be the standard of care and there was no standard regime for IP therapy that could be recommended. They concluded that further research using a recognised IV control arm and a more easily deliverable IP regime was required before this treatment became universally accepted as a standard component of care (Swart et al. 2008).

Treatment of relapsed disease

The management of relapsed disease depends on the site of relapse and the time since completion of initial treatment. Unfortunately, relapse is seldom manifested as an isolated mass that may be amenable to surgery. Ideally all these patients should be discussed within the MDT, so that the possibility of surgery is not missed. The mainstay of treatment is chemotherapy. If it has been longer than 6 months from completion of platinum based chemotherapy, then it is appropriate to rechallenge with a platinum based combination as there is a good chance of a further response to a platinum agent (Blackledge et al. 1989). Following ICON4, there is good evidence for rechallenging with a platinum-taxane combination, as this led to 7% improvement in survival at 2 years and an increase of 5 months in the median survival (Parmar et al. 2003). There is also emerging evidence for the use of other platinum based combinations, including gemcitabine (Pfisterer et al. 2006) and liposomal doxorubicin (Alberts et al. 2007). These combinations may be preferable in patients with residual taxane induced neurotoxicity and in patients not wishing to lose their hair a second time.

In patients with platinum refractory disease, the response rate to a number of agents is around 20–25%. Single agent topotecan and liposomal doxorubicin (caelyx) both have NICE approval in this setting (www.nice.org.uk). Gemcitabine is not approved in the UK, but is extensively used elsewhere. The choice of single agent in this setting depends on the patient's situation and the toxicity profile of the agent. Weekly paclitaxel has also been shown to have useful activity in this setting (Thomas and Rosenberg 2002).

Combination agents such as cisplatin-etoposide may have improved response rates in this situation (van de Berg et al. 2002), but toxicity and time in hospital are likely to be greater and so these treatments may have a more negative impact on quality of life, which is due particular consideration in this group of patients who have incurable disease.

Oral etoposide may have useful activity in these patients, but tends to be given third or even fourth line. For patients who have exhausted standard chemotherapy treatments, consideration could be given to a phase 1 trial if available. The endocrine agent tamoxifen has an approximately 10% response rate and is very well tolerated (Williams and Simera 2000).

Radiotherapy

Radiotherapy is now rarely utilised in the treatment of ovarian cancer. It can be useful for the management of vaginal bleeding due to tumour ulcerating through the vaginal wall and in the management of bony metastases and para-aortic lymphadenopathy. Historically, whole abdominal radiotherapy was used following surgery, but with the advent of effective chemotherapy this is no longer the case.

Monoclonal antibodies

Monoclonal antibodies are new agents that work by specifically targeting signalling pathways. These agents have the advantage of fewer systemic side effects and so tend to be well tolerated. In addition, they may be given with chemotherapy to potentiate the effect of the treatment.

Avastin (bevacuzimab) is a monoclonal antibody that targets vascular endothelial growth factor (VEGF) receptors. VEGF is important in angiogenesis – the formation of new blood vessels – and is involved in tumours developing their own blood supply. A GOG trial looking at the single agent use of this agent in platinum resistant patients demonstrated a 21% response rate (Cannistra et al. 2007). Another trial performed in a similar population showed a response rate of 16%, but was stopped prematurely due to an 11% bowel perforation rate (Cannistra et al. 2006). However, this agent is expensive and the risk of gastro-intestinal bleeding and perforation is a significant concern.

Germ cell tumours of the ovary

Germ cell tumours of the ovary are relatively rare, but it is important always to keep this diagnosis in mind in younger patients. These patients can be treated more conservatively at surgery and so fertility can be maintained. Pre-operative tumour markers αFP and βHCG are available within most hospitals at short notice and should be part of the pre-operative work-up in women of child-bearing age. These patients will require post-operative chemotherapy with two to four cycles of BEP (bleomycin, etoposide, cisplatin), which is fairly intensive in-patient chemotherapy but is generally curative.

Small cell carcinoma of the ovary

Small cell carcinoma of the ovary is a rare but extremely aggressive form of the disease. If the diagnosis is made before surgery, then chemotherapy is the main-stay of treatment and the most appropriate form of treatment is a platinum based regime, for example carboplatin-etoposide or in young fit patients ICE (ifosphamide, cisplatin, etoposide). These tumours tend to respond very rapidly to chemotherapy, but unfortunately remissions tend to be short.

Mixed Mullerian tumours

Some ovarian tumours may have mixed histology – carcino-sarcoma or mixed Mullerian tumours. These patients probably should be considered for regimes containing an anthracycline, either in combination with platinum and taxane or as sequential therapy.

Follow-up

The standard approach for follow-up is for initial 3-monthly visits for the first 2 years post-treatment, followed by 6-monthly visits until 5 years – at that point most units would go to annual follow-up until 10 years, when it is probably reasonable to discharge the patient to GP care. Follow-up can be either with gynae-oncology alone, with medical oncology alone or alternating visits between the two specialities.

Some units would use routine Ca 125 monitoring as a component of follow-up. Many patients are accustomed to Ca 125 testing at diagnosis or during the course of chemotherapy to monitor response to treatment. A normal result can be enormously reassuring (although, of course, not all tumours produce Ca 125), but if abnormal and the patient is asymptomatic, it can open a can of worms. A well patient is instantly turned into an unwell patient and then comes the dilemma as to whether or not it is appropriate to institute further treatment at that point. It is uncertain whether early treatment for relapse in those who are asymptomatic offers any benefit over waiting until patients become symptomatic. This is a complex issue and one that the OVO5 trial attempted to resolve – this trial has now closed to recruitment and patients are in follow-up. In patients with germ cell tumours, then serial monitoring of αFP and βHCG is mandatory.

There is little role for routine CT scanning, except possible in patients who have had fertility preserving surgery and in these patients trans-vagina USS may be considered. Most centres would reserve CT scanning for investigating worrying symptoms or clinical signs in a patient or for patients with rising tumour markers.

Follow-up appointments can be incredibly stressful for patients – they may see staff they never met during their treatment and have no rapport with, they are anxious about results and to be given the 'all-clear'. The presence in the appointment to the clinical nurse specialist can be very reassuring and provide an extra pair of ears and someone whom the patient can liaise with after the appointment if they have forgotten or misunderstood something. If further investigations are to be organised, doing this in a timely fashion where at all possible is helpful.

Palliative care issues in ovarian cancer
(See also Chapter 17 on 'Palliative Care')

Unfortunately, the majority of patients diagnosed with ovarian cancer will ultimately die from their disease. Symptomatic management can be particularly challenging in these patients, due to the presence of peritoneal disease, which can cause recurrent ascites, bowel obstruction and renal failure. The management of each of these particular scenarios will be briefly discussed. The involvement of a palliative care specialist in the MDT is invaluable.

Recurrent Ascites

Many patients presenting with advanced disease have some ascites and this can be a recurrent and distressing problem. Ascites gives rise to tense abdominal swelling, breathlessness – due to upward pressure on the diaphragm, poor appetite, nausea and vomiting and occasionally symptoms of bowel obstruction. Ascites is usually managed by drainage as required – if there is any concern about bowel obstruction (which may give rise to very similar symptoms) then the patient should first have an ultrasound to assess and identify a suitable position for drainage. There is some evidence for the use of loop diuretics (e.g. spironolactone, which may slow the re-accumulation of the fluid). If the ascites is a recurring problem and the requirement for drainage increases, then either a long-term indwelling drain or a peritoneal shunt may be considered. In these situations, it is helpful for the patients to have direct access to either the oncology ward or unit where the drainage is to be performed, to avoid unnecessary delays that can be distressing when they are very symptomatic. Very occasionally the fluid becomes gelatinous, which makes drainage very difficult. The other problem that may arise with multiple drainage is loculation of the fluid, which can make symptomatic relief difficult to achieve, although again USS guidance is useful.

Bowel obstruction

Bowel obstruction can occur either due to blockage by the tumour at one specific level or at multiple levels due to disseminated peritoneal disease. Patients present typically with colicky abdominal pain, vomiting, abdominal distension and absence of bowel movements. Patients should initially be considered for conservative management with adequate pain relief and anti-emetic delivered usually most efficiently by sub-cutaneous infusion. Buscopan may provide useful symptomatic relief if colicky pain and spasm is a feature. The use of steroids is controversial – it may decrease inflammation around the tumour and help to relieve the obstruction, but there is some concern that is may increase the risk of perforation (Feuer and Broadley 2003). Octreotide may also be useful for its anti-secretory properties and may reduce the intensity of nausea and frequency of vomiting (Ripamonti et al. 2000; Mercadante et al. 2000).

If the patient is generally fit, then surgery should be considered early, although it will benefit only selected patients and would not be deemed routine practice. Pre-operative CT is useful to assess whether or not there is more than one level of obstruction.

The majority of patients in this situation would require a stoma and it is essential they receive proper counselling and preparation for this.

Renal failure

Renal failure most typically arises due to ureteric obstruction. The obstruction may be overcome by insertion of stents that can either be inserted via the bladder (retrograde stenting) or via the kidneys (antegrade stenting). This may not be possible and in these situations the only option is nephrostomy tubes. This needs to be carefully considered and discussed with the patient, particularly within the context of the rest of the disease.

Future research

Ovarian cancer remains a difficult cancer to cure. Ongoing research using newer agents, such as the mono-clonal antibodies and tyrosine kinase inhibitors, may increase responses to chemotherapy and make remissions more durable. Due to their tolerability, they also bring the possibility of maintenance therapy in patients with relapsed disease.

The development of an effective screening test for ovarian cancer could save thousands of lives every year in the UK and several trials are ongoing.

Conclusion

Ovarian cancer is the commonest gynaecological cancer in the UK. Patients often present with non-specific symptoms leading to delay in diagnosis and hence more advanced stage at presentation affecting prognosis and should be managed by a specialised MDT. For the majority of patients, primary treatment consists of surgery and chemotherapy.

The mainstay of treatment for patients with relapsed disease is chemotherapy, although surgery may occasionally have a role. The majority of patients diagnosed with carcinoma of the ovary will die from their disease – palliative care issues in these patients include recurrent ascites and bowel obstruction.

Reflective points

- Ovarian cancer is often seen as a chronic disease, meaning that women may require many modes and lines of treatment. Consider the physical and psychological effect of diagnosis and recurrence.
- As there are more treatment options, there seem to be more complex palliative symptoms, including ascites and bowel dysfunction. Are there measures put in place to prepare women for these symptoms and do they have the information available to access relevant services to aid in their management.

References

Alberts, D.S., Liu, S., Wilczynski, S. et al. (2007) Phase III randomised trial of pegylated liposomal doxorubicin plus carboplatin versus carboplatin in platinum sensitive patients with recurrent epithelial ovarian cancer or peritoneal carcinoma after failure of initial platinum-based chemotherapy: Southwest Oncology group Protocol SO200. *Journal of Clinical Oncology* **25(185)**, 5551.

Blackledge, G., Lawton, F., Redman, C. et al. (1989) Response of patients in phase II studies of chemotherapy in ovarian cancer: implications for patient treatment and the design of phase II trials. *British Journal of Cancer* **59(4)**, 650–3.

Bookman, M.A. (2006) Gynaecologic Cancer Intergroup through the gynaecological oncology group: GOGO182-ICON5: 5-arm phse III randomised trial of paclitaxel (P) and carboplatin (C) versus combinations with gemcitabine (G), liposomal doxorubicin (D) or topotecan (T) in patients with advanced stage epithelial ovarian or primary peritoneal cancer. *Journal of Clinical Oncology* **4**, 4565, suppl_abs 5002.

Cancer Research UK. *UK Ovarian Cancer Incidence Statistics.* www.cancerresearchuk.org/cancerstats/type/ovary

Cannistra, S.A., Matulonis, R., Penson, R. et al. (2006) Bevacuzimab in patients with advanced platinum-resistant ovarian cancer. *Journal of Clinical Oncology* ASCO Annual meeting proceedings Part 1. **24**, No18S:5006

Cannistra, S., Matulonis, R., Penson, R.T. et al. (2007) Phase III study of bevacuzimab in patients with platinum resistant ovarian cancer and peritoneal serous cancer. *Journal of Clinical Oncology* **25**, 5180–6.

Chung, H.H., Hwang, S.Y., Jung, K.W. et al. (2007) Ovarian cancer incidence and survival in Korea 1993-220. *International Journal of Gynecological Cancer* **17(3)**, 595–600.

Cochrane Review (2007) *Intraperitoneal Chemotherapy for the Initial Management of Primary Epithelial Ovarian Cancer.*

Colombo, N., Guthrie, D., Chiari, S. et al. (2003) International Collaborative Ovarian neoplasm (ICON) collaborators. International Collaborative ovarian neoplasm trial 1 (ICON 1): a randomised trial of adjuvant chemotherapy in women with early stage ovarian cancer. *Journal of National Cancer Institute* **95(2)**, 125–32.

Feuer, D.J. and Broadley, K.E. (2003) Corticosteroids for the resolution of malignant bowel obstruction in advanced gynaecological and gastrointestinal cancer (Cochrane review). In: The Cochrane Library, Issue 1.

Franceschi, S., Parazzini, F., Negri, E. et al. (1991) Pooled analysis of three European case-control studies of epithelial ovarian cancer; III. Oral Contraceptive use. *International Journal of Cancer* **49(1)**, 61–5.

Hunter, R.W., Alexander, N.D. and Soutter, W.P. (1992) Meta-analysis of surgery in advanced ovarian carcinomas is maximum cytoreductive surgery an independent determinant of prognosis? *American Journal of Obstetrics and Gynecology* **16692**, 504–11

International Collaborative Ovarian Neoplasm Group (2002) Paclitaxel plus carboplatin versus standard chemotherapy with single agent carboplatin or cyclophosphamide, doxorubicin and cisplatin in women with ovarian cancer: the ICON 3 randomised trial. *Lancet* **360(93320)**, 505–15.

Jacobs, I., Oram, D., Fairbanks, J. et al. (1990) A risk of malignancy index incorporating Ca 125, ultrasound and menopausal status for the accurate preoperative diagnosis of ovarian cancer. *British Journal of Obstetrics and Gynaecology* **97(910)**, 922–9.

Junor, E.J., Hole, D.J., McNulty, L. et al. (1999) Specialist gynaecologists and survival outcome in ovarian cancer; a Scottish national study of 1866 patients. *British Journal of Obstetrics and Gynaecology* **106(911)**, 1130–6.

Mercadante, S., Ripamonti, C., Casuccio, A. et al. (2000) Comparison of octreotide and hyoscine butylbromide in controlling gastrointestinal symptoms due to malignant inoperable bowel obstruction. *Support Care Cancer* **8(3)**, 188–91.

Muggia, F.M., Braly, P.S., Brady, F.M. et al. (2000) Phase IiI randomised study of cisplatin versus paclitaxel versus cisplatin-paclitaxel in patients with suboptimal stage III or IV ovarian cancer: a gynaecologic oncology group study. *Journal of Clinical Oncology* **18(1)**, 106–15.

National Institute of Clinical Excellence (2003) *Guidance on the Use of Paclitaxel in the Treatment of Ovarian Cancer*. Technology appraisal no 55. London: The Institute.

Ozols, RF. (2007) Ovarian cancer: is dose intensity dead? *Journal of Clinical Oncology* **25(27)**, 4157–8.

Parmar, M.K., Ledermann, J.A., Colombo, N. et al. (2003) Paclitaxel plus platinum-based chemotherapy versus conventional platinum-based chemotherapy in women with relapsed ovarian cancer: the ICON4/AGO-OVAR2.2 trial. *Lancet* **361(9375)**, 2099–106.

Pecorelli, S., Odicino, F., Maisonneuve, P. et al. (1998) FIGO staging of gynaecological cancer. Carcinoma of the ovary. *The International Federation of Gynaecology and Obstetrics*. http://www.figo.org/content/PDF/staging-booklet.pdf

Pfisterer, J., Plante, M., Vergote, I. et al. (2006) Gemcitabine plus carboplatin compared with carboplatin in patients with platinum sensitive recurrent ovarian cancer: an Intergroup trial of the AGO-OVAR the NCIC CTG, and the EORTC GCG. *Journal of Clinical Oncology* **24(29)**, 4699–707.

Rebbeck, T.R., Lynchm, H.T., Neuhausen, S. et al. (2002) Prophylactic oophorectomy in carrieris of BRCA1 or BRCA2 mutations. *New England Journal of Medicine* **346(21)**, 1616–22.

Ripamonti, C., Mrcadante, S., Groff, L. et al. (2000) Role of octreotide, scopolamine butylbromide and hydration in symptomatic patients with inoperable bowel obstruction and nasogastric tubes: a prospective randomised trial. *Journal of Pain Symptom Management* **1(91)**, 23–34.

Rose, P.G., Nerenstone, S., Brady, M. et al. (2002) A randomised phase III study of interval secondary cytoreduction in patients with advanced stage ovarian carcinoma with suboptimal residual disease. *Gynaecologic Oncology Group Study*. [abstract]. American Society of Clinical Oncology.

Swart, A.M., Burdett, S., Ledermann, J. et al. (2008) Why IP therapy cannot yet be considered as a standard of care for the first-line treatment of ovarian cancer: a systemic review. *Annals of Oncology* **19(4)**, 688–95.

The Breast Cancer Linkage Consortium (1999) Cancer risks In BRCA2 mutation carriers. *Journal of National Cancer Institute* **15**, 1310–6.

Thomas, H. and Rosenberg, P. (2002) Role of weekly paclitaxel in the treatment of advanced ovarian cancer. *Critical Reviews in Oncology/Haematology* **44 (suppl.)**, S43–51.

Thompson, D. and Easton, D.F. (2002) Cancer Incidence in BRCA1 mutation carriers. *Journal of National Cancer Institute* **94(18)**, 1358–65.

van de Berg, M.E., van Lent, M., Buyse, M. et al. (1995) The effect of debulking surgery after induction chemotherapy on the prognosis of advanced epithelial ovarian cancer. Gynaecological Cancer Cooperative group of the European organisation for Research and Treatment of Cancer. *New England Journal of Medicine* **332(910)**, 629–34.

van de Berg, M.E.L., de Wit, R., van Outlen, W.L.J. et al. (2002) Weekly cisplatin and daily oral etoposide is highly effective in platinum pre-treated ovarian cancer. *British Journal of Cancer* **86**, 19–25.

Vasey, P. (2001) The Scottish Gynaecologic Cancer trials group. Preliminary results of the SCOTROC Trial: A phase III comparison of Paclitaxel-Carboplatin and Docetaxel-Carboplatin as first line chemotherapy for stage !c-IV epithelial ovarian cancer. *Proceedings of the American Society of Clinical Oncology* **20** (abstract 804).

Voest, E.E., van Houwelingen, J.C. and Nejit, J.P. (1989) A meta-analysis of prognostic factors in advanced ovarian cancer with median survival and overall survival as main objectives. *European Journal of Gynaecological Oncology* **2594**, 711–20.

Williams, C.J. and Simera, S. (2000) The Cochrane Collaborative reviews. Tamoxifen foo relapse of ovarian cancer. Cochrane database of systemic reviews 2000, issue 3.

Chapter 9

Cancer of the Ovary: the Patient's Perspective

Noeleen Young

In this chapter I aim to give an insight into the experiences of women with ovarian cancer, both from clinical knowledge and personal experience. As a health care professional, I thought I understood the experience of cancer both from study and listening to patients. As both carer and patient, I know that the experience is quite different.

There are many aspects of a diagnosis of cancer, cancer treatment and side effects that go unnoticed, but for the patient, and those close to them, they are an everyday reality and frustrating, debilitating and disheartening. The often advanced nature of the disease at diagnosis means that most women will face the real possibility of a premature death. The disease can therefore have a significant impact on women, who play an important role in family life, nurturing children, caring for the extended family and contributing to, or in some cases, earning the family income.

Both as an individual and as a family, we experience a number of different responses to a diagnosis and treatment of cancer, such as shock, disbelief, anger, fear, numbness, depression and devastation. Gail explains her experience:

> ...the whole time I sat there smiling and nodding; it felt as if I was watching this happen to someone else. It wasn't until I left the room and headed down the corridor that I broke down.
>
> The news that you have cancer can be difficult to absorb, it may not be expected and this shock and disbelief can 'block out' all that you are being told, it feels as if you are in a bubble, there is a shell around you that is fragile.

It is now recognised that the way in which the news is broken can have a lasting effect on both the patient and their family. The first thing that is said is often remembered and may be the only piece of information that is retained. Since the Cancer Plan (DH 2000), it has been identified that practice and technique are important and work has been undertaken to ensure that all staff working in cancer services have the opportunity to undergo training and assessment in breaking significant or bad news to patients. Hospitals now have policies for 'breaking significant or bad news' to ensure that all staff are aware of the correct procedure and the role of the clinical nurse specialist usually involves being

Women's Cancers, First Edition. Edited by Alison Keen and Elaine Lennan.
© 2011 Blackwell Publishing Ltd. Published 2011 by Blackwell Publishing Ltd.

present and supporting the patient at this time. From the patient's perspective, this is invaluable, as they know they are able to discuss the details with the nurse, once they have recovered from the initial shock. The clinical nurse specialist's presence when the news is broken also helps to create an understanding bond and a good working relationship with the patient and their family. It is quality not quantity that counts, being empathetic and positive, listening to what the patient understands and wants to hear, being perceptive to their needs whilst feeding back and giving unambiguous details. Positive thinking and reassurance is helped by a plan for the immediate future and patients value leaving the consultation with written details that enable them to discuss the diagnosis and treatment plan with their family. Patients need to understand enough information to make decisions, talk to their families and share their anxieties. They need to be able to make their own plans and come to terms with the diagnosis.

Ellie was age 3 when her mum, Susan, was diagnosed with ovarian cancer. Now at the age of 11, she can remember it well. She describes how she felt so sad, she had cried and she knew her dad had cried as well. She describes vividly how she wanted to stay with her mum in hospital; this experience is etched on her memory.

The impact of a diagnosis of a parent with cancer is immense, particularly when recovery is unlikely. Susan recalls:

> *When I was diagnosed with ovarian cancer, I was determined it would not change my life. I'd give it my best shot, but basically I'd remain the same. I'd pick up life where I left it before diagnosis. Oh, how wrong and naive I was.*

Being a mum and having cancer causes a lot of mixed emotions, concerns and worry. It can be very difficult to find the right way to support your children (whatever their age) when you are struggling to come to terms with the diagnosis yourself. Talking to your children about cancer can be very difficult and upsetting. It is a natural instinct to try and protect them from the situation by not discussing it with them. But even if adults do not tell them openly about what is happening, they will inevitably know that something is seriously wrong. Involving children and letting them know what is happening generally helps them cope better with a parent's illness. Just being honest with them is the most important thing and many families find they need professional help and support to achieve this.

For some, the problems can be very different. When you live alone and work full-time, the implications of time off work for treatment are numerous. Jill found that support and advice for her was not available when she was in this situation, as she did not fall into any of the benefits criteria. She therefore had no option but to continue with work during her chemotherapy treatment, as she could not afford to be without an income. 'No matter how ill you are, the bills still have to be paid.' There was no one to help her cope with the 'bad days', when it was 'sometimes too much effort to make a cup of tea'. Jill also expressed her anxiety about the cost of having cancer: 'unexpected prescriptions, taxi fares and parking costs'. Research by Owusu-Barnaby et al. (2006) found that the average cancer patient incurred 53 trips, costing them £325 during the course of their treatment and many patients were not made aware of the Hospital Travel Cost Scheme or the NHS Low Income Scheme. The same results of more than 1100 interviews showed that 91% of households suffered from a loss of income as a result of the cancer diagnosis and 70% of cancer patients experienced extra costs during treatment.

Women face a number of challenges when returning to work, especially when still experiencing side effects of chemotherapy, loss of hair, fatigue, loss of confidence and depression. Employers and employees may have misconceptions of cancer and can be unsympathetic to the woman's needs. Jackson et al. (2007) research identified that almost 100,000 people of working age are diagnosed with cancer each year and that getting back to work represents a huge milestone and financial security to them, yet two-thirds of people experienced difficulties in returning to work.

Women describe their journey from the diagnosis and treatment as both physical and emotional. They need to make changes to adjust their lifestyles. In terms of emotional changes there is worry and concern for the family, a feeling of loss of control and a sense of life being on hold. Frustrations and family upsets bubble up at a time when they are unable to cope and normal family routines are disrupted. Women are not just learning to cope with the diagnosis of cancer but also changes in their lifestyle and other life events, work, loss of a partner, parents who may be elderly, caring for children or a relative with a disability. At this stage, family life is usually busy and these would usually be considered normal life changes.

For some a diagnosis of cancer means a change in lifestyle, an opportunity to retire or move house. Susan decided that as soon as she felt well she would move nearer her family:

> *I was able to retire and take an early pension; as soon as I felt well enough I sold my house and moved. I now realise I should have done it years ago, and wonder if I would ever have had the courage to do it if life had gone on in the same way.*

However, others are less fortunate. Anne found her lifestyle changing when her cancer returned and she needed further treatment, as her partner 'disappeared at this point, unable to cope'. She was left feeling devastated and lonely. The stress and impact that a diagnosis of cancer can have on a family member is immense and the carer's needs are often overlooked. The partner may experience psychological distress and a poor quality of life because of the fear of losing a loved one. There are additional burdens in their life and there may need to be changes in the provision of care for children or elderly relatives. There is no certainty anymore, plans are abandoned and things that once would have been important become trivial.

There are changes in the woman's role in the family, if she is unable to carry out some of the routine family activities such as shopping, school runs, housekeeping, cleaning and cooking; this causes a shift in the family dynamics. Tensions arise and feelings of guilt occur related to not having enough energy to carry out the everyday tasks and therefore not fulfilling the role as mother and wife. Efforts are made to maintain a normal lifestyle for the children and in doing so some things need to be neglected or left undone. For example, it can be difficult to prepare food for others when you are nauseous from chemotherapy but in the normal lifestyle of the family this may well be the woman's role. Gwenda explains how her husband found it hard to cope and hated seeing her unwell, yet over time he learnt to manage with the changes.

In a study of 1751 patients by Jackson et al. (2006), they found that almost a third of patients reported that their relationship was under 'enormous' strain and 25% of people who had experienced difficulties separated from their partner as a result of the cancer.

At diagnosis, women are not only facing the anxieties around their own mortality because of the often advanced nature of the disease at presentation, but also having to make decisions or come to terms with the issues that are often not discussed, relating to sexuality, femininity, fertility and motherhood.

Lloyd (2005) observed that:

> *...surviving cancer and facing possible death changes us irrevocably. We cannot be the same people we were before diagnosis – our world has been turned upside down and although we may appear well, we have caught the first flicker of mortality out of the corner of our eye.*

Spirituality is often a neglected side of support for cancer patients faced with a potentially fatal disease. They need to assimilate the diagnosis into their senses and this changes how they view themselves and their future. Spiritual needs are often heightened by the fear of death and the mental anguish and pain that it causes. Spirituality is not only related to our religious beliefs but also to the relief from fears and worries, finding a purpose and meaning in life. When faced with a serious diagnosis, people often rearrange their priorities and find that relationships become closer. The thought of death brings life sharply into focus, often promoting examination of who we are and what we are doing with our lives and aspects of life become more meaningful. Some may find that their faith is challenged, whilst others ask if there is a God. These questions and concerns may go largely unrecognised by those around the patient, yet should be part of offering holistic care to the patient – caring for the body, mind and spirit.

These are complex issues and the disease and treatment have a real impact of the quality of life of both the woman and her family. When faced with these situations, women need good and clear communication about the disease in order to feel that they have some control and to be able to restructure their lives to cope with daily living. There are initial and immediate practical needs such as, who is going to care for the children, the elderly relative or disabled husband, for which they need support from family, friends or social services. In the initial stages following a diagnosis, life is structured around survival and treatment; however, as time goes on, anxieties often occur around womanhood, the sexual impact of the disease, and fertility. To help to deal with the psychological impact of the disease, women need to be able to access further support.

Hair loss has a real influence on women's lives, as it is a visible sign of the disease and its treatment. Anna felt that the loss of her long hair with the chemotherapy was a threat to her whole image and to her sexuality. She explains:

> *My hair got short and thin, but as it was winter, at least I could wear a hat. Initially I had been worried about losing my hair, but the chemo had lots of side effects, so it was just one of many things to cope with. It was frustrating more than anything, because I had to stand over the bin to brush my hair.*

The distress at the loss of hair is not only felt by the patient but by those who are caring for them. Their visual image of their loved one is no longer a reality and it takes time for that image to change. The hair loss reminds them of the distress, the treatment and the side effects that have been experienced. Trying to appear well and normal absorbs most women's thoughts. Gail comments 'I lost my hair, and wore hats, I could not find a wig I liked.' Anne said how 'during treatment I had brought two wigs as I did not feel confident to go around completely bald, even in front of my nearest and dearest.' Sue viewed hair loss as an opportunity, 'no expensive trips to the hair dressers', although the experience was different to what she expected:

It was the itching and the tenderness of the scalp, not the hair fall that were more of a nuisance. One night I even got out of bed to change my nightdress, which had become a sort of hair shirt.

A normal menopause for women is considered a private event, to be discussed and disclosed to those close to you. It happens over a period of time and is one of those unspoken taboos; women avoid disclosure, are embarrassed and try to maintain a normal and conventional image. For many women with gynaecological cancer, the surgery results in a surgical menopause; this event is instant and the hot flushes, night sweats, vaginal dryness and palpitations associated with menopause occur very soon following surgery. There is no time to adjust emotionally or physically to these changes. Women begin to mistrust their body and report being upset and distressed regardless of the circumstances, whether or not they have children or are in a relationship. Celia felt that it should not be called a menopause: 'Menopause is natural, but when you are young, it's not right, it's not natural or normal.'

Gynaecological cancers essentially affect parts of the body involved in the sexual act and fertility and studies have shown that these patients have a high risk of sexual and fertility sequelae. The loss of fertility is a distressing factor for women, even if their family is complete, as the choice has been taken away. Culturally and in the media, fertility is associated with being fruitful, productive and prolific, whilst infertility is associated with being barren, inadequate and useless. It is therefore generally felt that a complete woman is one that has the potential to be fertile and the loss of reproductive capability gives rise to feelings of grief, distress and bereavement for both the women and her family. For some of the younger women, it is the loss of their dreams or life-plan, their *raison d'être* for living; the goal posts have moved and they find that health care professionals underestimate the impact that this has, both emotionally and physically. Gail found that ovarian cancer changed her life when she was diagnosed with ovarian cancer at the age of 20. She describes the experience as very traumatic, but 6 years later she is married and planning to adopt children. 'I believe the experience has made me the person I am today and in a strange way I don't believe it was entirely negative, I survived to tell the tale.' Social perception is that menopausal women are aging and unappealing sexually. This impacts on and threatens the sexuality of the women who has undergone a surgical menopause. Their ability to dress and behave in a flirtatious way may be affected and this may impact on their personal relationships. Macmillan Cancer Support (2006) found that 43% found that their sexual relationship suffered. There are hidden losses in the relationship and within the family, a child they may never have, the experience of motherhood, confirmation of the union by having a family. There is a feeling of loss for the creative part of self and for the future of another generation experienced by grandparents. Anna, who was diagnosed aged 19 with ovarian cancer, expresses her thoughts: 'I am single at the moment and the fertility aspect is not something I dwell on. I hope when the right man comes along, it won't be a problem.' There have been times when she has been upset by what her illness took away from her but 'the reality is that I cannot conceive my own children and I have got used to that reality.'

Sexuality is defined as gender, personality, behaviour, appearance and sexual activity. Following treatment for cancer, many women experience some degree of sexual dysfunction or sexual morbidity, and this may present in a physical form such as vaginal dryness, vaginismus, anorgasmia, dyspareunia, fatigue, impaired bladder or bowel function, stoma formation or be related to the psychological impact of the disease resulting in a loss of libido and impaired sexual desire. Fear may play a role in the loss of desire; 'will it hurt, will it be normal?', and anxiety and depression certainly impact of sexual desire.

Sexual function and sexual needs are linked closely to the emotional need for love, closeness and caring. During the physiology of the sexual response, desire is the first phase of an encounter and may be inhibited by drugs such as antidepressants, tranquillisers and beta blockers. Alcohol in small amounts may increase desire as it lowers inhibitions, fear and guilt; however, in large amounts it decreases desire.

The excitement of the genital organs is a response to two sources – the brain and to touch; however, sexual excitement does not rise at a steady rate but in steps. During this phase, there is vasocongestion of the genitals and a sexual flush occurs, and the blood pressure, pulse and respiration are raised.

Labia minor become swollen and moist and open slightly and the clitoris becomes enlarged and erect. In the normal anatomy, lubrication of the vagina occurs at this stage; however, this may not occur in the menopausal woman and women therefore require advice about the most suitable vaginal lubricants for them to use. Nipples become erect and breasts enlarge and there is ballooning of the vagina and the uterus is lifted out of it normal position in the pelvis. These physical sensations are impaired for women who have had treatment for breast or a gynaecological cancer and further stimulation may be required. During the final phase of excitement, orgasm becomes inevitable for the male; however, for the female it is not, although for some this can give feelings of pleasure, fulfilment, well-being, harmony and relaxation, whilst for others, failure to reach orgasm results in feelings of discomfort, dissatisfaction and frustration. These tense irritable feelings can take some time to dissipate and repeated episodes can result in feelings of guilt and become a problem in the relationship.

Changes in body image may also be defined as a loss. The body image is concerned with two main factors, body perception and body attitude. Physical changes are not essential for a woman to experience an altered body image and women may experience an altered body image simply from the diagnosis of cancer. Western society places much emphasis on the 'perfect body', and even for the fit and healthy, media images can cause anxiety and concern. The body image is part of a woman's psychological self, self-concept, self-esteem and self-identity. It is this loss of social cultural self that can lead to a loss of social identity and role. For the woman with gynaecological cancer, disfigurement, mutilation, physical changes, surgical menopause, weight gain or loss and hair loss all cause psychological trauma as well as feelings of disgust, shame, guilt, grief and loss of fertility. Counselling or information with regard to sex and sexuality is not often offered and women say that they would like the support and information that a nurse can offer and they would like this to be initiated by the nurse. Successful counselling at this stage can overcome the physical and emotional problems that may have occurred due to the diagnosis of cancer, by teaching the women and her partner new skills that enable them to rediscover the art of love-making.

A diagnosis of ovarian cancer and the subsequent treatment is psychologically distressing and giving the necessary support cannot be as systematically organised as giving information. Patients who become highly psychologically distressed, perceive a low quality of life as a result of a fear of dying, worsening physical condition and side effects from treatment and this can affect their well-being and that of their carers. This experience can reduce the patient to a state of passive acceptance and increased vulnerability. Making choices and decisions about their treatment and care can be threatening and may make them feel guilty if the 'wrong' choice is made.

Emotional support involves spending time with another person, listening and talking about problems and concerns in a way that is helpful and reassuring. Emotional support involves elements of psychotherapy, which may range from dealing with issues actively to simply being someone to listen. There is a need for psychological support to be offered on an *ad hoc* basis, when a question or crisis occurs or when there is a need to talk. Scheduled appointments and discussions can give limited access to support, which requires maximum effort to attend. A range of people can contribute to the support network in primary and secondary care, family and friends, complimentary therapies, counsellors, charity help lines and support groups. The providers of support often benefit from some basic communication skills training and need not shoulder all the responsibility for the emotional care of their patients and their families. They should be able to access support from colleagues and introduce the patients to those services that are appropriate to their needs. The Cancer Reform Strategy (DH 2007) acknowledges the need to provide good psychological support services, as patients progress along their cancer journey, and identify key areas where support is required: patient experience and user involvement in shaping services; assessment of holistic needs at key stages; post-treatment requirements and survivorship.

Gwenda comments:

We have supported each other through thick and thin and have had wonderful friends who have been there for us. If I have ever felt low they have soon got me feeling positive again, which has really helped. We have laughed together and lived every day to the full.

Anne found she needed further support and she comments:

I try to remain positive and my mind is open to any other healing alternatives. I love to spend time with my family and dear friends who have been so supportive. I have a wonderful counsellor who is probably the only person I feel able to express my fears to.

Patients often discover practical methodologies that help them to cope. Gill found that her scrapbook of cards and documenting her journey helped her to cope:

The books contained every single card and message received during my illness, and so held a lot of emotional memories, but it was important to me that I captured it all to show how vital support had been to me and my family.

Families can find creating a scrapbook or box, particularly with young children, can help them to come to terms with the situation. The box can be decorated together and filled with mementos that are important to both, photos, a shell or fir cone collected on a walk, a piece of jewellery or an old perfume bottle. In the event of the death, this can then become a lasting treasure for the child.

Diaries are often valued by patients as a means of communication, either personally or as hand held records. They also provide the opportunity for a treatment plan or for goal setting. A small study by Ovacome with Southampton University found that writing about their experiences was beneficial for some patients, and can have a positive effect on their well-being; indeed, we can see that by the proliferation of books and articles related to personal experience in the media. There is something enduringly real about the written word, whereas the spoken word just hangs in the air for a brief moment and then is gone and can be quickly forgotten.

A support system and information giving that enables the patient to identify their own needs and help them to self manage living with cancer is imperative. As health care professionals and oncology nurses, there is more information and learning needed to be truly responsive to the issues surrounding a woman's needs when she is diagnosed with cancer. The Cancer Reform Strategy (DH 2007) recognises the need for patients to be enabled to take responsibility for their own care and to make choices when living with and beyond cancer. These choices are about the team or hospital where they are treated and they need good information to enable them to do so. The strategy also recognises the need to provide health care that supports and enables patients to resume a meaningful lifestyle. Gail said:

I don't believe it was an entirely negative time. I also feel that I was extremely lucky! Lucky that my cancer had been found and lucky that I had survived to tell the tale.

Anna comments that:

There were days when all I wanted to do was sleep, because I didn't want to think about what was going on and how rough I felt. But there were days when I'd feel absolutely brilliant and I'd go out and think, I'm alive and everything's so beautiful.

Acknowledgement

My thanks to all the women of Ovacome, who have given their permission for me to use their experiences and quotes, which make this chapter meaningful.

References

Canon Jayne Lloyd (2005) Touching lives: a service of encouragement for those affected by gynae-cological cancer. *The Journal of Health Care Chaplaincy* **Autumn/Winter**, 32–36.

Department of Health (2007) *Cancer Reform Strategy*.

Department of Health (2000) *NHS Cancer Plan*, 97 p.

Jackson, N., Dhearn, K. and Sparham, L. (2006) *Worried Sick: The Emotional Impact of Cancer. Macmillan Cancer Support*. April 2006 (available on www.macmillan.org.uk).

Macmillan Cancer Support (2007) *The Road to Recovery: Getting Back to Work*. November 2007 (available on www.macmillan.org.uk).

Ovacome Helpline: 0845 3710554. Admin line: 0207 299 6654 (Mon–Fri 9.00am–4.00pm) www.ovacome.org.uk

Owusu-Barnaby, A., Austin, K. and Fallows, A. (2006) Macmillan Cancer Support. *The Hidden Price of Getting Treatment*. June 2006 (available on www.macmillan.org.uk).

Chapter 10

Cancer of the Cervix

Ken Metcalf and Katherine McCarthy

Learning points

At the end of this chapter, the reader will have an understanding of:
- Human papilloma virus (HPV) and the cervix cancer screening programme
- The staging, and investigations for cervical cancer
- Fertility and sexual function
- Future research

Introduction

The cervix is the 'neck' of the uterus (Figure 10.1). It is the lowermost part of the uterus and projects into the vagina. The thick muscle bundles seen within the myometrium above rapidly decrease in size to make up only 10% of the tissue within the cervix. The rest of the tissue comprises connective tissue. The cervix is 3 cm long and can be divided into the supra-vaginal and vaginal portions. The tissue surrounding the supra-vaginal portion is called the parametrium. Posteriorly, the cervix is covered with peritoneum forming the Pouch of Douglas. The vaginal portion of cervix is covered by squamous epithelium, which becomes columnar at the external os leading into the cervical canal.

The cervical canal stretches to allow blood flow during menstruation and produces mucus that can either block or facilitate the passage of sperm during sexual intercourse. It widely dilates during parturition.

Epidemiology and aetiology

Cervical cancer is a cancer of the female reproductive tract and accounts for 2% of all female cancers. Cervical cancer may be asymptomatic or picked up through the NHS National Cervical Screening Programme (NHSCSP). Symptoms include post-coital,

Women's Cancers, First Edition. Edited by Alison Keen and Elaine Lennan.
© 2011 Blackwell Publishing Ltd. Published 2011 by Blackwell Publishing Ltd.

intermenstrual, post-menopausal bleeding or any persistent vaginal bleeding. It is usually slow growing and those most at risk are sexually active females between 30 and 50 years and over 85 years of age. In 2005, 2803 new cases were diagnosed in the UK, making it the 12th commonest cancer in women. After breast cancer, it is the second commonest cause of cancer in women under 35 years of age (Office of National Statistics 2005; Scottish Health Statistics 2008; Welsh Cancer Intelligence and Surveillance Unit 2008; Northern Ireland Cancer Registry 2008). The annual incidence rate in the UK is 8.4 per 100,000 females.

There has been an overall downward trend in incidence of cervical cancer since 1990, despite a small increase in the 1980s (Scottish Health Statistics 2008; Northern Ireland Cancer Registry 2008; Office of National Statistics 1999). This peak in incidence was in women aged 25–49 and has since declined. The most significant decline in incidence is seen in the 50–64 age groups. This decline in incidence is attributable to the introduction of the screening programme (NHSCSP) and so mostly affects Western countries. Worldwide, cancer of the cervix accounts for 1 in 10 of all female cancers and is the most common female cancer diagnosed in South Africa and Central America (Ferlay et al. 2004).

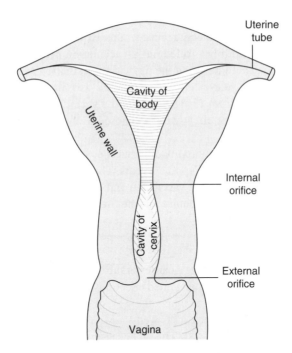

Figure 10.1   The normal cervix. From Nair and Peate (2009). Reproduced with permission from John Wiley & Sons Ltd.

Human papillomavirus (HPV)

Infection with human papillomavirus (HPV) has been identified as the major cause of cervical cancer. One large international study has demonstrated the prevalence of HPV amongst cervical cancers as greater than 99%, the highest ever attributable fraction identified for a specific cancer (Walboomers et al. 1999). After women become sexually active, usually in their mid-teens, infection with HPV peaks and most cases resolve spontaneously. Up to 80% of the population have been infected with HPV at some point. There are over 100 known strains of HPV; however, it is 16 and 18 that are the most oncogenic strains. Infection with these strains can lead to the development of high grade pre-invasive lesions (cervical intra-epithelial neoplasia) approximately 10 years later. If left untreated, the development of invasive disease usually occurs at 40–50 years of age (Nobbenhuis et al. 1999). This issue is complex; however, as infection with HPV may be systemic and not necessarily sexually transmitted, does not necessarily lead to cervical cancer and if cancer does develop, it may manifest soon or many years after HPV infection.

HPV vaccination

Two large studies have demonstrated a reduced incidence of pre-invasive cervical lesions in women vaccinated with anti-HPV vaccines, Gardasil (Merck) and Cervarix (GlaxoSmithKline) (Future 11 Study Group 2007; Frederick et al. 2004). Gardasil protects against oncogenic HPV strains 16 and 18 and also 6 and 11, which are known to cause genital warts. Cervarix protects against strains 16 and 18 only.

The Department of Health has rolled out a vaccination programme by consent for all girls aged 12–13 years to be given the Cervarix vaccination as a course of 3 injections over 6 months. A 2-year catch-up programme was also commenced in autumn 2008 to vaccinate all girls from 13–18 years, as the vaccination has been shown to be effective in females who have already been exposed to the virus (Future Study Group 11 2008).

The impact on incidence and mortality of cervical cancer as a result of the vaccination programme will not be known for up to 20 years. The other question mark is over how long females remain protected once vaccinated and whether booster immunisations are required. Current data suggests immunity may be lifelong.

Other risk factors

Cervical cancer is almost exclusively a cancer of the sexually active. Studies have shown that the presence of other sexually transmitted infections, herpes simplex and/or Chlamydia trachomatis with HPV infection increase the risk of development of cervical cancer (Zereu et al. 2007). Similarly, smoking is well known to increase the risk of developing cervical cancer (Stewart et al. 2008). This is because smoking impairs the function of local Langerhans cells within the cervix, which are responsible for clearing local infections.

An increased incidence of cervical cancer, amongst other cancers, is also seen in patients who are immunosuppressed because of HIV infection or due to medication. There is some evidence to suggest that use of the contraceptive pill for more than 5 years may increase the risk (McFarlane-Anderson et al. 2008).

Overall, women who become sexually active early, have frequent partners, have children young (before the age of 17), who live in a developing country and who smoke, are at the highest risk of developing cervical cancer. A Cochrane Review demonstrated that targeted health education for women regarding sexual behaviour did result in a reduced incidence of cervical cancer (Shepherd et al. 1999).

Screening and pre-diagnosis

The development of cervical cancer is preceded by a pre-invasive stage known as cervical intra-epithelial neoplasia (CIN). CIN I-III represents a spectrum of abnormal cells, which may progress into invasive disease over a period of time (Table 10.1). The NHSNCP was set up in 1967 in order to detect these abnormal cells before the development of malignancy. It involves a smear using a spatula (Papanicolaou test) or more recently, liquid based cytology (LBC). Smears are performed every 3 years up to the age of 50, then 5-yearly until 64 years. The programme used to start from 20 years of age; however, it has recently changed to 25 years of age in England. This was due to the low risk of developing cervical cancer before 25 years of age and the high risk of invasive procedures performed as a result of transient infection with human papillomavirus (HPV). In Northern Ireland and Wales, the screening age is still 20–64 years and in Scotland it is 20–60 years. Approximately 1 in 10 smears are reported as abnormal. This includes smears that are inadequate and need to be repeated and smears that demonstrate CIN I-III.

Table 10.1   Classification of CIN.

CIN I – mild dysplasia
CIN II – moderate dysplasia
CIN III – severe dysplasia/ carcinoma *in situ*

Telling the patient they have an abnormal smear

All smear results are reported to patients by letter or phone. Anyone with an abnormal result should be invited to see their GP for a discussion. Many women assume that an abnormal smear means that they have cancer. As they are usually asymptomatic, this comes as an enormous shock and there is a great deal of anxiety involved. 'Early warning cells' is a better way to present the scenario to a patient than 'precancerous lesion.'

Discussions about the influence of HPV infection, if it has been reported, may make the woman feel as if she is accused of being promiscuous and responsible for the abnormal result. Similarly, it may make some women question the fidelity of their partners, if in a long-term relationship. Reassurance should be given that this may not necessarily have been transmitted sexually.

Management of abnormal smears

Patients with CIN I are usually requested to have a repeat smear in 6 months. Some abnormalities resolve within this time frame, particularly if the woman gives up smoking. A test for CIN II or III requires referral for colposcopy. A colposcope is a lighted magnifying instrument that enables assessment of certain features of the cervix and aids in making a precise diagnosis and planning treatment. The usual recommendation at this stage is to remove the affected area by a loop excision using diathermy. This is called a large loop excision of transformation zone (LLETZ). The transformation zone is the area on the cervix where glandular epithelium from the cervical canal changes into squamous epithelium, which covers the vaginal cervix. It is the site where most abnormalities are seen. It can be done in the out patient clinic under local anaesthetic or in theatres at a later stage, under general anaesthetic.

This form of treatment is successful for 4 out of 5 women. If abnormal cells remain, the patient may undergo surveillance colposcopy in 6 months or a repeat LLETZ. If all is well at this point, annual smear tests are recommended, (normally for 9 years), and then the patient may be discharged to the NCSP. If the patient develops another abnormal smear, discussions on further management will consider a repeat LLETZ or hysterectomy. The feasibility of this latter option will depend on the patient. It is more of a straightforward option for the post-menopausal women than it is for the younger woman who wishes to have children. Patient preference is the key issue in this scenario, and a 'watch and wait' approach may be adopted.

CGIN

Cervical glandular intra-epithelial neoplasia (CGIN) is a less common cause of an abnormal smear. It is atypia of the glandular/columnar cells within the cervix, as opposed to CIN, which affects the squamous cells. It is classified as high or low grade, with high grade incorporating adenocarcinoma *in situ*. If left untreated, high grade CGIN will progress to adenocarcinoma in 1–14 years. Treatment for CGIN, as for CIN, is LLETZ. If the margins from the specimen are not clear, a further LLETZ may be indicated. Due to the difficulties in identifying invasion, it is advisable to follow the patient up in the colposcopy clinic.

Fertility issues

Nulliparous women undergoing LLETZ procedures may be concerned about their risks of future fertility. There is no risk of reduced fertility when undergoing one or two procedures, however, there is an increased risk of miscarriage in the second trimester of pregnancy. This is due to an incompetent cervix and the risk increases with the size of the loop excised. If there is any concern, the woman may have a pelvic scan early in pregnancy to assess the length of her cervix. A decision is then taken whether or not to place a stitch in the cervix (cerclage) to prevent the cervix opening prematurely and carry the pregnancy to full term.

Women who have had more than two LLETZ procedures and are still troubled by abnormal smears will need to discuss the issue of possible hysterectomy. This may be deeply traumatic for a woman who desires to have children and has not done so. The problem is compounded by the fact that she does not actually have cancer yet. Depending on the histology, it may be possible to allow her to complete her family, under close surveillance, and then perform the hysterectomy. Sometimes, however, the woman may not

Table 10.2   FIGO (2009 Federation for Gynaecology and Obstetrics) – staging of cervical cancer.

Stage 0		Carcinoma *in situ*
Stage I		Confined to cervix
	IA	Diagnosed microscopically ≤5 mm and largest extension >7 mm
	IAI	Stromal invasion <3 mm and extension of ≥7 mm
	IA2	Stromal invasion of >3 mm not >5 mm, with an extension of not >7 mm
	IB	Clinically visible lesions limited to the cervix or pre clinical cancers greater than stage IA
	IB1	Clinically visible lesions ≤4.0 cm in greatest dimension
	IB2	Clinically visible lesion of >4.0 cm in greatest dimension
Stage II		Invasion beyond the uterus but not to the pelvic wall or lower third of the vagina
	IIA	Without parametrial invasion
	IIA1	Clinically visible lesion ≤4.0 cm in greatest dimension
	IIA2	Clinically visible lesion N 4 cm in greatest dimension
	IIB	Parametrium involved
Stage III		Spread to pelvic side wall or lower vagina and/or includes hydronephrosis or non functioning kidney
	IIIA	Involves lower third of vagina but no pelvic sidewall
	IIIB	Involves pelvic sidewall and/or hydronephrosis or non-functioning kidney
Stage IV		Cancer spread to distant organs

be in circumstances that will allow her to do this. In this scenario, options such as egg freezing and surrogacy need to be discussed prior to further definitive treatment.

Classification and staging

Patients with suspected cervical cancer are referred urgently to a colposcopy clinic (within 2 weeks). Suspicious features include white epithelium after staining with acetic acid solution, abnormal blood vessel patterns, abnormal surface contour or presence of a large lesion. A biopsy is then taken for histological diagnosis. This may involve taking the whole lesion, if small, by a loop excision. If it is a larger lesion, only a representative sample needs to be taken for diagnosis.

Once the diagnosis of malignancy has been made, the tumour needs to be accurately staged in order that treatment can be planned. The Federation Internationale de Gynecologie et d'Obsterique (FIGO) staging of cervical cancer is clinical and is made before treatment has begun (Table 10.2) It involves examination of the cervix (including colposcopy), endocervical curettage, hysteroscopy, cystoscopy, proctoscopy, intravenous urography (IVU) and X-ray examination of the lungs and skeleton. In practice, most centres use CT scans to assess for metastatic spread to the chest and abdomen and

Table 10.3   5-year survival statistics for cervical cancer.

Stage	5 year survival (%)
0	100%
IA	95%
IB	80–90%
IIA	70–90%
IIB	60–70%
III	40%
IV	20%

Table 10.4   5-year survival rates of cervical cancer according to age.

Age at diagnosis	5 year survival (%)
15–39	80%
40–49	70%
50–59	60%
60–69	50%
70–79	35%
80–99	20%

an MRI to assess the pelvic tumour (although these modalities are not essential criteria in the FIGO staging). MRI scans have been shown to be superior to CT scans and clinical examination in assessment of local spread of tumour and local lymphadenopathy (Patrick et al. 1997).

It is essential that each patient is accurately staged pre-treatment, in order that they receive the appropriate treatment. Studies from the early 1990s have shown that in some centres up to 10% of patients were incorrectly staged. These patients then underwent conservative surgery and later required salvage surgery or radiotherapy (Jackson et al. 1997). Similarly, studies have shown that staging of cancers performed at teaching hospitals with specialist oncological support have a higher adequacy of staging rate compared with district general hospitals with no oncological support (Wolfe et al. 1996).

Survival

The number of cervical cancer deaths in the UK has been in decline since the 1970s. The mortality rate is 2.4 per 100,000 females and is nearly 70% lower than it was 30 years ago. This is attributable to the introduction of the NHSCSP. Overall, 68% of all women diagnosed with cervical cancer will be alive at 5 years and 66% will be alive at 10 years. This ranges from an approximate 100% survival for stage 0 cancers to less than 20% for stage IV cancers (Table 10.3) (Coleman et al. 1995). The age of the patient also affects survival. Generally, a younger woman has a better prognosis (Table 19.4) (Coleman et al. 2004). This is because younger women tend to present at an earlier stage due to the NHSCSP. Similarly, fitter patients who are able to withstand intensive treatment regimes also tend to have a better prognosis.

Treatment

Treatment of cervical cancer is dependent on the stage of the tumour.

Surgery

Stage 0 and IA disease is amenable to excision by LLETZ. With tumours that invade to a depth of less than 3 mm, the risk of positive lymph nodes is 1%. This rises to 4% for tumours that invade 3–5 mm. In this scenario, a discussion should take place with the patient regarding the need for a pelvic lymphadenectomy, which can be performed laparoscopically. Removal of these lymph nodes can provide useful prognostic information and, if enlarged, may fulfil a therapeutic role. Radical hysterectomy is not indicated in this stage of disease, as there is no parametrical involvement. Fertility is preserved with these treatment options.

Studies have shown that surgery or radiotherapy are equally effective in the treatment of stage IB disease (Landoni et al. 1997). Younger patients with small stage IB1 tumour, who wish to preserve their fertility, may be offered a trachelectomy and pelvic lymphadenectomy. Trachelectomy involves removal of the cervix and upper vagina and the remaining uterus is then sutured onto the vagina and a purse string stitch is placed at the new opening. This is a fertility sparing option and many successful pregnancies have been reported (Shepherd et al. 1998). This procedure is usually carried out vaginally or abdominally and is centralised to large, specialist cancer centres. A pelvic lymphadenectomy is also recommended for this stage of tumour and this may be carried out laparoscopically prior to the trachelectomy.

For women who do not wish to preserve their fertility, the options include radical hysterectomy, bilateral salpingo-oophrectomy and lymphadenectomy or radical radiotherapy, (sometimes with concomitant chemotherapy). Recommendations are that such surgery should be performed by specialist gynaecological oncologists in cancer centres, as this results in the best 5-year survival (Wolfe et al. 1996; Scheidler et al. 1997). The outcomes of both treatment options are similar; however, surgery is generally recommended as radiotherapy is associated with an increased long term morbidity including dyspareunia, cystitis and diarrhoea. Pelvic irradiation in younger, pre-menopausal women patients also results in premature menopause and subsequent infertility.

Wertheim's radical hysterectomy

This operation forms a central part of the management of cervical cancer. It is generally performed as an open procedure; however, some centres have begun to offer it laparoscopically (Pellegrino et al. 2009). Long-term results and oncological outcomes of this method are not known.

A radical hysterectomy differs from a simple hysterectomy in that the uterine vessels are ligated close to their origin, ureters are exposed up to the bladder, parametrial tissue is excised, 2 cm of upper vagina is taken and a pelvic lymphadenectomy performed. It is associated with an increased morbidity compared to a simple hysterectomy (Table 10.5). Ovaries may be preserved in younger women, due to the low incidence of metastases to the ovary.

It may still be necessary to administer radiotherapy after a patient has undergone radical surgery, if close or positive resection margins are reported on the histological specimen or if lymph node spread is shown. The morbidity associated with radical surgery and

Table 10.5 Morbidity associated with a radical hysterectomy for cervical cancer.

Haemorrhage
Ureteric dysfunction, stricture or fistula due to de-vascularisation
Urinary tract infection
Bladder dysfunction due to inadvertent nerve damage
Vesico-vaginal fistula
Lymph collection within pelvis – may require formal drainage
Lymphoedema of the legs
Inadvertent damage to obturator, genitofemoral, femoral or perineal nerves
Dyspareunia (painful intercourse)

radiotherapy is very high and so careful planning with the patient needs to take place to minimise this risk. Adjuvant radiotherapy has been widely used in patients who have undergone a radical hysterectomy and have positive nodes. Results demonstrate that whilst this may reduce the risk of a pelvic recurrence, there is no increase in long-term survival (Newton 1975; Soisson et al. 1990).

Chemo radiation

This represents the mainstay of treatment for tumours stage IIB and above. A study performed in 1999 demonstrated that concurrent use of platinum-based chemother-apy with radiotherapy was associated with a significant increase in survival and progression-free survival in women with stage 1B-IVA cancers compared with radi-otherapy treatment alone (Rose et al. 1999). However, studies since have shown that giving chemotherapy and radiotherapy together, whether cisplatin is used or not, still results in an improved overall survival (Green et al. 2005). This is thought to be due to one agent sensitizing the other or a systemic cytotoxic effect. Cisplatin is now the cytotoxic agent of choice and radiotherapy involves external beam and intra-cavity brachytherapy, (internal radiotherapy treatment). The morbidity associ-ated with having both treatments together is higher than either treatment alone (Table 10.6). Fortunately, it is generally not associated with hair loss and most side effects are short term.

Table 10.6 Morbidity associated with chemoradiation for cervical cancer.

Nausea and vomiting
Neutropenia/sepsis
Acute renal failure
Haemorrhagic cystitis
Ototoxicity
Infertility
Diarrhoea/proctitis
Long-term risk of developing acute leukaemia

Recurrent disease

For patients with recurrent disease, pelvic exenteration surgery may be an option. This surgery is highly specialised and may involve diversion of the urinary and gastro-intestinal tracts. It should only be considered in patients with node negative disease and those fit enough to withstand the procedure. Some centres have reported reasonable 5-year survival rates with morbidity rates of approximately 2–4% (Robertson et al. 1994; Shepherd et al. 1994; Morley et al. 1989). Full counselling needs to given if this option is taken, as it has a major impact on the patient's quality of life and is associated with high levels of morbidity.

For most patients with recurrent disease, radical surgery is not an option. If the patient has been treated with surgery alone, radiotherapy is usually the next line of treatment. In previously irradiated patients, treatment options are more limited and would involve palliative symptom relief. Chemotherapy may be an option, similarly, for distant metastases, management usually comprises palliative control. Painful bony metastases, for example, are well controlled by radiotherapy. Unfortunately, most women with recurrent disease die 7–10 months later. There is a need, therefore, for more effective treatment strategies in this area.

Follow-up

Most patients are seen 2–3 weeks after surgery or 6–8 weeks at the end of chemo radiation. Thereafter, it is normal to be seen every 3 months for a year by the surgeon, oncologist or a combination of the two. Each visit usually involves a vaginal examination, other investigations are individualised according to symptoms or clinical findings.

It is well known that attending hospital follow-up appointments induces a lot of anxiety in patients. Some patients also view such appointments as being given the 'all clear' until the next visit is due. This can represent a false sense of reassurance for the patient and may lead them to leave any worrying symptoms until they are due to come and see the doctor. It should always be explained carefully to the patient that they should bring forward their appointment if they experience any new onset of pelvic pain, bleeding or dyspareunia.

Sexual intercourse after treatment for cervical cancer

Resuming sexual intercourse after surgery or chemo-radiation needs to be discussed. Women may feel anxious about this and reassurance needs to be given. It is advisable to wait 6 weeks after surgery, allowing the vagina to heal. For women having radiotherapy, they can, if they so wish, have intercourse during the period of their treatment. Women need to be reassured that they will not make things worse by resuming intercourse, nor can they pass anything on to their partner. They may simply not feel like resuming their sex life and this is normal too. Surgical removal or irradiation of the ovaries induces the menopause, which can add to the loss of libido. Similarly, radiation can cause vaginal dryness, dyspareunia and a narrowing of the vagina (virginal stenosis). Women should routinely be given the opportunity to discuss these important issues and be guided on the use of hormone replacement therapy (HRT), vaginal oestrogen, vaginal lubricants and the use of vaginal dilators.

Future research

Preventative strategies

Cancer Research UK is currently undertaking a study looking at the effects of a dietary supplement containing diindolymethane (DIM) on mildly abnormal smears. DIM is a naturally occurring substance found in broccoli, sprouts and cabbage and is thought to prevent the progression of mild dyskaryosis to cervical cancer. The study involved 3000 women with mildly abnormal smears, taking either DIM or a placebo for 6 months. Smears were taken at the start and end of treatment and the study closed in December 2007 (Cervical Randomized Intervention Study Protocol – CRISP). Results are awaited.

Surgery

Much interest is currently focused on the developments of laparoscopic surgery in the treatment of cervical cancer. Currently, a few centres worldwide are offering a total laparoscopic radical hysterectomy for the treatment of early stage cervical cancer with comparable complication rates to the open approach (Zakashansky et al. 2008). There is also research into the use of robotic surgery in radical hysterectomy. This may be performed laparoscopically or vaginally with theoretical advantages of 3D vision and tremor reduction (Ramerez et al. 2008). Initial studies demonstrate that it is feasible and safe; however, long-term oncological outcomes are not known.

Chemotherapy

Current guidelines for treatment of advanced/recurrent cervical cancer involve use of agents carboplatin and paclitaxel. Unfortunately, there is no evidence to show these agents improve overall survival. The cytotoxic agent topotecan has been licensed for use in advanced or recurrent cervical cancer. Its use in combination with cisplatin was currently under review by the National Institute of Clinical Excellence (NICE) for potential use in the UK (October 2009). One study has shown that it is the only treatment to demonstrate an improvement in overall survival in recurrent cervical cancer (Long et al. 2005). However, it is associated with a higher incidence of febrile neutropenia compared with the use of cisplatin alone. It is also thought that prior use of cisplatin may reduce the effectiveness of subsequent use of cisplatin and Toptecan in combination. Similarly, there is currently interest in biological agent Erlotinib (Tarceva), which works by inhibition of the epidermal growth factor receptor. One study presented at the 2008 American Society of Clinical Oncology (ASCO) annual meeting demonstrated improved complete response rates when Erlotinib was used in combination with cisplatin and radiotherapy, compared to standard chemoradiation treatment (Ferreira 2008). Further study results are awaited.

Conclusion

Overall, the incidence and mortality of cervical cancer are in decline. The treatment for the disease varies of course, depending on stage at diagnosis. For women who have chemotherapy and radiotherapy in combination, the toxicities are variable but can be life changing and long term. Offering on-going supportive follow-up with a view to monitoring and helping to manage these potential long-term problems is very important. The introduction of the HPV vaccination programme should further contribute very significantly to the reduction in burden of this disease on society.

Excerpts from patient diary following confirmation of cervix cancer

Cervix cancer, that dreaded disease. The one everyone has been talking about. The one that's a sexually transmitted disease! And I've 'caught' it. How could this happen. I'm 36, met my husband when I was 19 and only had 2 other 'flings' before him? I feel dirty and don't want anyone to know.

As the consultant was talking to me about treatments I've only ever heard about – chemotherapy and radiotherapy. What do they mean, what will they do to me, how will I feel? Sickness was mentioned, fatigue, vaginal stenosis (whatever that may mean), diarrhoea, cystitis-like symptoms. I won't lose my hair though! I suppose that is a bonus. But will I be cured? Will I see my children grow up; so many scary thoughts crowd into my head, I couldn't concentrate on the doctor's words. I looked at my husband, Dave, he looked close to tears, he looked scared, and that frightened me more than anything. The nurse looked at me and seemed to sense how I felt. She reached out her hand and held mine. I could cry; such a relief.

The doctor chose her words carefully – we 'aim' to cure; not we 'will' cure. That was so telling, I really might die; this might really be it.

Next came my planning appointment – I was placed on a hard X-ray table in a cold open room. The table was raised so high, I couldn't see the people who were doing the measuring and planning of my radiotherapy treatment. They moved me around and made tiny tattoos on my skin to make sure that they treat me in the right place each time.

Another first the radiotherapy – it's a relief, just like an X-ray. The radiographers are professional and kind. The music playing in the background was 'All by myself' – how ironic is that, I plan to take my I-pod next time. Only 24 more treatments to go.

Chemotherapy started the day after radiotherapy. I was even more afraid. My best friend came with me; we were quiet together for the first time ever. Sitting, waiting, not knowing what it might feel like. It felt like any other 'drip', no different, just cold liquid going into my vein. Liquid that would shrink my cancer. Lots of information, lots to remember, pills to take when I got home.

Have got into a pattern of daily radiotherapy, weekly chemotherapy, and the weekends free. It's not too bad really apart from diarrhoea, not being able to eat fruit and veg and the tiredness. I feel very loved, and cared for. So many kind people. The school have been incredible; they have really looked after the girls and made sure that they have someone they can talk to outside of the family. My friends and neighbours have been fantastic. Meals made, rotas to take and collect children from school organised; and the willingness to listen to me whenever I want to talk. I had no idea that people could be this kind. Dave has been incredible – I knew already that he loved me, know I know just how much.

Reflective points

- Consider the woman's experience of cervical screening leading onto investigations and eventually cancer diagnosis.
- Think about the psychological impact on the woman and the effect on sexual function and fertility.

References

Coleman, M.P. et al. (1995) *Cancer Survival Trends in England and Wales, 1971–1995 Deprivation and NHS region.* London: The Stationery Office.

Coleman, M.P. et al. (2004). Trends and socioeconomic inequalities in cancer survival in England and Wales up to 2001. *British Journal of Cancer* **90(7)**, 1367–73.

Ferlay, J. et al. (2004) GLOBOCAN (2002) *Cancer Incidence, Mortality and prevalence Worldwide.* IARC CancerBase No. 5, Version 2.0. Lyon: IARC Press.

Ferreira, C.G. (2008) Erlotinib combined with cisplatin and radiotherapy for patients with locally advanced squamous cell cervical carcinoma: a phase II trial. Presented at ASCO meeting.

Frederick, P.J. and Huh, W.K. (2004) Evaluation of the interim analysis from the PATRICIA study group; efficacy of a vaccine against HPV 16 and 18.

Future II Study Group (2007) Quadrivalent vaccine against human papillomavirus to prevent high-grade cervical lesions. *New England Journal of Medicine* **10,356(19)**, 1915–27.

Future II Study Group (2008) Prophylactic efficacy of a quadrivalent human papillomavirus (HPV) vaccine in women with virological evidence of HPV infection. *Journal of Infectious Diseases* **196(10)**, 1438–46.

Green, J.A., Kirwan, J.J., Tierney, J. et al. (2005) Concomitant chemotherapy and radiation therapy for cancer of the uterine cervix. *Cochrane Database of Systematic Reviews*, Issue 3.

Jackson, S., Murdoch, J., Howe, K., et al. (1997) The management of cervical cancer within the southwest region of England. *British Journal of Obstetrics and Gynaecology* **104**, 140–44.

Landoni, F., Maneo, A., Columbo, A. et al. (1997) Randomised study of radical surgery vs radiotherapy for stage IB–IIA cervical cancer. *Lancet* **350**, 535–40.

Long, H.J., Bundy, B.N., Glendys, E.C. et al. (2005) Randomised phase III trial of cisplatin with or without topotecan in carcinoma of the uterine cervix: a gynaecologic group study. *Journal of Clinical Oncology* **23(21)**, 4626–33.

McFarlane-Anderson, N., Bazuare, P.E., Jackson, M.D. et al. (2008) Cervical dysplasia and cancer and the use of hormonal contraceptives in Jamaican women. *BMC Women's Health* **30(8)**, 9.

Morley, G.W., Hopkins, M.P., Lindenauer, S.M. et al. (1989) Pelvic exenteration, University of Michigan: 100 patients at 5 years. *Obstetrics and Gynaecology* **73**, 34–43.

Nair, M. and Peate, I. (Eds) (2009) *Fundamentals of Applied Pathophysiology: An Essential Guide for Nursing Students*. Chichester: Wiley-Blackwell.

Newton, M. (1975) Radical hysterectomy or radiotherapy for stage I cervical cancer. A prospective comparison with 5 and 10 year follow-up. *American Journal of Obstetrics and Gynecology* **123**, 535–40.

Nobbenhuis, M.A., Walboomers, J.M., Helmerhorst T.J. et al. (1999) Relation of human papilloma-virus status to cervical lesions and consequences for cervical-cancer screening: a prospective study. *Lancet* **354**, 20–5.

Northern Ireland Cancer Registry (2008) *Cancer Registrations in Northern Ireland, 2005.*

Office of National Statistics (2005) *Cancer Statistics registrations: Registrations of Cancer Diagnosed in 2005*, England. Series MB1, No.36.

Office for National Statistics (1999) Cancer 1971–1997. London: Office of National Statistics.

Patrick, J. and Winder, E. (1997) *Cervical Screening: A Practical Guide for Health Authorities*. Publication No. 7. Sheffield: NHSCSP;.

Pellegrino, A., Vizza, E., Fruscio, R. et al. (2009) Total laparoscopic radical hysterectomy and pelvic lymphadenectomy in patients with Ib1 stage cervical cancer: analysis of surgical and oncological outcome. *European Journal of Surgical Oncology* **35(1)**, 98–103.

Ramirez, P.T., Soloman, P.T., Schmeler, K.M. et al. (2008) Laparoscopic and robotic techniques for radical hysterectomy in patients with early stage cervical cancer. *Gynecological Oncology* **3(Suppl 2)**, S21–4.

Robertson, G., Lopes, A., Beynon, G. et al. (1994) Pelvic exenteration: a review of the Gateshead experience 1974–1992. *British Journal of Obstetrics and Gynaecology* **101**, 529–31.

Rose. P.G., Bundy, B.N., Watkins, E.B. et al. (1999) Concurrent cisplatin-based radiotherapy and chemotherapy for locally advanced cervical cancer. *New England Journal of Medicine* **340**, 1144–53.

Scheidler, J., Hricak, H., Yu, K.K. et al. (1997) Radiological evaluation of lymph node metastases in patients with cervical cancer. A meta-analysis. *JAMA* **278**, 1096–101.

Scottish Health Statistics (2008) Scotland: ISD.

Shepherd, J.H., Ngan, H.S., Neven, P. et al. (1994) Multivariate analysis of factors affecting sur-vival in pelvic exenteration. *International Journal of Gynaecological Cancer* **4**, 361–70.

Shepherd, J.J., Peersman, G. and Napuli, I. (1999) Interventions for encouraging sexual lifestyles and behaviours intend to prevent cervical cancer. *Cochrane database of Systematic Reviews 1999*, Issue 4.

Shepherd, J.H., Crawford, R.A.F. and Oram, D.H. (1998) Radical trachelectomy: a way to preserve fertility in the treatment of early cervical cancer. *British Journal of Obstetrics and Gynaecology* **105**, 912–6.

Soisson, A.P., Soper, J.T., Clarke-Pearson, P. et al. (1990) Adjuvant radiotherapy following radical hys-terectomy for patients with stage IB and IIA cervical cancer. *Gynecological Oncology* **37**, 390–5.

Stewart, S.L., Cardinez, C.J. et al. (2008) Surveillance for cancers associated with tobacco use – United States 1999–2004. *MMWR Surveillance Summary 5* **57(8)**, 1–33.

Walboomers, J.M., Jacobs, M.V., Manos, M.M. et al. (1999) Human papillomavirus is a necessary cause of invasive cervical cancer worldwide. *Journal of Pathology* **189**, 12–9.

Welsh Cancer Intelligence and Surveillance Unit (2008) *Cancer Registrations in Wales 2005s.*

Wolfe, C.D., Tilling, K., Bourne, H.M. and Raju, K.S. (1996) Variations in the screening history and appropriateness of management of cervical cancer in South East England. *European Journal of Cancer* **32A**, 1198–204.

Zakashansky, K., Bradley, W.H. and Nezhat, F.R. (2008) New techniques in radical hysterectomy. *Current Opinion in Obstetrics and Gynaecology* **20(1)**, 14–9.

Zereu, M., Zettler, C.G., Cambruzzi, E. and Zelmanowicz, A. (2007) Herpes simplex virus type 2 and Chlamydia trachomatis in adenocarcinoma of the uterine cervix. *Gynecological Oncology* **105(1)**, 172–5.

Chapter 11

Cancer of the Endometrium

Ellen Bull and Robert Woolas

Learning points

At the end of this chapter, the reader will have an understanding of:
- Risk factors, presentation and incidence of endometrial cancer
- The importance of clinical staging and histopathology in determining the treatment plan
- Future therapies

Introduction

Endometrial cancer accounts for the highest proportion of gynaecological malignancies in developed countries (Ferlay et al. 2004; Traina et al. 2004). Also referred to as womb cancer, cancer of the corpus uteri and uterine cancer, this malignancy is the fifth most common amongst the female population in the UK, with 6000 cases diagnosed annually. This accounts for 4% of all female cancers in the UK (Cancer Research UK 2006). Within gynaecological malignancies, endometrial cancer remains second only in incidence to ovarian cancer.

Incidence

Endometrial cancer predominately occurs in post-menopausal women. In 93% of cases, women are over 50 years of age, with the peak incidence being 60–69 years (Cancer Research UK 2006). Rates decline slowly after 70 years of age. However, in 2000, 116 women under 45 years of age developed endometrial cancer (Farthing 2006). Although relatively low in incidence, pre-menopausal occurrence can involve significant morbidity, such as infertility and premature menopause. Overall, this disease carries a 75% cure rate with current therapy. However, there is speculation that future incidence may increase in the elderly as life expectancy increases (Southcott 2001).

Women's Cancers, First Edition. Edited by Alison Keen and Elaine Lennan.
© 2011 Blackwell Publishing Ltd. Published 2011 by Blackwell Publishing Ltd.

Risk factors

Long-term oestrogen exposure is the most common risk for the development of endometrial cancer (Maidens et al. 2005). This may be through physiological means, such as obesity, or synthetic, such as hormone replacement therapy (HRT). Obesity creates an increase in circulating oestrogen leading to an increased risk of endometrial adenocarcinoma (Pavelka et al. 2004). Unopposed oestrogen HRT was a significant aetiological factor, although recent years have seen a universal introduction of combined therapies, which should minimise this risk (Woolas and Oram 1994). Other factors include obesity and associated conditions such as diabetes and hypertension, anovulatory menstrual cycles and tamoxifen usage. Tamoxifen usage is known to stimulate endometrial proliferation, therefore the guidance for women on tamoxifen should be to report any abnormal vaginal bleeding immediately (Maidens et al. 2005). Unopposed oestrogen exposure due to tamoxifen can lead to a variety of factors, including nulliparity, low parity, early menarche, late menopause (after 52 years of age), anovulation and polycystic ovary disease, all of which are related to unopposed oestrogen exposure.

Genetic factors include hereditary non-polyposis colon cancer (HNPCC) syndrome. This should be suspected with early age onset tumours, but fortunately the condition is rare.

Presentation

Abnormal vaginal bleeding is the most common presenting symptom and is easily identified in the post-menopausal woman. In pre-menopausal women there may be persistent bleeding, oligomenorrhea and unusually heavy periods, menometrorrhagia. This can often lead to a diagnostic delay due to the many other causes of these symptoms in younger women.

In post-menopausal women, (defined as a year without a mense), any abnormal bleeding is investigated as a potential malignancy and guidance recommends urgent investigation. However, post-menopausal bleeding (PMB) does not necessarily indicate a malignancy, with only 15% of women presenting with PMB being diagnosed with endometrial cancer (Hacker 2005).

Pathophysiology

Hyperplasia (precursor lesions)

Endometrial hyperplasia is described as an overgrowth of the endometrial lining within the uterus. This is due to prolonged unopposed oestrogen stimulation of the endometrium (Figure 11.1). This histological change is not technically malignant, but is considered at risk of developing into a malignancy and may co-exist adjacent to a malignant area. (Paniscotti, in Moore 1997). Endometrial hyperplasia refers to the histopathological state of the glands and stroma and is categorised as simple, complex and atypical. The progression rate of simple and complex hyperplasia to a malignancy is relatively low, at 1 and 3%

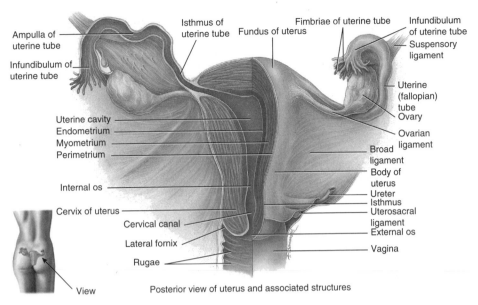

Figure 11.1 Ovaries and uterus with associated structures. From Tortora and Derrickson (2006). Reproduced with permission from John Wiley & Sons, Ltd.

annually, respectively. However, when atypia is also present, the risk of malignancy is significantly more. Progression occurs in 8% with simple atypia and 29% with complex atypia (Paniscotti, in Moore 1997).

Grade and cell type

Histopathological examination of the degree of differentiation and the tumour cell type is very important, as this determines management and likely prognostic outcomes.

Classification of endometrial cancers

- Endometrioid adenocarcinoma
- Mucinous carcinoma
- Serous carcinoma
- Clear cell carcinoma
- Undifferentiated carcinoma
- Squamous cell carcinoma

Endometrioid adenocarcinoma accounts for 85% of all endometrial cancers (Woolas and Oram 1994). The other adenocarcinomas, as listed above, are rarer and all behave slightly differently. Adenocanthomas comprise benign squamous metaplasia and adeno-carcinoma and tend towards being well differentiated. Mucinous carcinoma of the endometrium carries a similar prognosis to endometrioid carcinoma. Adenosquamous lesions contain malignant squamous elements usually poorly differentiated and are associated with extra uterine spread. Serous carcinomas tend to have virulent behaviour and peritoneal surface involvement.

Serous, clear cell and squamous cell and undifferentiated carcinomas all carry poor prognostic outcomes.

However, histological type must be evaluated together with tumour type, degree of myometrial invasion, local extension and extra uterine spread (Woolas and Oram 1994). The first two can be obtained from the pre-operative biopsy specimen and imaging may help identify the other features.

Surgical staging of endometrial cancer was classified in 1988 by the International Federation of Gynaecology and Obstetrics (FIGO) Table 11.1. Surgico-pathological evaluation remains the principle method of establishing the extent of disease. This accounts for the configuration of Table 11.1 and gives a stage of disease from where management is decided and overall prognosis can be assessed.

Table 11.1   FIGO (2009) staging of cancer of the endometrium.

Stage I	Tumour confined to corpus uteri IA – No or less than half myometrial invasion IB – Invasion equal to or more than half the depth of the myometrium
Stage II	Tumour invades cervical stroma, but does not extend beyond the uterus
Stage III	Local and regional spread of the tumour IIIA – Tumour invades the stroma of the corpus uteri and/or adenexae IIIB – Vaginal and/or parametrial involvement IIIC – Metastases to pelvis and/or para-aortic lymph nodes IIIC1 – Positive pelvic nodes IIIC2 – Positive para-aortic lymph nodes with or without positive pelvic lymph nodes
Stage IV	invasion of bladder and/or bowel mucosa and/or distant metastases IVA – Tumour invasion of bowel and/ or bladder mucosa IVB – Distant metastases, including intra-abdominal and/or inguinal lymph nodes

Diagnosis

Most gynaecological hospital departments now have a specialist post-menopausal bleeding service. Clinics such as these perform one-stop ultrasound examination, pipelle biopsies and hysteroscopy providing timely referral and diagnostic pathways. Because of the proximity of the probe to the endometrium, trans-vaginal ultrasound is more accurate than the trans-abdominal route. Most women can tolerate this procedure. The purpose of both approaches is to measure the thickness of the endometrium. Generally an endometrial thickness of 5 mm or less is highly unlikely to be malignant (negative predicative value 99%). If the endometrial thickness is over this, other investigations will be initiated. A pipelle biopsy can be performed in the outpatient clinic if tolerated. This is a small cannula, which passes through the cervix into the endometrium and a random sample of endometrium is aspirated. This is examined for cancer cells or evidence of hyperplasia in the pathology laboratory. The sensitivity of pipelle for the detection of cancer is in the order of 70%.

Therefore, if this is inconclusive, not tolerated or symptoms persist, a further investigation of hysteroscopy (passing a telescope into the uterus often under general anaesthetic) and dilatation and curettage (visually directed biopsy) will be required. This involves sending the endometrial lining to the histopathology laboratory to examine for evidence of cancer.

Once the diagnosis is established, complete assessment for extent of disease is necessary. Recent practice has included an abdominal and pelvic MRI or CT scan to assess for myometrial invasion and lymphadenopathy. Use of MRI in establishing metastatic disease in this cancer remains debatable amongst the gynae-oncology speciality. The American College of Obstetricians and Gynaecologists in 2005 stated MRI and CT were unnecessary, as the surgeon should be prepared to resect macroscopic disease evident at operation.

Staging

Staging for endometrial cancer was updated by FIGO (Table 11.1) from clinical to surgo-pathological in 1988. This included new data affecting prognostic outcomes. The implication is that surgery is necessary to accurately stage an endometrial cancer. Whilst this increased accuracy of staging and subsequent management encourages individualisation of appropriate treatment schedules, it has to be balanced. Highly interventional procedures must be offset with risk of mortality and potential morbidity. Omission of surgical staging risks under- or over-treatment of endometrial cancer patients, and may lead to unnecessary morbidity from external beam radiotherapy and a worse long-term prognosis (Pavelka et al. 2004).

Exceptions for surgical staging include grade 1 endometrioid adenocarcinoma associated with atypical endometrial hyperplasia, because this has a good prognosis regardless, and some women are at increased risk of mortality due to co-morbidity (ACOG 2005). The NHS Cancer Plan (2000) and Clinical Outcome Guidance (policy documents from the UK) have positively impacted on staging and management with sub-specialist surgeons now operating on most patients. Women with endometrial cancer significantly benefit from the multi-disciplinary team (MDT) discussion. This discussion before management and treatment is decided, debates the issues arising from clinical findings, taking into account co-morbidity and psycho-social influences and all the varying nuances of an individual's case.

In summary, pre-, peri- and post-operative evaluation is mandatory for safe and effective management.

Pre-operative factors

The histological subtypes described have a clear influence on prognosis. Thus, pathological analysis can further determine nuances to treatment to optimize both morbidity and survival.

Grade

Histological differentiation is an important factor in prognosis. Cells are usually graded in four categories, well differentiated, moderately and poorly differentiated and undifferentiated. Well differentiated, a mutated cell that still has features identifiable as to its origin, generally carries a better prognosis than moderately or poorly differentiated tumours. In addition, undifferentiated, being unidentifiable in origin, carries a poor prognosis due to the multiple mutation of the cancer cell.

Performance status

Endometrial cancer occurs predominantly in the elderly age group and has epidemiological predispositions to co-morbid conditions that preclude extensive surgical endeavour. High risk disease often occurs in the elderly who may have other co-morbidities or lower performance status that make it more difficult to tolerate adjuvant treatment (i.e. chemotherapy or radiotherapy).

Post surgical features

Myometrial Invasion

The myometrium is the muscle layer of the uterus. If the cancer has spread halfway or more through this layer, there is a significant risk of the cancer having escaped the uterus. Myometrial invasion is one of the biggest indictors of prognosis in endometrial cancer. The degree of myometrial invasion is an essential aspect of the histological report and is influential in the prescription of post-operative radiotherapy.

Cervical invasion

The cancer in the uterus is examined to determine any spread into or near the cervix uteri. If the cervix has evidence of spread, this will be discussed at the MDT. Other indicative factors will determine treatment overall, but in isolation, this may mean adjuvant brachytherapy (internal radiotherapy treatment).

Peritoneal cytology

Cytological inspection of the fluid sluiced around the peritoneal area intra-operatively is performed to check for evidence of stray cancer cells. Cancer cells detected in the washings (fluid used to irrigate the pelvic cavity at the outset of surgery) indicate metastatic spread outside the uterus. This immediately upgrades the cancer to IIIA. However, in the absence of other metastatic spread, the potential for adjuvant treatment for women with positive cytology is discussed in the MDT environment and further discussed in the outpatient setting with the patient.

Prognostic factors in endometrial cancer

- Age
- Differentiation
- Uterine Size
- Histopathological subtype
- Ploidy
- Pre operative serum Ca 125 level
- Myometrial Invasion
- Lymphovascular space involvement
- Oestrogen and progesterone receptor
- Her2 neu status
- Cervical involvement
- Peritoneal cytology
- Lymph node metastasis
- Pelvic or distant metastasis (Woolas and Oram 1994, updated 2010)

Lymph nodes

Positive pelvic lymph nodes are associated with a 45% 5-year survival (Woolas and Oram 1994). Positive para aortic nodes are indicative of high chance of metastatic spread into the pelvic-nodal chain, adnexal disease and outer third of myometrium invasion (Woolas and Oram 1994). Retroperitoneal lymph node assessment is a critical component of surgical staging associated with increased survival (ACOG 2005). Sixty-two percent of women with positive pelvic lymph nodes have para aortic metastasis and 17% of high risk cases have para-aortic metastasis alone (Creaseman et al. 1987).

Surgical treatment

Approximately 55% of patients with endometrial cancer will have surgical intervention at some point of their trajectory (Groenwald 1997; Nattress and Lancaster 2005). Surgery remains the mainstay of curative treatment for this cancer type. Once the likelihood of endometrial cancer is established, the necessary investigations are completed, and a staging MRI-CT will obtain an indication of nodal status. A discussion will ensue to decide on the appropriate treatment. In many cases, a laparotomy, total abdominal hysterectomy, bilateral salpingoopherectomy and lymph node dissection are conducted. However, just as obesity is a risk factor for this disease, it is also a risk factor for surgical morbidity. Pavelka et al. (2004) report morbidly obese women were less likely to undergo lymph node evaluation than ideal body weight women. Multiple factors were given to explain this, a more favourable stage and histology in obese women and increased technical difficulty in the obese population. Pavelka et al. further clarified that obese women were more likely to have a lower grade histology than ideal weight women.

Pelvic surgery in the obese population can be challenging, requiring more operative time and resulting in increased blood loss, although other intra-operative complications were not significantly increased when compared to ideal body weight counterparts (Pavelka et al. 2004).

A randomised controlled trial has been performed by the Medical Research Council (MRC) to assess the impact of removing lymph nodes. Outcome data suggested that the removal of lymph nodes as a standard procedure was not beneficial to the prognosis. However, appropriate and complete surgical staging can spare the patient unnecessary exposure to radiotherapy.

Frozen section has been evaluated in peri-operative surgical decision-making, although it may not be accurate at predicting deep myometrial invasion or other poor prognostic features in a minority of patients (Pavelka et al. 2004).

Fertility-sparing options (see also Chapter 14 on "Fertility")

Fertility preservation techniques in gynaecological cancer have become an increasing issue in recent years. Societal changes have led to later childbearing. A cancer diagnosis in childbearing years brings the added complicated dimension of fertility preservation in addition to offering optimal prognosis and cure. Selection invariably relies on meticulous staging and early stage disease. This is most often seen in cervical cancer. In endometrial cancer, this is relatively new ground. Initially a firm diagnosis must be established. A young woman with complex atypical hyperplasia will face difficult decision-making. Hysterectomies performed for complex atypical hyperplasia will confirm invasive disease in approximately 30% of cases (Farthing 2006). Therefore fertility preservation in this scenario carries a risk of future malignancy. MRI imaging can be employed to further determine myometrial invasion but detection rates stand at 90% (Farthing 2006), leaving an uncomfortable feeling of doubt. Endometrial cancer in a young woman can also mean a more aggressive disease, or a genetic aetiology such as HNPCC. Early stage IA disease responds successfully to hormonal treatment and it is possible to consider the use of progestin in well-differentiated stage IA disease. This treatment alone will not have long-term implications for fertility. Evidence for treatment efficacy exists but is limited (Imai et al. 2001). However, the option and risks must be emphasised to women who want to consider fertility sparing options. Morice et al. (2005) describe two cases of carefully selected patients with early stage disease for fertility preservation. In this scenario, the surgical implications are precise histopathological evaluation of all extra-uterine disease, including peritoneal washings. The ovaries were preserved and chemotherapy and brachytherapy employed, respectively. Both patients were disease free. The authors conclude conservative management can be possible with careful evaluation of disease status using a laparoscopic approach, which also reduces adhesions and potentiates future fertility.

Adjuvant treatment

The MDT will discuss the surgical specimen analysed by the histopathologist and the washings analysed by the cytologist. This evidence will determine the stage of cancer. This, in conjunction with the performance status, leads to a management plan, of either further adjuvant treatment, i.e. radiotherapy and/or chemotherapy, or follow-up alone. What is discussed and decided here is then discussed with the woman in the clinic and can usually occur within two weeks of surgery. This is obviously a very anxious time, as results are awaited to confirm diagnosis and prognosis. This discussion, especially if adjuvant treatment is required, should be held with the gynaecological oncologist and the clinical nurse specialist together.

The concept of adjuvant treatment should have been discussed as a possibility before surgery. The degree of likelihood can be discussed according to the clinical evidence available before surgery. Psychological preparation for pending adjuvant treatment is important to allay distress, and maintains trust in the professional-patient relationship.

Radiotherapy can be used as adjuvant treatment, to optimise cure, or to palliate in advanced or recurrent disease. Administered to the whole pelvis, abdomen and/or intravaginally, radiotherapy treatment may cause significant morbidity. Varying symptoms occur according to the area being treated. In the pelvis this includes sore skin, diarrhoea and fatigue in the short term, and vaginal stenosis, infertility, and menopause in the long term. External beam radiotherapy has traditionally been used where evidence of likely metastases exists. However, to date there is still no conclusive evidence that this is beneficial to survival. The PORTEC and ASTEC trials appear to support this conclusion. Local recurrence is most likely to occur in the vaginal vault area; hence the intravaginal radiotherapy is specifically administered to this high risk area.

Cytotoxic chemotherapy

Chemotherapy for endometrial cancer was traditionally given for palliative intent and control of symptoms. Accrued survival data for women with endometrial cancer suggests that 30% of patients actually have advanced disease (stages IIIC or IV). These individuals are clearly candidates for systemic treatment. However, advanced age is interrelated to the presence of adverse pathological features at the time of diagnosis and this in turn mitigates against the use of toxic therapies due to the concurrent co-morbidities of the individuals concerned. Furthermore, although the light microscopic features of endometrial tumours are not dissimilar to those of their ovarian counterparts, the sensitivity to established chemotherapeutic regimens appears less than that of ovarian cancer. The situation is further compounded by the relative infrequency with which the problem arises amongst women who are fit to consider cytotoxic chemotherapy. This requires multicentre evaluation to reach meaningful conclusions.

The best expected results with current cytotoxic chemotherapy are a median progression-free survival of 9 months and an average median survival of less then 1 year (Elit and Hirte 2002). In recent years, the role of chemotherapy used mainly in the adjuvant setting in endometrial cancer has widened, in part due to enhanced staging of extra pelvic disease. The use of Carboplatin and Paclitaxel for more advanced disease administered prior to radiotherapy in primary treatment scenarios has become more commonplace. The addition of drugs such as epirubicin to this regimen for sub-types such as clear cell can enhance 5-year survival.

The use of Topotecan in endometrial cancer is being evaluated, with weekly topotecan having anti-tumour activity in some small research samples (Triana et al. 2004). More research in this area is required.

Endocrine therapy

The relationship between oestrogen and the genesis of endometrial cancer, in particular the endometrioid subtype, has long been established. As with breast cancer, this leads to the possibility that endocrine manipulation therapy may have a role in influencing prognosis. Most well differentiated endometrial tumours will express high concentrations of oestrogen and progesterone receptors and anecdotal evidence suggests the possibility of treating measurable metastatic deposits with high dose progesterone and obtaining significant remissions. However, these are exactly the least likely tumours to metastasise and recur and therefore the majority of fatal cases are endocrine receptor negative. Nevertheless, the low toxicity profile of endocrine treatment means that it should be considered for all cases of known metastatic or recurrent disease and measurement of the receptor status via immunocytochemistry on the histopathology specimen is now widespread. An empirical prescription carries the risk of some morbidity through fluid retention and cardiovascular problems, but is significantly less than the application of cytotoxic chemotherapy to these individuals (Woolas et al. 1993).

The use of local delivery of progesterone has also been considered in women who are unfit to undergo hysterectomy (Dhar et al. 2005; Nattress and Lancaster 2005). This appears to have a holding action on some tumours, perhaps allowing women to be medically optimised for surgery without detriment to progression of their disease.

Novel therapeutic agents

'Targeted' therapy is the term applied to those agents that have been developed in response to the increasing knowledge of molecular biology. They are designed to address particular molecular targets within the cell that are known to be involved in the cellular mechanisms that support cancer progression (Gemill and Idell 2003). Cancer is a genetic disease, and the cell receives instruction regarding cell division or protein synthesis from extra-cellular messengers such as cytokines. The process by which cells transmit the information through the cell to the DNA is known as signal transduction. Many of the newest agents have some aspect of signal transduction as their target. Targets may include the growth factor receptors on the cell membrane. Others are protein kinase inhibitors and therefore target protein synthesis pathways. Other agents are those termed 'gene therapy', where a section of DNA from a virus is used as a vector to insert codons beside known oncogenes or active portions of the DNA in an attempt to switch the production of certain proteins off. If a tumour suppressor gene is absent from a cell, gene therapy may be a consideration to introduce the gene into the cellular genetic material to switch on production.

Many of these newer agents are monoclonal antibodies, where the monoclonal antibody is the mode by which the receptor is accessed on the cell membrane. It is generally known that tumours require a blood supply for continued growth – the molecular process of angiogenesis. If drugs can be developed to block the production of the capillaries in tumours, disease progression can theoretically be halted. This is the basis for a new range of drugs attacking cellular receptors such as vascular endothelial receptor or anti-

VeGF. The emerging discoveries of the role of matrix metalloproteinases is a further example where drugs are being developed to interfere with a known cellular process involved in metastatic development. Increasing knowledge of the role of cytokines in tumour promotion and progression has meant the introduction of drugs such as interferon and interleukin.

Positive experience with these agents in other tumours may yet be extrapolated to enhance survival prospects for women.

Follow-up

Follow-up for cancer remains relatively set in a pattern of 3-monthly for 2 years, tailing down to 4- and 6-monthly, then annually with discharge at 5 years. This differs between centres. It is not necessary to perform vaginal vault smears, as the evidence base for this endeavour is scanty but it has been shown that vaginal vault smears to evaluate recurrent endometrial tumour are not helpful and can be confusing in their interpretation amongst those women who have undergone pelvic radiotherapy.

Recurrent disease

Endometrial cancer overall has an excellent 70% 5-year survival rate. Local recurrence in the upper vagina can be successfully treated with intracavity radiotherapy if not given previously, and surgical options can be discussed if disease is found to be local after CT and MRI scans. However, if extra pelvic disease is found, the only option is to control it systemically with chemotherapy. However, regimens are toxic and the benefit vs treatment toxicity must be discussed at the MDT and with the patient. Relief of symptoms and psycho-social support remains a priority in recurrent disease.

Life after treatment

In recent years, as treatment efficacy improved, one could argue that cancer, for some, is a chronic illness as opposed to a life threatening disease. Although cure remains a primary focus (Quigley 1989), quality of life issues have come to the forefront. Cancer management is constantly reviewed, but always in terms of treatment. It has only been relatively recently that consequences of survival have become an area to consider. Surviving malignancy is not an easy task for many, as the same level of support, teaching and rehabilitation that was offered earlier in the illness often reduces (Mcaffery 1991). If health professionals understand a women's experience of endometrial cancer following surgery, effective supportive strategies in the rehabilitation phase can be planned.

The limited quantity of morbidity research in gynaecological malignancies has been highlighted in many studies (Lamb 1985; Gamel et al. 2000), who focus on sexuality. Auchincloss (1995) discusses other issues for gynaecological cancer survivors, mortality issues, and self-perception, aging, menopause and fertility and relationship issues.

Conclusion

Endometrial cancer is a disease that affects the population of older women with significant co-morbidities, which have consequent impact on our ability to develop more effective strategies for curative treatment. The great majority of patients present with post-menopausal bleeding and are therefore diagnosed early. Many will be cured by simple hysterectomy and bilateral salpingo-oophorectomy alone.

The application of adjuvant therapy has been traditional rather than evidence based and is currently under scrutiny in terms of both its morbidity and equivocal impact on survival. Quality of life for women with this disease remains a woefully under-investigated area, as the majority will be long-term survivors.

The condition is prevalent amongst elderly women and those with a Western lifestyle and therefore we can expect these problems to magnify in coming decades.

Endometrial cancer: the patient's perspective

This narrative and the following poem were written by a woman who had been treated for endometrial cancer.

I don't consciously dwell on having had cancer or the hysterectomy or the internal radiotherapy. However, I cannot deny, nor do I try to, that all of that is now an integral part of my life. As such, I am aware (and have been for some time) that underlying all my being there are now two main themes: first of all, heartfelt gratitude both because the cancer was caught in time (as far as we know) and also for the caring nurses who make such a difference to patients and, secondly, terror that the cancer might someday reappear to the detriment of my life and that of those around me.

Once having experienced that awful moment of finding out I had cancer, I can never forget the feelings that went with it. Yes, I heard the consultant telling me that I was lucky in that the cancer was early and that it could probably be removed once and for all. Rationally, I accepted everything he was saying. I knew it to be true. But at the same time, my internal emotion was screaming, 'I'm going to die ... now, soon. Peter will be left without me. He'll be bereft.' I was in emotional shock for a long time ... maybe even now, some 17 months since I first heard the diagnosis. I was so afraid.

But now, to balance things with equal intensity, I always have the thought that 'I'm alive!' ... and, believe me, that always brings up a well of emotion, the stark reality of life vs death. It has helped me put a lot of things into perspective. I really value now what I thought I had lost forever. No doubt having (over)emotional patients makes doctors and consultants somewhat uncomfortable. However, to the patient, it's a uniquely personal thing – the patient has experienced thoughts of their own life vs their own death in an intimately personal way. It would be helpful if the doctors and consultants better understood the power of the emotion that the patient may still carry with them, no matter how long ago the diagnosis/operation took place. Personally, I don't think it is something I want to lose. It makes me a better, more caring person myself. (Anon)

The Check-up

He said don't be so emotional,
Learn to toe the middle line,
He'd had a look as usual,
And everything was fine.

How could he know the thoughts I had,
Of when the cancer came,
And now how glad I was to know,
It would … probably … stay away.

To him one of many,
To me only ever one,
That gap between life and death,
Lived again and again and again.

So tears trickled out,
As I found myself reliving,
Moments when I thought I'd die,
And kindnesses and thanksgiving.

He's uncomfortable, that much I see,
But doesn't he know it's now all part of me?
Don't be afraid, just let me get it out,
These emotions are valid I almost hear myself shout.

Without the feelings remembered from before,
There'd be less of a person … a smaller inner core.
And so, for that reason, I won't let them go,
These heights and these depths that affected me so.

And just when I wonder if I'm out of step,
The nurse leans over and I hear her say,
A comment of feeling and caring support,
She understands, now I'll go away …
Reaffirmed.

(Anon)

A woman's feelings when diagnosed with endometrial cancer.

Reflective points

- As the use of adjuvant radiotherapy in many cases is based on tradition rather than evidence, how would you assist patients in making an informed decision?
- In your area of practice, are there services available to support patients (particularly the elderly) to be discharged safely into their home following major surgery for endometrial cancer?
- What should be the follow-up plan for this group of patients?

References

American College of Obstetricians and Gynaecologists (ACOG) 2005 Management of Endometrial Cancer. ACOG Bulletin No. 65. *Obstetrics and Gynaecology* **106**, 413–25.

Auchincloss, A. (1995) After Treatment psychosocial issues in gynaecologic cancer survivorship. *Cancer* **(Suppl Nov 15), 76(10)**, 2117–24.

Cancer Research UK (2006) http://info.cancerreserchuk.org/cancerstats/types/uterus/incidence 1–6

Creaseman, W.T., Morrow, C.P., Bundy, B.N., Homesly, H.D., Graham, .J.E. and Heller, P.B. (1987) Surgical pathologic spread patterns of endometrial cancer. A Gynaecologic Oncology Group Study. *Cancer* **60(Suppl 8)**, 203–41. (level 1–2).

Dhar, K.K., Needihan, T., Koslowski, M. and Woolas, R. (2005) Is levonorgestrel intrauterine system effective for treatment of early endometrial cancer? Report of four cases and review of the literature. Gynecologic Oncology **97**, 924–7.

Elit, L. and Hirte, H. (2002) Current status and future innovations of hormonal agents, chemotherapy and investigation agents in endometrial cancer. *Current Opinion in Obstetric and Gynaecology* **14**, 67–73.

Farthing, A. (2006) Conserving fertility in the management of gynaecological cancers. *British Journal of Obstetrics and Gynaecologists.* **113**, 129–34.

Ferlay, J., Bray, F., Pisani, P. and Parkin, D.M. (2004) GLOBOCAN 2002: *Cancer Incidence, Mortality and Prevalence Worldwide*. Lyon: IARC Press.

Gemill, R. and Idell, C.S. (2003) Biological advances for new treatment approaches. *Seminars in Oncology Nursing* **19(3)**, 162–8.

Gamel, C., Hengeveld, M. and Davis, B. (2000) Informational needs about the effects of gynaecological cancer on sexuality; a review of the literature. *Journal of Clinical Nursing* **99**, 678–88.

Groenwald, S.L., Hansen Frogge, M., Goodman, M.and Henke Yarbro, C. (1997) *Cancer Nursing Principles and Practice.*, 4th edn. Boston MA: Jones and Bartlett.

Hacker, N.F. (2005) Uterine cancer In: J.S. Berek and N.F. Hacker (Eds) *Practical Gynecologic Oncology* 4th edn. Philadelphia: Lippincott Williams & Wilkins.

Imai, M., Jobo, T., Sato, R., Kawaguchi, M. and Kuramoto, H. (2001) Medroxyprogesterone acetate therapy for patients with adenocarcinoma of the endometrium who wish to preserve the uterus – usefulness and limitations. *European Journal of Gynaecological Oncology.* **XXII(3)**, 217–20.

Lamb, M. (1985) Sexual dysfunction in the gynaecologic oncology patient. *Seminars in Oncology Nursing* **1(1)**, 9–17.

Maidens, J., Natress, K. and Lancaster, T. (2005) Gynaecological Cancer Care. *A Guide to Practice*. Melbourne: Ausmed Publications.

Morice, P., Fourchette, V., Sideris, L., Gariel, C., Duvillard, P. and Castaigne, D. (2005) A need for laparoscopic evaluation of patients with endometrial carcinoma selected for conservative treatment. *Gynecologic Oncology* **96**, 245–8.

Moore, G.J. (1997) *Women and Cancer. A gynaecological oncology nursing perspective*, 1st edn. Boston MA: Jones and Bartlett.

Nattress, K. and Lancaster, T. (2005) *Gynaecological Cancer Care. A guide to practice*. Melbourne: Ausmed publications.

Panniscotti (1997) *Women and Cancer. A Gynecologic Nursing Perspective*. (G.J. Moore (Ed.). Boston MA: Jones and Bartlett.

Pavelka, J.C., Ben-Shachar, I., Fowler, J.M. et al. (2004) Morbid obesity and endometrial cancer: surgical, clinical and pathologic outcomes in surgically managed patients. *Gynecologic Oncology* **95**, 588–92.

Quigley, K.M. (1989) The adult cancer survivor: psychosocial consequences of cure. *Seminars in Oncology Nursing* **5(1)**, 63–9.

Southcott, B.M. (2001) Carcinoma of the endometrium. *Drugs* **61(10)**, 1395–405.

Tortora, G. and Derrickson, B. (2006) *Principles of Anatomy and Physiology*, 11th edn. Chichester: Wiley-Blackwell.

Triana, T., Sabbatini, P., Aghajanian, C. and Dupont, J. (2004) Weekly topotecan for recurrent endometrial cancer: a case series and review of literature. *Gynecologic Oncology* **95**, 235–41.

Woolas, R., Hammond, I.G. and McCartney, A.J. (1993) Endometrial Cancer before age 35 and subsequent use of hormone replacement therapy Journal of *Obstetrics and gynaecology* **13**, 468–70.

Woolas, R. and Oram, D. (1994) *Management of Endometrial Cancer*. The Yearbook of the Royal College of Obstetricians and Gynaecologists.

Chapter 12

Cancer of the Vagina

Sandra Tinkler

Learning points

At the end of this chapter the reader will have an understanding of:
- Incidence and aetiology of vaginal cancers
- Staging and clinical presentation
- Treatment options including prognosis

Introduction

Vaginal neoplasms are very uncommon and over 80% are secondary. Metastatic spread occurs either from direct extension of adjacent organs or from distant sites through the lymphatic system or bloodstream. Primary vaginal cancers account for only 2% of all female genital malignancies and squamous cell carcinoma is the commonest histology type.

The most common clinical presentation is with abnormal vaginal bleeding, but pain and a palpable mass can also occur. Most patients with clinical symptoms have locally advanced disease. Around 20% of patients are asymptomatic and present with an abnormal Papanicolaou test (PAP) smear.

Treatment of vaginal cancers is based on clinical stage, tumour size and location, and any prior therapies. Management options include surgical excision (± reconstructive surgery); radiotherapy (brachytherapy, external beam therapy or both) with or without concomitant chemotherapy; or a combination of surgery and radiotherapy.

Prognosis for early stage vaginal cancers is relatively good, with a 75% 5-year survival for stage I disease. However, it is poor for advanced tumours, with less than 20% of patients with stage IV disease surviving 5 years. With improvements in treatment techniques, including technological advances allowing more targeted radiotherapy and the addition of concomitant cisplatin chemotherapy, it may be possible to improve the outcome for patients with locally advanced disease.

Women's Cancers, First Edition. Edited by Alison Keen and Elaine Lennan.
© 2011 Blackwell Publishing Ltd. Published 2011 by Blackwell Publishing Ltd.

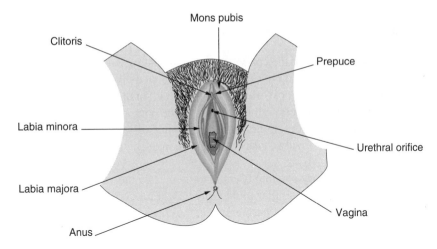

Figure 12.1 Female external genitalia. From Nair and Peate (2009). Reproduced with permission from John Wiley & Sons Ltd.

Figure 12.1 shows the female external genitalia.

Vaginal malignancies are rare and approximately 80% of these are metastatic from other sites. Primary vaginal cancers account for only 1–3% of female genital neoplasms (Percorelli 2003; Hellman et al. 2004).

Aetiology and pathology

Pre-invasive lesions (VAIN) (vaginal intraepithelial neoplasia)

Carcinoma *in situ* of the vagina (VAIN) occurs much less commonly than a similar entity in the cervix or vulva. Vaginal carcinoma *in situ* can progress to invasive disease in a similar way to that occurring in the cervix or vulva. It is most common in the upper third of the vagina. Around 50–75% of patients with VAIN have a history of cervical (CIN) or vulval (VIN) intraepithelial neoplasia, which may have been present many years earlier. An abnormal PAP smear is usually the first indication of VAIN.

Invasive cancers

Metastatic tumours

The most common primary sites include endometrium, cervix, bowel or bladder. If a tumour involves both the cervix and vagina, then it is classified as cervical tumour with vaginal extension. To be classified as a primary vaginal tumour, the cervix needs to be uninvolved or absent. An isolated vault recurrence after hysterectomy for endometrial cancer is one of the more common occurrences and can be potentially curable with radiotherapy. Treatment is otherwise that of the primary tumour.

Primary vaginal cancers

Squamous cell carcinomas are the commonest histological variant and have a mean age of onset at 60–65 years. The pattern of spread is dependant on the location of the tumour within the vagina. They occur most often in the upper third of the vagina when the pattern of spread is similar to that of cervical cancer, i.e. to the obturator and iliac lymph nodes and then to the para-aortic nodes. If the tumour occurs in the lower vagina, then its pattern of spread is similar to that of vulval cancers, i.e. to the inguinal nodes and then to the deep pelvic nodes.

The aetiology of primary squamous cell carcinomas of the vagina is poorly documented, but is thought to be similar to that of cervical cancers including early age at first intercourse, multiple sexual partners and smoking (Daling et al. 2002) There is also a strong link with Human Papilloma Virus (HPV), as in carcinoma of the cervix.

Other less common histological variants include melanoma and adenocarcinoma. The latter is rare but important because of its link with *in-utero* exposure to diethylstilboestrol and its presentation in young women. The former is important, as it is often relatively unresponsive to radiotherapy and is therefore best treated with surgery.

Staging

Gynaecological malignancies are often staged using the FIGO classification but the TNM staging system, although less used in the UK, is an acceptable alternative (Table 12.1).

Table 12.1

TNM	Vagina	FIGO
T1	confined to vaginal wall	I
T2	extension to paravaginal tissues	II
T3	extension to pelvic side wall	III
T4	involvement of bladder or rectum, extension beyond the pelvis	IVA
N1	regional lymph node metastases	–
M1	distant metastases	IVB

In addition to a clinical examination (usually under anaesthesia), radiological investigations are used to stage the patient and to determine the most appropriate treatment. A CT scan of the abdomen, pelvis and usually the chest is done to assess local involvement and distant metastases. An MRI scan of the pelvis is often also done, as it can provide more detailed information on the primary tumour and is especially helpful if surgery is being considered. A tissue diagnosis is essential before radiotherapy, chemotherapy or radical surgery is undertaken.

Pre-diagnosis

Women who have pre-invasive disease are usually asymptomatic and VAIN is identified by an abnormal PAP smear.

Abnormal vaginal bleeding is the most common presenting symptom of invasive vaginal cancer, usually post-menopausal bleeding. If the woman is pre-menopausal then inter-menstrual or post-coital bleeding may be the first symptom. Unfortunately this symptom is often associated with a locally advanced lesion. A vaginal discharge can be an earlier symptom and it may or may not be bloody. However, even with this non-specific symptom, an identifiable lesion can usually be seen.

Urinary symptoms such as frequency, dysuria and haematuria are more likely with tumours arising from the anterior vaginal wall. They are, however, common symptoms in women generally, especially after the menopause. They are often due to a urinary tract infection. Vaginal cancer would be a rare diagnosis in a woman who presented to her GP with these symptoms. However, persistent or recurrent urinary symptoms should always be investigated further if they fail to settle with conventional treatments such as antibiotics. Urinary retention is rare in women due to a short urethra, and if present should always initiate further investigations as there could be a serious underlying cause. It would be an indication of a locally advanced tumour if due to vaginal cancer.

Rectal symptoms, for example bleeding or discharge are much less common but could occur with a tumour arising or involving the posterior vaginal wall. Again, vaginal cancer would be a very rare cause of these symptoms.

Management

All patients should be under the care of a multidisciplinary team involved in the treatment of gynaecological malignancies. The team would include a gynaecologist specialising in malignancies, an oncologist(s) (specialising irradiation and chemotherapy), a specialist radiologist, and a clinical nurse specialist. Treatment is dependant on the stage and location of the tumour, in addition to any associated conditions. However, vaginal cancer is rare and therefore treatment needs to be individualised. That said, there are some generalisations and guidelines that can be formulated. The first is that radiotherapy is the mainstay for treatment of vaginal cancer, except for very early small tumours.

Stage 0/VAIN

The treatment of choice for these pre-invasive tumours is surgical excision.

Stage I / II

Small superficial tumours (<5 mm)

Treatment choices include surgery (the preferred option, if possible), intracavity radiotherapy or interstitial radiotherapy. Intracavity radiotherapy is the insertion of a radiation sources into a body cavity, in this case the vagina. Interstitial radiotherapy is the introduction of a radioactive source directly into the tumour/tissues using needles or wires. Both of these radiotherapy techniques apply a concentrated high dose of radiation to a small area, thereby maximising the dose to the tumour and minimising the toxicity of treatment.

Upper 2/3 tumours

If the tumour is small, then surgical excision ± reconstruction may be an option if technically feasible. However, this is often not possible and radiotherapy is the mainstay of treatment for these tumours. The lymphatic drainage and spread of upper vaginal tumours is similar to that of cervical tumours and therefore their treatment with radiotherapy is also similar.

Radiotherapy is given in two parts. The first is external beam therapy using a linear accelerator. This allows treatment of the primary vaginal tumour and the pelvic lymph nodes together. The pelvic lymph nodes are treated prophylactically, even if they are not enlarged on imaging, because of the risk of microscopic spread. A total dose of between 45 and 50.4 Gy in 25 to 28 daily fractions is commonly used. This part of the treatment therefore takes 5–6 weeks to complete, usually as an outpatient travelling daily to the radiotherapy department. Four radiation fields are usually used to concentrate the highest radiation dose in the middle, creating a square or rectangular 'box' of high dose. Modern radiotherapy techniques allow a more precise tailoring of the volume of the dose for the patient to be treated by using irregular shaped fields, thereby shielding out normal areas at the edges.

The second phase of the treatment is determined by the size and position of the remaining tumour and the anatomy of the patient. The most effective treatment is with brachytherapy if technically possible, as this allows the radiation dose to the tumour to be maximised by using a localised high dose, thereby limiting the toxicity to the surrounding normal structures. This technique is only possible with relatively small tumours. Therefore, a substantial reduction in size of the larger tumours is necessary by the end of the external beam therapy, if this technique is to be successfully used. It is also very dependant on the anatomy of the patient, including whether or not she still has her uterus, as well as the position and accessibility of the tumour. A total tumour dose of around 75 Gy or more can be achieved using this technique.

Use of intracavity brachytherapy (radiation therapy in which a cylindrical container holding a radioactive substance is placed into the vagina for a prescribed length of time) would usually only be of therapeutic value if there was only minimal residual tumour at the end of external beam radiotherapy, as the high dose treatment zone only extends to about 5 mm beneath the vaginal mucosal surface. Where there is a larger tumour at the vaginal vault, in a patient who still has an intact uterus, use of an intra-uterine tube as well vaginal sources may increase the high dose volume sufficiently to be able to adequately treat the residual disease.

It is possible in some patients to boost the tumour dose using a radioactive implant. This would allow a higher dose at greater depth beneath the surface and could therefore treat thicker tumours. Accessibility in the confined space of the vagina can be the greatest challenge and is easiest the lower down the vagina the tumour is located.

If brachytherapy is not possible, then a conformal boost using external beam radiation is used. This involves treating only the tumour with a very small margin (usually ~1 cm) and taking the radiation dose up to around 65 Gy, or more if possible. The dose limiting structure is the rectum, part of which is usually within the high dose volume due to its proximity to the vagina (being separated only by millimetres). A maximum of 65 Gy in total to this structure is usually set to limit long-term morbidity. Therefore, the total dose of radiation to the tumour using this technique is usually less than can be achieved using brachytherapy.

The higher the radiation dose the greater the chance of eradicating the tumour, but the greater the risks of long-term damage to the surrounding normal structures. If the total dose of radiation is lowered, the risk of later side effects on the normal tissues is lowered, but also so is the chance of cure of the tumour. There is no 'cut off' whereby below a certain dose of radiation no toxicity is seen and above which all tumours are cured. Consequently, we choose an 'optimal' dose where the cure rates and toxicity are both acceptable. We therefore know that about 5–10% of patients will get moderate or severe late toxicity.

The early/acute side effects of radiotherapy to this area include tiredness, diarrhoea, cystitis and perineal skin redness or breakdown. Side effects usually start about 2 weeks into a radiation course and peak around week 4. They stay at this level until treatment is finished and then gradually settle down. The long-term/late side effects of radiotherapy to the pelvis include bowel damage, bladder damage, vaginal dryness and stenosis (narrowing of the vagina). This treatment will also induce a premature menopause and infertility in younger patients. There is also a very high incidence of psycho-sexual dysfunction, as well as the physical issues of vaginal dryness and stenosis.

Lower one-third tumours

The lymphatic drainage of the lower vagina is similar to that of the vulva, going first to the inguinal nodes and then the deep pelvic nodes. The mainstay of treatment for these tumours is also radiotherapy, but the location of the beams needs to include the inguinal nodes. This entails a rather large radiation field and usually opposed anterior and posterior fields are used with shielding at the edges if possible. The lower deep pelvic lymph nodes are routinely included, but not the higher pelvic nodes, as the area treated would be too great. A dose of around 45 Gy in 25 fractions is commonly used, with a boost to the tumour either with an implant or a conformal boost as above.

The side effects of this treatment are similar to above but the perineal skin reaction is almost inevitable and more severe. Bladder and/or urethral irritation are also more likely. Some patients may need strong analgesics to get them through the latter part of the course of radiation. Sometimes hospital admission is needed for symptom control.

Concomitant chemotherapy

The use of chemotherapy during external beam radiotherapy is now extensively used in cervical cancers as well as those tumours arising elsewhere in the body, for example head and neck, oesophagus, anus, etc. Its use has not been explored in randomised clinical trials in vaginal cancer, as this is a very rare tumour and there would be insufficient patients with the condition to derive meaningful data in a reasonable timeframe. On the basis of evidence from other tumour sites, especially cervical cancer, its use has 'evolved' to include vaginal cancers.

The commonest regimen used is weekly cisplatin chemotherapy at a dose of $40\,mg/m^2$ (max 70 mg). It is most often given before that day's radiation treatment and thereby acts as a radiation sensitiser as well as a chemotherapeutic agent. Radiation sensitisers are drugs which, when given before a fraction of radiation, increase the effects of the radiation. If it is given after a fraction of radiation, this effect is not seen. These drugs are often but not always chemotherapeutic agents, and the dose needed as a radiation sensitiser is usually much less than that needed to produce active chemotherapeutic effects.

Concomitant chemotherapy is known to increase the acute toxicity of radiation, and this has been well documented in many tumour sites. Studies on the late toxicity of this combined treatment, for example in patients with cervical cancers, have not shown an increase in adverse late side effects. However, these late effects are poorly documented, as the information is harder to retrieve months or years after the treatment has taken place. The increased effectiveness of concomitant chemo-radiotherapy evident in long-term control of many tumour sites has been shown in many studies. However, that this is achieved without a similar increase in late toxicity has not yet been conclusively demonstrated. Nevertheless, this combined management is now well established in many tumour sites and is widely considered to be the 'gold standard' of treatment.

Stage III / IVA

Treatment for patients with these advanced stage tumours is similar to that described above, with radiation as the primary modality. As the tumour is more advanced, the volume to be treated will be larger and the side effects potentially more likely and possibly more severe. If there is evidence of bowel or bladder involvement, then there is a risk of a fistula forming between the vagina and bowel or bladder as the tumour shrinks with treatment. Both are very unpleasant, but a recto-vaginal fistula is probably the most distressing for the patient, and if this occurs, a defunctioning colostomy is indicated. A vesico-vaginal fistula can be more difficult to manage and the extent of surgery needs to be individualised. Radical surgery in the form of an extenteration (removal of the pelvic contents, i.e. bladder and/or rectum and/or uterus and vagina) may be considered in exceptional circumstances – when disease is localised and cure is thought to be an option. Such heroic surgery is, however, rarely appropriate.

Stage IVB

Patients who present with metastatic disease are incurable and treatment should be aimed at palliation to optimise quality of life. It can consist of a short course of radiotherapy if local pelvic symptoms are a problem. Surgery also has a place in palliation, for example a defunctioning colostomy if a recto-vaginal fistula is present. Even in a patient with a very limited life expectancy, the latter surgery can be very worthwhile due to the extremely distressing symptoms and the relative ease and simplicity of the procedure.

Palliative chemotherapy is also an option to temporarily reduce symptoms. Active chemotherapeutic regimens would include carboplatin and paclitaxel, cisplatin ± other agents, for example paclitaxel and methotrexate. The side effects of these drugs must, however, be balanced against the potential benefit to the patient.

The most important aspect of care of these patients with advanced disease and limited life expectancy is good quality palliative care to minimise symptoms and maximise quality of life.

Prognosis

Survival of patients with a vaginal metastasis will depend on the primary site of the tumour. If it is an isolated vault recurrence of an endometrial cancer following hysterectomy, then radiotherapy has a 'salvage' cure rate of over 70%. Survival of primary vaginal cancers is dependant on the stage of disease at presentation (Table 12.2) (Creasman 2005; Creasman et al. 1998; Frank et al. 2003; Mock et al. 2003).

Table 12.2

FIGO Stage	Survival
I	70–80%
II	50–60%
III	30–40%
IV	<20%

The future

Radiation treatment techniques are improving, with more accurately targeted beams. This primarily reduces toxicity but may ultimately allow an increase in radiation dose and therefore higher cure rates. Conformal external beam therapy is already commonplace with the advent of MLCs and computer software programmes. IMRT is well established as a technique worldwide and is becoming much more widely available in many UK centres. This allows shielding of areas inside the radiation field, as well as at the edges. The use of conformal techniques to shape brachytherapy treatments is also possible and very effective but is currently only available in a small number of centres in the UK. It is very time consuming and labour intensive, but its use is set to increase over the next few years.

Perhaps the biggest change to UK practice in gynaecological radiotherapy is the need to decommission the low/medium dose rate selectron machines by the end of 2009. These are used to administer brachytherapy in the majority of UK centres. Most centres are likely to change to high dose rate (HDR) technology, and many have already done so. This will bring a number of benefits and challenges. The main benefit to the patient is that the procedure can be carried out as an outpatient, because treatment only takes minutes rather than hours, but two or three treatments are needed instead of one.

However, the most effective management is to avoid the need for treatment at all. Prevention of some vaginal tumours may be achieved by the introduction of vaccines against HPV. Immunisation programmes against the common strains of HPV, as an attempt to prevent cervical cancers, are already underway worldwide, including one recently started in the UK.

Conclusion

Vaginal cancer is uncommon and the majority of women present with metastatic disease. Patients most commonly present with vaginal bleeding, pain and sometimes a palpable mass. Treatment often involves a combination of surgery, chemotherapy and radiotherapy. Advances in radiation therapy and the developments of vaccination programmes will improve the outlook for women with this rare cancer.

Vaginal cancer: the patient's perception

I can say that I had prepared myself to be informed, at some stage in my life, that I had gynaecological cancer. Strange as this may sound, but my gynaecological history, since the age of 21, had followed a pattern of cervical and vaginal cell abnormality, laser treatment and cone biopsies, with results ranging from 'nothing abnormal detected', through to CIN1-111 and VIN 1-111, but never malignancy.

At the age of 49 years, when vaginal cancer WAS diagnosed, I initially felt a sense of calm and ability to face the challenge of my planned chemotherapy and radiotherapy during the following five weeks... or so I thought.

My initial thoughts turned to my family, husband (who I had took in a rather blasé way on recollection) and children ages 19 and 20 years. And my mother, who had been recently bereaved. How would they take the news and cope? I had always been able to protect my children from distress, or at the very least, be there to offer them comfort and support. Now the tables were being turned and they would see ME as being vulnerable ... something I had never wanted to put them through, but had little choice. My husband was far more anxious than I was, but my entire family supported me throughout, for which I will be eternally grateful. At least I had a strong and constant support system of family and friends.

I planned to take my treatment 'in my stride' and deal with each day as it presented itself. I consider myself to be of strong character......however, the challenge of chemotherapy and radiotherapy would prove far greater than I had anticipated. I naively thought that I would be able to combine treatment with employment and managed, in the initial 2 weeks, to sustain weekly chemotherapy and daily radiotherapy, whilst working 4 hours a day, 5 days a week. This routine finally took its toll, leaving me with fatigue, a sense of failure and occasional bouts of feeling low. I found my frustration increasing, as I wanted to achieve my daily goals (as I had always done), but quickly had to come to terms with the restrictions my treatment caused and to take life at a very much slower pace, listening to what my body was telling me.

Chemotherapy and radiotherapy are two words commonly used in our society today but they are treatments (although lifesaving) that can have a destructive effect on the body and its systems. Generally it was not the treatment that I found problematic, but the side effects of it. Very often these were inevitable and refusing treatment was not an option I contemplated, as my prognosis was good. In addition, I felt an increasing sense of loss of control over what was happening to my body.

Five weeks of daily radiotherapy (25 sessions) sounded quite daunting initially, especially as each visit involved a round trip of 60 miles from my home to the hospital. However, both myself and my husband adjusted fairly quickly to that routine and it became the norm (even though some days I had to muster up all my willpower to make the journey, as I felt tired and nauseous). I took pride in the fact that I did not miss one session of radiotherapy. The relaxed environment of the radiotherapy department, together with the sense of camaraderie amongst the various individuals receiving treatment over the same 5-week period. made the experience valuable. My husband found this a great source of support too.

I felt quite anxious about chemotherapy, after the first session really. On my first visit, I was made to feel comfortable in an easy chair, along with five other cancer patients (each one undergoing a different treatment) and browsed through a magazine whilst my intravenous treatment was being administered. This took approximately 2 hours, after which I was able to go home. It was during the days following that I noticed how pale I was becoming and generally tired, although this had a cumulative effect as treatment progressed. I seemed to have picked up strength by the fifth day, had one day feeling reasonable before returning to hospital on the seventh day for the next week's dose... and so the cycle continued I was aware of how I would be feeling by the end of each treatment and this contributed to my apprehension. A little knowledge can be a bad thing! My husband sat with me for each chemotherapy visit, which was a welcome distraction. The impact of having a chemical injected into my body became a growing concern for me (combined with my positive thought that this was going to destroy my cancer) and I was not at all convinced that I could successfully see the 5 weeks' of chemotherapy through. Rather a mixed bag of emotions.

During my treatment I spent rather more time than I would have liked as an inpatient on the cancer ward, where I had the privilege of sharing my emotions with fellow cancer patients. My treatment seemed to pale into insignificance, compared to the journey of other individuals whose lives were affected by cancer....some very much younger than myself, and, on more than one occasion I reminded myself how lucky I was. I can understand why some people decide not to receive treatment and indeed met a few on the ward.

The forced separation from my husband and children was difficult to face when I was in hospital, again the feeling that I had abandoned them.

Now, with my treatment finished and 3-monthly reviews with my consultant oncologist taking place, I am able to move forward. I must admit that now I look back over those events with similar sentiments to child birth. Time is a great healer and it feels as if I have been caught in a time warp for the periods of my illness, a hazy dream. I am amazed at how my body is getting stronger, the fact that I can manage three days a week at work. Because of my character, I do have to set realistic goals and try to be more patient with myself. I struggle with this still.

As for answering the question often ask myself... 'What if the cancer returns?'

I would be prepared to receive further treatment. The explanations, the information, and support received from all members of the Health Care Team involved in my treatment and care was second to none and remains ongoing.

Reflective points

- Consider the differences in management in early stage presentation and late presentation of vaginal cancer.
- How would you retain privacy and dignity for a women undergoing radiotherapy for vaginal cancers?

References

Creasman,W.T. (2005) Vaginal cancers. *Current Opinion in Obstetric and Gynaecology* **17**, 71–76.

Creasman, W.T., Phillips, J.L. and Merck, H.R. (1998) The National Cancer Data Base report on cancer of the vagina. **83**, 1033–1040.

Daling, J.R., Madeleine, M.M., Schwartz, S.M. et al. (2002) A population-based study of squamous cell vaginal cancer: HPV and cofactors. *Gynecologic Oncology* **84**, 263–270.

Frank, S.J., Jhingranm A., Levenback, C. and Eifel, P.J. (2003) Definitive treatment of vaginal cancer with radiation therapy (abstract 116). International *Journal of Radiat. Oncol. Biol. Phys.* **57(suppl)**, S194.

Hellman, K., Silfversward, C., Nilsson, B. et al. (2004) Primary carcinoma of the vagina: factors influencing the age at diagnosis. The Radium Lermmet series 1956–96. *International Journal of Gynaecolical Cancer* **14**, 491–501.

Mock, V., Kucera, H., Feliner, C. et al. (2003) High dose rate (HDR) brachytherapy with or without external beam radiotherapy in the treatment of primary vaginal carcinoma: long-term results and side effects. *International Journal of Gynaecol. Biol. Phys.* **56**, 950–957.

Nair, M. and Peate, I. (Eds) (2009) *Fundamentals of Applied Pathophysiology: An Essential Guide for Nursing Students*. Chichester: Wiley-Blackwell.

Percorelli, S. (Ed.) (2003) FIGO annual report on the results of treatment in gynaecological cancer. *International Journal of Gynaecologic Obstetrics* **83(Suppl 1)**, 27–40.

Chapter 13

Cancer of the Vulva

Beccy Hoddinott Isaac and Lisa Young

Learning points

At the end of this chapter the reader will have an understanding of:
- The incidence and risk factors associated with vulval cancer
- The types of vulval cancers and associated presenting symptoms
- The staging and grading of vulval cancers
- The prognostic factors and treatment options available
- The side effects of treatment
- The management of recurrent disease
- Follow-up strategies and future research

Introduction

Cancer of the vulva undoubtedly affects a woman's emotional health. Such a diagnosis causes physical change to the genital area, which is often exacerbated by surgical/radiation treatment.

Vulval cancer patients may experience mood swings, anger, depression, fear of recurrence and death. Women with vulval cancer have very articulately spoken of their feelings, and here is a small representation:

I felt mutilated...no longer female...I had no shape to my external genitalia, only a deformed and hollow space where my labia and clitoris once were, from the base of the pubic hair line there was nothing, just a crude opening. (Anon)

My diagnosis made me feel numb...I couldn't cope with my emotions, nor could my partner...it was a struggle...I felt a loss of control, shameful and worthless...I felt alienated and assaulted by my surgery. (Anon)

Women's Cancers, First Edition. Edited by Alison Keen and Elaine Lennan.
© 2011 Blackwell Publishing Ltd. Published 2011 by Blackwell Publishing Ltd.

Such women spoke of the support gained from their clinical nurse specialist (CNS), doctor, support groups and friends/family. Emotional support decreases feelings of isolation and distress and maximises life quality (Stead et al. 2007).

Anatomy and physiology of the normal vulva

The term vulva is the collective name for the female external genitalia. The anatomy of the vulva and perineum is outlined in Figure 13.1.

The vulva is covered by squamous epithelium. The mons pubis is a mound of fat anterior to the pubic symphysis covered by coarse pubic hair. The labia majora are two prominent folds of skin, also covered by pubic hair, which extend from the mons pubis on either side of the vestibule. The vestibule is the area into which the entrance to the vagina and urethra opens. The labia majora merge with each other anterior to the anus. As the female equivalent of the scrotum, they consist of fat and areolar tissue and have many sebaceous glands on their surface. The labia minora are two small folds of skin devoid of pubic hair, which are enclosed by the labia majora and also contain many sebaceous glands. At the top of the vestibule they divide and surround the clitoris. The clitoris is the female equivalent of the penis and is a small mass of erectile tissue and nerves. It is capable of enlargement when stimulated and enhances sexual excitement in the female (Tortora and Derrickson 2008).

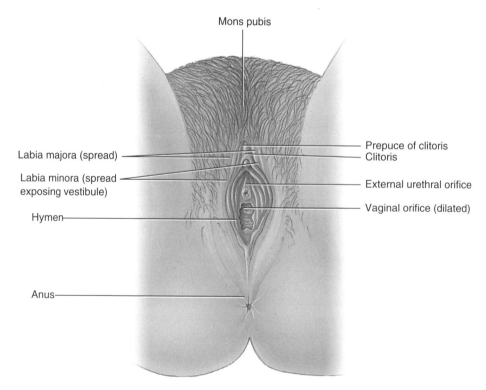

Figure 13.1   The external anatomy of the vulva and perineum. From Tortora and Derrickson (2008). Reproduced with permission from John Wiley & Sons, Ltd.

The vaginal orifice takes up the greater part of the vestibule and is partially covered by the hymen (mucous membrane). The hymen is often separated during first sexual intercourse but can be separated by other means. The urethral orifice lies anterior to the vaginal orifice and posterior to the clitoris. On each side of the vaginal orifice lie the Bartholin's glands (greater vestibular glands), which produce mucous supplying lubrication during sexual intercourse. There are a number of lesser vestibular glands opening into the vestibule, including the para-urethral glands. These are the female equivalent to the prostate.

Lymphatic drainage

Lymph is made from interstitial fluid, which flows through the lymphatic system, eventually returning to the circulatory system. During this process the lymph is filtered of particulate through lymph nodes. The lymph nodes are small and encapsulated nodules and are located throughout the lymphatic system. The lymphatic drainage of the vulva is primarily via the inguinal nodes in the groin, then draining into the deep femoral nodes situated along the femoral artery, vein and nerve. Drainage from central structures of the vulva, such as the clitoris, is to both sides of the groin (Figure 13.2).

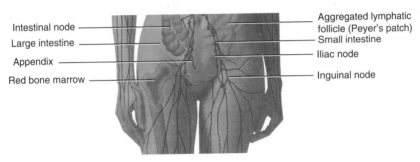

Figure 13.2   Lymphatic drainage of the pelvis. From Tortora and Derrickson (2008). Reproduced with permission from John Wiley & Sons, Ltd.

Incidence

Vulval cancer is rare, with 1000 new cases per annum in the UK. This accounts for less than 1% of all cancers and for 6% of all gynaecological cancers (Cancer Research UK 2008). The European age-standardised incidence rate of UK vulval cancer is 2 per 100,000 female population. Rates are less than 1 per 100,000 for women aged 25–44 years, increasing to 3 per 100,000 aged 45–64 years, reaching 14 per 100,000 if aged over 65 years (Cancer Registration in England 2004).

Risk factors

Human Papilloma Virus

HPV is clearly associated with vulval squamous cell carcinoma. Interestingly, 70% of squamous cell vulval cancers contain HPV DNA (Madeleine et al. 1997). This clearly is suggestive of viral causation. HPV infection is particularly linked to vulval neoplasm in younger women. Genital warts (associated with HPV type 6 and 11), also increase vulval cancer risk.

Human Immuno Virus

A dampened down immune response from HIV infection is linked to an increased vulval cancer risk.

Vulval intraepithelial neoplasia

VIN is a squamous intraepithelial vulval lesion, which shows dysplasia with varying amount of atypical cells. The base epithelial membrane remains intact; hence the lesion is not described as invasive. Nevertheless, it does possess the ability to invade. VIN I is the mildest form, VIN II is the intermediate form and VIN III is most severe form and includes carcinoma *in situ*.

There are thought to be two types of VIN – HPV-related and lichen-sclerosis-related. Reducing the amount of HPV, by a vaccination programme, ought to deliver a reduction in VIN rates (Cancer.org 2007).

A history of CIN or cervical cancer incurs ten times the vulval cancer risk (Cancer Research 2007).

Iatrogenic immunosuppression

Penn, in 1986, noted vulval cancer risk is augmented 100-fold following a renal transplant. This is due to the effect of immuno-suppression agents, which are prescribed to prevent transplant-organ rejection.

Smoking

Smoking is commonly known to be cancer-causing, and in the case of vulval cancer, increases invasive malignancy risk 3-fold and of carcinoma *in-situ* 6-fold (Cancer Research 2007). The risk increases proportionally alongside both intensity of smoking and number of years spent smoking (Daling et al. 1992). Women infected with HPV have a much higher risk of developing vulval cancer if they also smoke (Cancer org 2008).

Age

Vulval cancer risk increases in line with age. Vulval malignancy is primarily a disease of women aged over 50 years, although is certainly not unique to this cohort.

Lower socio-economic status

This group are more prone to engage in lifestyle activities attributable to an increased risk of vulval cancer, such as smoking, earlier age of first sexual contact and less years spent in education (Brinton et al. 1990).

Prevention

Studies have shown that vulval cancer can be avoided by delaying first sexual contact (to minimise HPV exposure), and by not smoking (Madeleine et al. 1997; Kagie et al. 1997; Kanye et al. 1997). It is also thought that using a barrier-method of contraception may avoid virus transmission, although clearly this does not protect against all skin-to-skin contact.

Regular gynaecological awareness reduces the risk of an undiagnosed malignant lesion. It is important for a woman to be aware of her genital area, recognise abnormalities and seek advice appropriately.

Vulval self-examination is a simple process. This should be performed regularly, ideally completed once a month and in between menses. In essence, vulval skin changes need to be looked out for, and may take the form of increased pigmentation, whitened areas, lumps and bumps or blisters/ulcers, which fail to heal. Symptoms such as itching, soreness and discomfort that are persistent, need to be checked out by a medical practitioner. There are excellent guides to vulval self-examination widely available to women, in health care settings such as the GP practice and also on-line (VACO 2003, accessed June 2008).

UK HPV vaccination commenced in September 2008, to girls aged 12 and 13 years. There are two HPV vaccines available, Gardasil™ and Cervarix™ (Reuters 2007). In June 2008, the British government ruled to offer Cervarix as part of a vaccination programme, which disappointed many women's health campaigners, as Cervarix does not offer the equivalent comprehensive quadrivalent cover of Gardasil. A trial looking at HPV vaccination in VIN has shown some response, and further study is indicated.

Types of vulval cancer

Squamous cell carcinomas (SCC)

Ninety per cent of vulval cancers are squamous, forming slowly and often preceded by VIN. SCC spread locally and metastasises to the groin and then the pelvic nodes (Cancer.org 2006).

Verrucous carcinomas

These have a wart-like appearance, are a slow-growing SCC type and as a rule are associated with good prognosis (Rosmanich et al. 1989).

Malignant melanomas

These account for 4% of vulval cancers and develop from pigment-producing cells (Weinstock 1994).

Lichen sclerosis (LS)

This is a chronic vulval skin condition, which presents as flat, white and/or glistening patches (Perrett et al. 2003).

LS causes skin itching, thinning and scarring. This can make sexual intercourse difficult and has the potential to have a detrimental affect on a woman's self-esteem. Between 1–2% cent of women with LS will develop vulval cancer, whereas 60% of vulval cancer patients will also have LS (Perrett et al. 2003).

Basal cell carcinomas

These are rare, developing from deep basal layers and are related to sun damage.

Paget's disease

This occurs when adenocarcinoma cells spread from glands across the skin. This is a non-invasive cancer originating from apocrine or epithelial stem cells. This is a rare condition affecting mainly menopausal women. Paget's can present as a red scaly area (likened to eczema), which itches. Paget's can recur, hence close follow-up by a gynae-concologist is advocated.

Merkell cell tumours (MCT)

Neuroendocrine carcinomas are very rare, originating from cells just below skin and in hair follicles. They present as firm, painless shiny lumps of skin with a red/blue tinge and most commonly occur between the ages of 60 and 80 years. MCT grow fast, often metastasising to regional nodes, liver, bone and lungs.

Sarcomas

These represent less than 2% of vulval cancers and commence in connective tissue cells. These are fast growing with rapid haematogenous/lymphatic metastatic spread. Leiomyosarcomas and rhabdomyosarcomas begin in the muscle layer; angiosarcomas begin in blood vessels (artery, vein, capillary) cells. Sarcomas develop at any age and are firm and nodular to touch.

Adenocarcinoma

A small proportion of vulval cancer develops from vulval glands, for example Bartholin's glands.

Presenting symptoms

- Constant vulval itching/pain
- Burning upon micturition
- Vaginal discharge/bleeding unrelated to menses
- Ulcerated/lumpy vulva
- Change in vulval skin colour

Management

Referral to a specialist gynaecological cancer surgeon is advocated, for careful vulval examination to identify abnormal vulval skin, possibly with a colposcope. A targeted biopsy or series of punch biopsies over a larger area will follow. To enable accurate staging, the clinician will request a series of tests, including radiological imaging, Magnetic Resonance Imaging (MRI)/Computer Aided Tomography (CAT))/Positive Emission Topography (PET) scan), blood test, chest X-ray (CXR) and possibly an examination under anaesthesia (EUA) to assess local disease progression.

Staging and grading of cancer of the vulva

Staging

Cancer of the vulva is usually staged according to the International Federation of Gynaecology and Obstetrics system (FIGO 2009), in which stage I is the earliest stage and stage IVB is the most advanced (Table 13.1). This is a surgical staging method in

Table 13.1 FIGO (2009) staging of cancer of the vulva.

Stage	Features
Stage I	Tumour confined to the vulva
IA	Lesions 2 cm or less in size confined to the vulva or perineum with stromal invasion 1.0 mm* or less, no nodal metastasis
IB	Lesions >2 cm or with stromal invasion >1.0 mm, confined to the vulva or perineum, with negative nodes
Stage II	Tumour of any size with extension to adjacent perineal structures (1/3 lower urethra, 1/3 lower vagina, anus) with negative nodes
Stage III	Tumour of any size with or without extension to adjacent perineal structures (1/3 lower urethra, 1/3 lower vagina, anus) with positive inguino-femoral lymph nodes
IIIA	(i) With 1 lymph node metastasis (≥5 mm), or (ii) 1–2 lymph node metastasis(es) (<5 mm)
IIIB	(i) With 2 or more lymph node metastases (≥5 mm), or (ii) 3 or more lymph node metastases (<5 mm)
IIIC	With positive nodes with extracapsular spread
Stage IV	Tumour invades other regional (2/3 upper urethra, 2/3 upper vagina) or distant structures
IVA	Tumour invades any of the following: (i) upper urethra and/or vaginal mucosa, bladder mucosa, rectal mucosa or fixed to pelvic bone, or (ii) fixed or ulcerated inguino-femoral nodes
IVB	Any distant metastasis including pelvic lymph nodes

*The depth of invasion is defined as the measurement of the tumour from the epithelial-stromal junction of the adjacent most superficial dermal papilla to the deepest point of invasion.

which clinical assessment of lymph node status is limited and therefore pathological assessment is needed to determine accurate lymph node involvement.

Current research is looking at sentinel node identification during surgery to reduce the number of unnecessary lymphadenectomies, thus reducing potential morbidity.

A study by Lavenback et al. (2001) concluded that using iosulfan blue dye injection alone could identify sentinel nodes in more than 95% of patients with vulval cancer. However, this study failed to identify the sentinel node in 2 out of 12 patients who proved to have metastatic disease. However, this study did not have any false-negative results.

A study by Martinez-Palones et al. (2006) aimed to determine the usefulness of sentinel node biopsy in early stage vulval cancer. They concluded that sentinel node identification is feasible in early stage vulval cancer and may be considered a possible alternative to inguino-femoral lymphadenectomy.

Grading

Cancer cells are graded according to how closely they resemble normal morphology. The more the cells resemble normal cells, the lower the grade. The lower the grade, the slower the cancer is likely to grow and metastasise. Stage and grade of tumour is used when making decisions regarding the most appropriate treatment. There are usually three grades of tumour:

- Grade 1 – low grade or 'well-differentiated', looking very similar to normal cell morphology
- Grade 2 – medium grade or 'moderately-differentiated', looking more abnormal that Grade 1 cells
- Grade 3 – high grade or 'poorly-differentiated' and are very unlike normal morphology.

Prognostic factors

Prognostic factors include FIGO stage, tumour size, depth of invasion, grade and numbers of nodes involved and are all highly predictive of survival. Increased stage of disease indicates a poorer prognosis and patients with positive nodes are more likely to experience early recurrence than those with negative nodes. Bilateral lymph node involvement is also indicative of a worse prognosis than unilateral involvement. Higher-grade tumours are more likely to involve deep tissue invasion, again indicating a poor prognosis (Blake et al. 1998; Stehman and Look 2006).

Following complete surgical resection of primary invasive squamous cell cancer of the vulva, a 5-year survival rate of 75% and 10-year rate of approximately 58% should be expected. If a patient is diagnosed with negative nodes, then the overall survival rate can be as high as 90%; however, this figure drops to approximately 40% if there is nodal metastasis.

In tumours of less than 2 cm, the incidence of nodal spread is approximately 10–15% and in around 30% of patients undergoing surgery, positive nodes will be found.

If one node is positive then the 5-year survival rate is likely to be 94%, reducing to approximately 80% if two nodes are positive. If three or more nodes are positive, then there is a high risk of pelvic metastases, which greatly reduces the 5-year survival rate to 0–25% (Blake et al. 1998; Satmary et al. 2003).

Treatment

Once a diagnosis of vulval cancer has been confirmed, patients should be referred to the specialist gynaecological oncology team at a Cancer Centre for treatment (Department of Health 1999). The DH advocates that surgery should be the 'mainstay of treatment, irrespective of the age of the woman…. and should only be carried out by gynaecological surgeons who specialize in this work' (DH 1999: p. 48).

Choosing the best surgical treatment for each patient involves balancing the important need to maintain sexual function with the need to remove all of the cancer. The surgical intent is to have maximal clearance with good margins, whilst at the same time removing only what is absolutely necessary. This approach involves wide local excision (WLE) of the tumour, with at least a 1 cm margin of normal cells (Blake et al. 1998; Wojtowicz et al. 2001; Satmary et al. 2003; Stehman and Look 2006; Cancerbacup 2008).

Early stage disease with less than 1 mm invasion should be managed with WLE; if invasion depth is between 1 and 5 mm, then surgical treatment should also include ipsilateral groin node dissection. This radical local excision of the tumour reduces the psychosexual morbidity for the patient; local recurrence occurs in approximately 10% of patients, regardless of whether a radical vulvectomy was performed or not (Crawford 2002).

Management of advanced disease (Stages III and IV) often involves radical vulvectomy or a variation of pelvic exenteration and vulvectomy. These surgical techniques aim to completely resect the tumour but are often unsuccessful in curing these patients, especially if the tumour was bulky and/or positive groin nodes were present. Pelvic exenteration may involve removing the bladder (anterior exenteration), rectum (posterior exenteration), and total exenteration includes clearance of all the contents of the pelvis. Total exenteration involves gastrointestinal and urinary tract diversion, leaving the patient with stomas (Blake et al. 1998).

Side effects post surgery

Due to the movement towards less extensive surgical procedures, post-operative complications and resultant morbidity have become less problematic (Stehman and Look 2006). However, side effects following surgery remain significant and affect approximately 50% of patients. These include short-term effects such as post-operative infections/wound breakdown, sepsis, lymphocysts and long-term effects such as leg lymphoedema, stress incontinence and psychosexual distress (Wojtowicz et al. 2001; Gaarenstroom et al. 2003; Golding and Wright 2006; Stehman and Look 2006).

Stehman and Look (2006) describe several techniques to attempt to restore the appearance and function of the vulva after radical local excision. These include using flaps of skin from the thigh and the buttock to cover skin and tissue defects.

For early stage cancers, primary radiotherapy to the groin is considered to reduce the morbidity following surgical groin dissections, especially lymphoedema. However,van der Velden et al. (2005) concluded from their Cochrane Review that there is insufficient evidence that radiotherapy works as well as surgery for early stage vulval cancer and results in a higher level of recurrences.

Lymphoedema

Lymphoedema is an accumulation of lymph within the tissues, which can cause swelling. Lymphoedema may result from damage to or removal of the lymph nodes. Lymphoedema can lead to tissue fibrosis, an increased risk of infection and can have a negative impact on a patient's physical and psychological well-being (Lymphoedema Support Network 2003; Lymphoedema Framework 2006).

The Lymphoedema Framework (2006), a UK based research partnership, aims to increase the profile of lymphoedema and improve standards of care; their model for best practice advocates that those patients with lymphoedema should receive a 'co-ordinated package of care and information appropriate to their needs'. This should include both a holistic and multidisciplinary approach including exercise, swelling reduction, skin care, risk reduction and pain/psychosocial management.

Patients at an increased lymphoedema risk should receive education about risk reduction and the early signs of swelling. Many cancer centres will have access to a lymphoedema clinic and patients with early signs of lymphoedema should be referred for management advice and/or further education. The LSN provides written information and support for patients with lymphoedema and offers a network of UK support groups.

Chemo/Radiotherapy

Radiation therapy is often used pre-operatively in patients with bulky tumours, in order to reduce their size and as such improve resectability. Administering a chemotherapeutic agent such as Cisplatin or 5-Fluoracil (5FU) concurrently with the radiation, in order to sensitise the radiotherapy response, has proved to be beneficial (Wojtowicz et al. 2001). A 2006 Cochrane Review concluded that neo-adjuvant chemoradiation reduces tumour size and improves the chances of surgical resection in women with initially inoperable primary tumours or fixed lymph nodes. However, it also stated that side effects of this treatment were considerable (van Doom et al. 2006). These include the effects of radiotherapy as discussed later in this chapter and the specific chemotherapeutic agent effects such as nausea and vomiting, changes to appetite, temporary alopecia and immunosuppression. Anecdotally, the radiotherapy-specific side effects appear in some cases more severe in patients being treated with concurrent chemotherapy.

Adjuvant radiotherapy

Adjuvant radiotherapy to the groin and pelvis is offered to patients who have been found post-operatively to have positive groin nodes following inguino-femoral lymphadenectomy (Clifford Chao et al. 1999). A recent Cochrane protocol for review stated that there is no consensus on which patient group should receive adjuvant radiotherapy (van der Velden et al. 2005). Some believe that adjuvant radiotherapy should be offered to patients when more than one or two positive lymph nodes are found; others include the breakthrough of the capsule as an indicator for adjuvant radiotherapy (van der Velden et al. 2005).

Side effects of radiotherapy

Radiotherapy to the vulva and groin causes general side effects such as diarrhoea and tiredness, and can also cause other specific side effects:

- Skin reactions – vulval soreness and breakdown
- Cystitis
- Diarrhoea
- Alopecia of the pubic hair
- Vaginal stenosis

Treatments are available to reduce the impact of these side effects and the CNS or specialist radiographer will discuss the use of vaginal dilators to reduce the risk of vaginal stenosis, the long-term impact on sexual function and ability to undergo full vaginal examination during follow-up.

Recurrent disease

Local recurrence

In 85–90% of patients, local recurrence does not occur following adequate primary treatment. A large proportion of these recurrences will occur on the vulva and many are amenable to further surgical resection (Clifford Chao et al. 1999; Stehman and Look 2006). Clifford Chao et al. (1999) state that recurrences after surgical resection remain potentially curable and must be treated aggressively with radiotherapy.

Groin recurrence

Up to a third of recurrences will occur in the groins and unfortunately carries a poor prognosis. Radical excision of groin recurrences appear to have some benefit if the femoral vessels are not involved (Hopkins et al. 1990). Chemoradiation following excision could also be beneficial (Stehman and Look 2006) or radiotherapy alone (Wojtowicz et al. 2001).

Distant recurrence

Distant recurrences are detected in fewer patients and pelvic recurrences are rare, but they are associated with a dismal prognosis. Chemotherapy has not been extensively studied in this group of patients nor proved to be of any value, thus there is no standard systemic chemotherapy for metastatic disease. These patients may be suitable for clinical trials. Chemotherapy agents such as cisplatin, methotrexate, cyclophosphamide, bleomycin and mitomycin C, have shown a partial response of only 10–15% with duration of a few months (Wojtowicz et al. 2001). Stehman and Look (2006) advocate a palliative approach to this patient group, recommending local measures for symptomatic recurrent lesions.

Follow-up

The purpose of this is to check for recurrence, but can also address treatment side effects. The patient's CNS can advise how to adjust to life following cancer and how to remain healthy. Follow-up is individualised depending upon cancer type, lifestyle and the patient's wishes (Cancerbacup 2008).

Future research

Research can compare existing therapies and find improved anti-cancer therapies. Here are some examples of new technologies, which have a potential application in the treatment of cancer of the vulva.

Photodynamic therapy

This involves injecting patients with a light-sensitive chemical absorbed by cancer cells. The cancer cells are exposed to a special light, with the aim of cell destruction.

HPV vaccines

The role of HPV vaccination against VIN needs further research; with the aspiration it will be as successful as against cervical intraepithelial neoplasia (CIN).

Oncogenes

Oncogenes control cell growth. Further research is needed to investigate gene therapy, with the aim of replacing damaged genes with normal healthy genes.

Treatment improvements

Trials to determine the safest most effective way of combining radiotherapy, surgery and chemotherapy are running. Studies looking at Intensity Modulated Radiotherapy (IMR) continue.

Anti-viral creams

These stimulate the immune system to fight viruses. Imiquimod™ stimulates cells to produce Interferon to combat HPV.

Conclusion

Vulval cancer is a highly distressing disease that without doubt affects a women's physical, social and emotional being. Early detection with vulval self-examination is a simple process and one that should be encouraged in all women. Surgery is the primary treatment, but radiotherapy and chemotherapy also have a role to play. However, all treatment is difficult, with acute and long-term side effects requiring health care professionals to have specific insight into the specialist needs of this group of patients.

Cancer of the vulva: Sue's story

Sue is 58 and had a wide local excision, a left sided lymphadenectomy (removal of groin nodes on left side), followed by 5 weeks of daily radiotherapy. This is her response to a question about whether she has 'got back to normal' after her cancer treatments.

I've been thinking about whether or not I've got back to my normal self since my cancer treatment. I finished my radiotherapy 9 months ago. Physically I would say that I have felt very well and I have managed to go on holiday as well; I'm able to do some of the things I could do before. I swim 50 lengths of my local pool 3 times per week. I run most days; physically I never thought that I would get back to doing all that I can do but I can, and that feels good. I still get tired, but then I work three days per week now, I do a stressful job, so I think that is not really surprising. I do feel different though; I am a different person to what I was 18 months' ago. I have been through an awful lot and I think that I have learnt a lot about people and myself. I am still continuing to come to terms with what has happened to me. Because it takes a long time.

Then I have counselling every month, which has helped tremendously. It wasn't just the cancer that affected me, my mum dying of cancer and the difficulties with my daughter's behaviour that made everything seem worse and more difficult to cope with. I think that I'm still working through it. But I feel quite together actually, despite all that I've been through. I feel that emotionally I am coping quite well. Sex is difficult – painful – it's not like it was, it's still not, it's never going to be; it's difficult to think about it. It's never going to be like it was, I feel as though I think that's changed. There is a lack of desire. I associate sex now with something, not pain exactly, but more discomfort I suppose. I think that having sex as we get older changes anyway, your desire, especially women, I think there's a biological thing, and most women are not so keen. It may not necessarily be all due to what I've been through, some of it may have happened any way.

One of the reasons I do all of the running and swimming (I didn't used to do it when I was young, in my 20s). I didn't start this until my 30s or so, because you sort of accept it. You realise when you get into your 30s that you have to do something, because otherwise everything's going to fall apart, so you have to start looking after your body. I do need to go to work and I do need to be active and have an interest in things. So, I don't feel that I feel differently as a woman because of the cancer, no, maybe I would if I'd had breast cancer.

I've learnt so much about myself; I've learnt that I'm strong. I am now more patient and more understanding and I try to be nice to people. I try to think about what people might have gone through. I think that I'm a fighter, I've been right down at the bottom, feeling hopeless and helpless and low. I've never felt helpless before. I felt that my life was completely out of control and I absolutely hated it and I've never felt like that before. Not being able to do anything, and desperately wanting to do just the normal things. So I suppose I have more insight into how it feels to feel really helpless and not to know what's going to happen. I'm the sort of person who likes to plan my life and have control, so I know what it's like and it's horrible. I now appreciate people more. I don't know what's going to happen down the road, I really don't so it's made me a more compassionate person and a more understanding person with other people's problems really.

Reflective points

- Consider the impact of a diagnosis of vulval cancer on relationships.
- How can you meet the psychosocial needs of a women diagnosed with this cancer?
- Consider the late effects of vulval cancer. What strategies can be put in place to address concerns?

References

Blake, P., Lambert, H. and Crawford, R. (1998) *Gynaecological Oncology: A Guide to Clinical Management.* Oxford: Oxford Medical Publications.

Brinton, L.A. et al. (1990) Case-control study of cancer of the vulva. *Obstetrics and Gynaecology* **75(5)**, 859–866.

Cancer Research UK Stats: 2008.

Cancer Registration in England (2004) Office for National Statistics.

Clifford Chao, K.S., Perez, C.A. and Brady, L.W. (1999) *Radiation Oncology: Management Decisions.* Philadelphia: Lippincott-Raven.

Crawford, R.A.F. (2002) Recent advances in gynaecological oncology surgery. In: P.J. O'Donovan and E.G.R. Downes (Eds) *Advances in Gynaecological Surgery*, London: Greenwich Medical Media Ltd, pp. 147–154.

Daling, J.R. et al. (1992)_Cigarette smoking and the risk of anogenital cancer. *American Journal of Epidemiology* **135(2)**, 180–189.

DH (1999) *Improving outcomes guidance for women with gynaecological cancers.* London: The Stationary Office.

van Doom, H.C., Ansink, A., Verhaar-Langereis, M. and Stalpers, L. (2006) Neoadjuvant chemoradiation for advanced primary vulvar cancer. *Cochrane Database of Systematic Reviews* Issue 3, Art. No. CD003752.

FIGO (2009) Revised FIGO staging for carcinoma of the vulva, cervix and endometrium, *International Journal of Gynecology and Obstetrics* **105**, 103–104.

Gaarenstroom, K.N., Kenter, G.G., Trimbos, J.B. et al. (2003) Postoperative complications after vulvectomy and inguinofemoral lymphadenectomy using separate groin incisions. *International Journal of Gynecological Cancer,* **13**, 522–527.

Golding, J. and Wright, S. (2006) delivering patient-centred cancer care in gynaecology. In: S. Jolley (Ed.) *Gynaecology: Changing Services for Changing Needs*, Oxford: John Wiley & Sons, pp. 185–207.

Hopkins, M.P., Reid, G.C. and Morley, G.W. (1990) The surgical management of recurrent squamous cell carcinoma of the vulva, *Obstetric Gynecology* **75**, 1001–5.

Kagie, M.J. et al. (1997) HPV infection in squamous cell carcinoma of the vulva, in various synchronous epithelial changes and in normal vulval skin. Gynaecology Oncology **67(2)**, 178–83.

Kanye, M.J. et al. (1997) HPV infection in SCC of the vulva in various synchronous epithelial changes and in normal vulval skin. *Gynaeoncology*. **67(2)**, 178–83.

LSN (2003) *Lymphoedema Support Network,* London.

Lavenback, M.D., Coleman, R.L., Burke, T.W., Bodurka-Bevers, D, Wolf, J.K. and Gershenson, D.M. (2001) Intraoperative lymphatic mapping and sentinel node identification with blue dye in patients with vulval cancer. *Gynaecological Oncology* **83(2)**, 276–81.

Lymphoedema Framework (2006) *Best Practice for the Management of Lymphoedema*. International Consensus. London: Medical Education Partnership Ltd.

Madeleine, M.M. et al. (1997) Cofactors with HPV in a population-based study of vulvar cancer. *Journal National Cancer Institute* **89(20)**, 1516–23.

Martinez-Palones, J.M., Perez-Benavente, A., Diaz-Feijoo, B., et al. (2007) Sentinel lymph node identification in a primary ductal carcinoma arising in the vulva. International Journal of Gynecological Cancer **17(2)**, 471–7.

Penn, I. (1986) Cancers of the anogenital region in renal transplant patients. *Analysis of 65 cases. Cancer* **58(3)**, 611–16.

Perrett, C.W. et al. (2003) *The molecular biology of lichen sclerosis and the development of cancer in lower genital tract neoplasia*. London: RCOG Press.

Rosmanich, A., Briones, H. and Espinoza, A. (1989) Verrucous carcinoma of the vulva. *Review Chil. Obsetrics Gynaecology*. **54(6)**, 390–393.

Satmary, W., Memarzadeh, S., Smith, D.M. and Barclay, D.I. (2003) Pre-malignant and malignant disorders of the vulva and vagina. In: A.H. De Cherney and L. Nathan (Eds) *Current Obstetrics and Gynecologic Diagnosis and Treatment*, 9th edn, New York: McGraw-Hill Professional, pp. 879–93.

Stead, M. et al. (2007) Psychosexual function and impact of gynae cancer. *Best Practice and Research, Clinical Obstetrics and Gynaecology* **121(2)**, 309–320.

Stehman, F.B. and Look, K.Y. (2006) Carcinoma of the vulva. *Obstetrics and Gynaecology*, **107(3)**, 719–33.

Tortora, G.J. and Derrickson, B.H. (2008) *Principles of Anatomy and Physiology,* 12th edn., Oxford: John Wiley & Sons Ltd.

van der Velden, J., Ansink, A. and Stalpers, L. (2005) Adjuvant radiotherapy for all stages of vulvar cancer, (Protocol), *Cochrane Database of Systematic Reviews,* 3, Art. No. CD005345.

Weinstock, M.A. (1994) Gynaecology: malignant melanoma of the vulva and vagina in the population-based estimates of survival. *American Journal of Obsetrics and Gynaecology*. **171(5)**, 1225–1230.

www.cancerorg/docroot/CRI/content?CRI_2_4_2X

GlaxocervicalshotapprovedinAustralia.www.reuters.com/article/health-SP/idUSL2149778820070521) Reuters 21 May 2007.

Wojtowicz, M., Khong, H.T. and Khleif, S. (2001) Vulvar cancer. In: J. Abraham and C.J. Allegra (Eds) *Bethesda Handbook of Clinical Oncology*. London: Lippincott Williams & Wilkins, pp. 225–230.

Useful websites

www.cancerbackup.org.uk/cancertype/vulva/precancerous conditions/vulvaintraepithelialneoplasm.
www.cancerhelp.org.uk
www.cancerresearchuk.org
www.emedicine.com/derm/topic234.html
www.thegcf.org
www.jotrust.co.uk/about_cervical_cancer/hpv.cfm
www.mayoclinic.com
www.merck.com
www.nature.com/nm/journal/v7/n4/full/nm0401_388a.html
www.NCI.co.uk
www.tellheraboutit.com
www.VACO.org
http://www.vaco.co.uk/vacofrontpage/VACO%20VSE%20April%202008.pdf
www.vulavrhealth.org/LS/lichenhtml.
www.wcn.co.uk

Chapter 14

Fertility and Cancer in Women

Susan Ingamells, C. Basu, J. Tucker and A. Umranikar

Learning points

At the end of this chapter the reader will have an understanding of:
- Normal fertility process
- The extent of fertility issues in women with cancer
- The impact of cancer and cancer treatment on fertility
- The effects of pregnancies on cancer
- Modern techniques to preserve fertility
- Specific womens cancers and their effect on fertility

Introduction

Over recent years, the advances in cancer treatment in women and girls have been paralleled by advances in fertility preservation and reproductive technology. Whilst chemotherapy, radiotherapy, surgery and stem cell treatments have improved the survival of young female patients with cancer, many have gone on to experience fertility problems as a direct result of the cancer treatment. These problems include ovarian failure, premature menopause, recurrent miscarriage, premature delivery, cervical stenosis and implantation failure. In addition, the social and psychological impact of the resulting infertility places a high burden on the women who survive their cancer treatment. Today, many of these women can be helped to have their own child using the assisted reproductive techniques that allow for cryopreservation of embryos, oocytes and ovarian tissue. Many others will benefit from donor gamete treatment, surrogacy or adoption. In addition, improved knowledge about the nature of cancers has allowed surgical developments to improve survival rates, whilst also retaining natural fertility options.

The incidence of cancer in women of reproductive age is 49.2 cases per 100,000 women, with gynaecological cancers accounting for approximately 10% and cancer of

Women's Cancers, First Edition. Edited by Alison Keen and Elaine Lennan.
© 2011 Blackwell Publishing Ltd. Published 2011 by Blackwell Publishing Ltd.

the breast accounting for 14%. In total, just less than 8000 women aged 15–40 years will be diagnosed with a cancer each year. In addition, 1400 children less than 15 years of age will be diagnosed with cancer each year and of these, 75% will survive through to adulthood. The number of women of reproductive age who have received cancer treatment is rising, along with the success of the oncology treatments.

Knowledge of the fertility options for a woman with a diagnosis of cancer is essential to her holistic care. An understanding of the issues with conception, after cancer treatment, centres on the ovarian reserve and the impact of both age and cytotoxic treatments on the function of the ovary. This chapter aims to give an overview of the current fertility treatments available to women of reproductive age with cancer. It will outline the specific treatments and highlight the issues relating to specific malignancies.

Normal ovarian development

In a human female, germ cells migrate into the ovary during development *in utero*. By 6 months gestation, 7 million germ cells are located in the ovaries. Just before birth, the germ cells stop dividing mitotically and enter their first meiotic division becoming primary oocytes. By entering meiosis, the primary oocytes are no longer able to divide and as a consequence, by the time of birth, a woman has all the oocytes within her ovaries that she will ever have. If these oocytes are lost or damaged as a result of surgery or exposure to X-irradiation or cytotoxic drugs, they cannot be replaced from stem cells.

The primary oocytes subsequently form primordial follicles and then further development of the oocyte ceases. From puberty onwards, the primordial follicles are recruited and the development of the oocyte and meiosis continues. The primordial follicle can remain in the arrested state for 50 years, until a signal to resume development is received.

Just after birth, large numbers of the meiotically arrested oocytes die for reasons that are unclear, so that only 1–2 million oocytes remain. This number continues to decline throughout a woman's life and reaches very low levels at the time of the menopause.

Ovarian reserve

The ovarian reserve refers to the total number and quality of primordial follicles remaining in a woman's ovaries. The primordial follicles have two functions, as they contain the gametes and steroidogenic cells. Loss of the primordial follicles through natural aging or ovarian tissue destruction leads to a decline in both fertility potential and hormone production, resulting in premature menopause. The poor correlation between the chronological age and menstrual characteristics to reproductive age and fertility potential has led to the development of ovarian reserve tests for use in the fertility clinic. Reduced ovarian reserve is related to treatment cancellation and poor IVF outcome, so prior knowledge of the likely ovarian reserve can assist in optimising treatment and providing a realistic expectation of outcome.

Table 14.1   Ovarian reserve tests.

Ultrasound	Ovarian volume
	Antral follicle count
	Ovarian stromal blood flow
	Uterine dimensions
Biochemical	Early follicular levels:
	• Follicle stimulating hormone (FSH)
	• Lutinizing hormone (LH)
	• Oestradiol
	• Inhibins
	• Anti Mullerian Hormone (AMH)
	Ovarian stimulation tests
	• Gonadotrophin agonist stimulation test
	• Clomiphene citrate challenge test

Ovarian reserve tests are either based on analysis of biochemical markers or ultrasound parameters (Table 14.1). A combination of tests is usually needed, as no one test is entirely predicative. Basal Follicle Stimulating Hormone (FSH) is the most commonly used biochemical test, as it is readily available and cheap. It is an indirect measure of ovarian reserve, but the inter-cycle variability limits its usefulness. Observational studies have shown an association between elevated day 3 oestradiol levels and decreasing numbers of oocytes and pregnancy rates in IVF programmes (Licciardi et al. 1995). Studies in an assisted reproduction population show that women with a low day 3 cycle inhibin B concentration had a poorer response to ovulation induction and decreased likelihood of achieving pregnancy, compared with women with higher day 3 inhibin B levels (Seifer et al. 1997). Anti Mullerian hormone (AMH) is produced by the granulosa cells of the ovary. Levels of AMH decline with increasing age and are directly correlated with antral follicle counts and ovarian response in IVF cycles. AMH levels are stable throughout the menstrual cycle and can be easily analysed, making AMH a reliable and convenient test of ovarian reserve (Gruijters et al. 2003).

Dynamic ovarian reserve tests can be used to detect reduced ovarian reserve. In practice, they are rarely used now that good data is available on the reliability and predictive value of AMH. The clomiphene citrate challenge test is the most commonly used and involves the administration of 100 mg of clomiphene citrate on days 5–9 of the menstrual cycle and analysis of the FSH levels on days 3 and 10 of the menstrual cycle. Women with a normal ovarian reserve will have FSH levels in the normal range on day 10, whilst those with reduced ovarian reserve will have highly elevated levels on day 10.

Routine ultrasound can be used to measure parameters such as ovarian volume, antral follicle counts and ovarian stromal blood flow. Ovarian volume and reproductive outcome do appear to be correlated with small ovarian volume (<3 cm) being associated with poor ovarian response in IVF cycles (Singh et al. 2005). Ultrasound counts of the number of follicles of less than 10 mm diameter in the early follicular phase is known as the antral follicle count (AFC). This number is assumed to be related to the cohort of growing follicles and also to the ovarian reserve. There is a gradual decline in AFC with age, and AFC counts have been shown to be useful estimates of ovarian reserve (Yong et al. 2003).

Cancer treatments and the ovary

The ovaries and uterus may be damaged by radiotherapy or chemotherapy.

Radiotherapy

Radiotherapy effects on the ovary

The human oocyte is sensitive to relatively low doses of radiation. The extent of the damage depends on the dose and the age of the patient (Thomson et al. 2002). A radiation dose of less than 2 Gy is enough to destroy 50% of the oocyte population (Sonmezer and Oktay 2006). The younger the patient, the higher the number of germ cells present and the higher the dose of radiation required to sterilise the patient. Radiotherapy induces ovarian failure by causing DNA damage to the ovarian follicles, resulting in a significant depletion of the follicular pool. It is possible to predict how long after treatment ovarian failure will occur, by the use of a modified model of natural oocyte decline (Wallace et al. 2005), enabling clinicians to offer advice regarding future fertility.

Secondary effects on the ovary are seen when high dose cranial irradiation is given in the treatment of brain tumours, which may lead to gonadotrophin deficiency and result in delayed puberty or amenorrhoea.

Radiotherapy effects on the uterus

There is a significant risk of damage to the uterus from abdominal or pelvic irradiation and women conceiving following such treatment are considered a high risk pregnancy (Critchley et al. 1992). Pregnancy complications noted are early pregnancy losses, pre-term labour and intrauterine growth restriction. These effects are due to impaired uterine growth and blood supply. Irreparable damage may occur when a pre-pubertal uterus is irradiated, as it is more vulnerable to radiation than a mature uterus. Scattered radiation also has effects on ovaries and uterus, although this is less than direct radiation. Pelvic, abdominal or total body radiation is likely to have the greatest damaging effects on the ovary and the uterus. Use of lead shields has been known to reduce the harmful effects of radiation by 70%.

Chemotherapy

Damage to the ovary from chemotherapy is related to age at time of treatment, the type and combination of chemotherapeutic drugs and the cumulative dose of drugs used. Ovarian damage is directly proportional to age, as younger women have a larger follicular reserve at the initiation of treatment. In one study, resumption of menses occurred in 22–56% of women under the age of 40, as compared to less than 11% in the over-40 group (Wallace et al. 2003). The ovaries are particularly susceptible to damage from alkylating agents (Whitehead et al. 1982). Studies have shown that women receiving cyclophosphamide have a 4- to 9-fold greater risk of premature ovarian failure (Meirow and Nugent 2001; Byrne et al. 1992). Some chemotherapeutic drugs can cause an irreversible reduction of ovarian reserve, leading to amenorrhoea and premature ovarian failure.

Fertility drugs and risk of cancer

Considerable debate has arisen regarding the safety of fertility treatment and whether the use of fertility drugs increases the risk of ovarian cancer. The 'incessant ovulation' theory postulates that the cycle of damage and repair that occurs in the ovary with repeated ovulation may lead to DNA damage and potentially cause cancer (Fathalla 1971). Therefore, the concern has been that by causing super-ovulation, fertility drugs may increase this risk. Early studies which led to anxiety studied few patients, and subsequent studies have not reported the same association. Infertility itself is a risk factor for ovarian cancer.

Most recently, Jensen et al. (2009) have carried out a large cohort study of infertile women referred to Danish clinics over a 25-year period. They concluded that there is no association between the use of fertility drugs and ovarian cancer, even in women who had undergone ten or more cycles. This is an important study and included much greater numbers than previous studies; however, even larger numbers will need to be followed to exclude the possibility of a small increase in risk. Nonetheless, the study is reassuring that fertility drugs do not significantly increase the risk of ovarian cancer. This is important, given the increased numbers of women seeking fertility treatment. Although breast cancer is a hormone dependant malignancy, drugs used for IVF treatment have not been shown to have any association with breast cancer (Antoniou et al. 2003).

Effect of pregnancy on cancer

Generally women with a good prognosis following cancer treatment are still advised to delay pregnancy for at least 2 years. This is because any recurrence is more likely to happen in the first 2 years and pregnancy will undoubtedly make management more difficult. Delaying pregnancy helps to ensure that women who conceive are in a better prognostic group. In women with localised breast cancer, Ives et al. (2007) found that early conception 6 months after completing treatment was unlikely to reduce survival. However, with more extensive breast cancer, a 5-year survival of 54% was reported in women with an end of treatment to pregnancy interval of less than 6 months, as compared to 78% in end of treatment to pregnancy interval between 6 months and 2 years, and 100% in those who waited for over 5 years.

Preserving fertility in women with cancer

With modern treatment regimes, high rates of survival from cancer are achieved, but this is frequently at the cost of ovarian failure. Conventional fertility treatment has little to offer women with reduced ovarian function, because the efficacy of fertility drugs is dependent on adequate ovarian reserve.

Assisted reproduction techniques prior to cancer treatment are indicated where there is a high chance of inducing ovarian failure. It is contraindicated where the woman is clearly terminally ill or if the risks of the procedure outweigh the benefits. Women need to be fully counselled regarding the processes involved and potential outcomes, so that they are able to give informed consent. It is important that this aspect is not overlooked when time is of the essence. The options for fertility in women of reproductive age are listed in Table 14.2.

Table 14.2 Fertility options for women undergoing cancer treatment.

In vitro fertilisation with embryo cryopreservation
In vitro fertilisation with oocyte cryopreservation
Ovarian tissue freezing
Ovarian tissue transposition
Donor eggs
Surrogacy
Adoption
Childlessness

IVF with embryo cryopreservation

IVF and embryo cryopreservation is used before initiation of chemotherapy for women with cancer, but cannot be used in all situations. It involves ovarian stimulation for multi-follicular development, oocyte retrieval and embryo creation for future use. There is the need for involvement of the male partner, or donor semen in the absence of a partner. A conventional controlled ovarian stimulation cycle using gonadotrophin agonist down-regulation can take several weeks to prepare the ovaries for oocyte retrieval and for some cancers it may not be advisable to delay the onset of chemotherapy. Newer protocols using GnRH antagonists provide shorter cycle lengths and more flexibility. Of concern with some cancers, notably breast, is that tumours may be stimulated by the high levels of oestrogen that occur with ovarian super-ovulation. Current regimes use aromatase inhibitors in conjunction with ovulation induction agents to reduce the levels of oestrogen (Oktay et al. 2004). This does not appear to compromise oocyte numbers or embryo quality and there is no increase in the cancer recurrence rate when compared with controls. An alternative option in hormone dependant cancers is natural cycle oocyte aspiration, *in vitro* maturation and cryopreservation of embryos. The advantage is that this form of treatment minimally interferes with the primary disease. The success rate reported with natural cycle is lower than hormonally stimulated cycles, as only one or two oocytes are retrieved.

Oocyte cryopreservation

Cryopreservation of oocytes is technically much more difficult than freezing embryos, but overcomes the need for a partner. This method has a lower success rate than embryo cryopreservation, as freeze-thawing causes damage to the oocytes, resulting in a 3- to 4-fold lower success rate of live births per frozen oocyte than standard IVF.

The first pregnancy resulting from cryopreserved oocytes in a cancer survivor was reported by Yang et al. (2007). With conventional freezing techniques, only a few hundred births have been reported worldwide. With the recent development of vitrification techniques that result in better survival rates, oocyte storage is likely to become more established as a method of preserving fertility (Kuwayama et al. 2005). This process still requires ovarian super-ovulation and, therefore, the time restrictions discussed above will apply.

Ovarian tissue banking

Ovarian tissue storage, in which ovarian cortical slices containing the primordial follicles being cryopreserved, is a controversial developing technology. The primordial follicles are less susceptible to cryo-injury than oocytes or embryos. It avoids the need for ovarian stimulation, does not delay the initiation of cancer treatment, does not require a male partner and can be used in pre-pubertal girls. Two live births have now been reported from frozen ovarian tissue that has been regrafted (Donnez et al. 2004; Meirow et al. 2007). The tissue is re-implanted as an autograft, either into a site in the pelvis (orthotopic) such as the ovarian cortex of the residual ovary, or into the medulla of the other ovary (Sanchez et al. 2008). Alternative sites of implantation (heterotopic), the forearm and anterior abdominal wall, have also been used. Ovaries have been seen to regain their functional capacity after transplantation. It is not yet possible to assess how effective this treatment will be, as there are still many technical difficulties to overcome. One possible risk is transplantation of malignant cells when re-grafting ovarian tissue. Research continues in this area.

Ovarian tissue transposition

Surgical transposition of ovaries (oophoropexy), involving the laparoscopic repositioning of ovaries away from an intended radiation field, is suggested for women who need radiotherapy. It gives patients an opportunity to retain their ovarian function and attempt future pregnancies. The ovaries are transposed to a level above the pelvic brim to minimize the radiation exposure. What remain unknown are the unavoidable radiation effects on the ovary due to scatter radiation.

Donor eggs

Unfortunately, assisted conception technologies will not be successful or available to all women undergoing cancer treatment and some survivors may wish to access donor eggs in order to have a child. Success rates are good if the egg provider is young, but suitable sources of eggs are limited in the UK, due to HFEA rules governing anonymity and payments. Some patients will seek treatment with donor eggs provided by a family member, but this can cause social difficulties for the resulting child. In many other countries, donor eggs are in plentiful supply and patients may need to travel to other parts of the world to secure suitable treatment.

Surrogacy

Women who have received uterine irradiation or a hysterectomy have no option other than surrogacy if they wish to have their own genetic child using stored oocytes or embryos. In a surrogacy arrangement, a women will carry a child for another woman and surrender the child at birth. It is known as host or gestational surrogacy when the woman carries a genetically unrelated child conceived in an IVF programme. Surrogate mothers are entitled to receive reasonable expenses, but not to be paid. In the UK, host surrogacy is regulated by the Human Fertilisation and Embryology Authority and can only be practised in licensed IVF centres. The actual surrogacy arrangement is a private agreement between the commissioning couple and the surrogate host. After the birth of the child, a parental order is required in order for the commissioning couple to become the legal parents of the child. The parental order cannot be issued until the child is 6 weeks of age, but parental responsibility can be assigned earlier if a parental responsibility agreement is signed.

Women's cancers and the specific factors affecting fertility

Cancer and the uterus

Cancer of the endometrium is primarily a disease seen in women belonging to the perimenopausal and post-menopausal age group. It is the fourth most common cancer in women in the UK, accounting for 5% of all female cancers. Young women in the reproductive age group at risk of developing endometrial cancer are those with polycystic ovarian syndrome (PCOS), those with a genetic predisposition to the development of endometrial cancer or those with oestrogen secreting ovarian tumours. Most of the risk factors for endometrial cancer share a common underlying aetiology of unopposed oestrogenic stimulation of the endometrium without the protective effect of progestins. Unopposed oestrogens lead to a greater proliferation of the endometrium, as compared to the stroma causing endometrial hyperplasia and subsequent risk of malignancy. Less than 5% of cases occur in women under the age of 40. The common histological type is endometrioid carcinoma, which has a favourable outcome with 93% survival at stage I grade 1 tumour. Conservative treatment with progestins, although in experimental stages, is an option for patients who wish to retain their fertility potential. Few studies have been published involving use of progesterone (medroxyprogesterone acetate) in endometrial cancer. The reported resolution rate has been between 50 and 80%, with 30–40% recurrence rate. Twenty-nine pregnancies have been reported after treatment (Wang et al. 2002; Seli and Tangir 2005).

Primary surgery is fundamental in achieving a cure for early stage disease. Total abdominal hysterectomy with bilateral salpingoophorectomy with peritoneal washings is the recommended treatment for stages I and IIa. Women may wish to preserve gametes prior to the surgery and those doing so will need to make use of a surrogate host in order to use those gametes in the future.

Endometrial cancer in pregnancy is extremely rare. Most cases are diagnosed as result of persistent irregular bleeding after a miscarriage, or a termination of pregnancy or in the post-partum period. Only 30 cases have been reported so far (Acheson 2008), with endometrioid carcinoma being the most common histological type observed.

Ovarian cancer and fertility

Ovarian carcinoma is the fifth most common malignancy in women in the UK. Only those women with early stage disease have any option of future fertility, as advanced disease would indicate surgery leading to a pelvic clearance. Women with early stage I disease tend to be younger and may wish to have the option of fertility in the future. In women of less than 40 years of age, most ovarian cysts or masses will be due to benign causes such as endometriosis or functional cysts. For these women, it is reasonable to initially offer a unilateral oophorectomy combined with surgical staging. If the cyst is subsequently found to be malignant, adjuvant chemotherapy would be recommended for stages IB or IC of the disease. The adjuvant chemotherapy may further reduce their fertility potential in the future. Women refusing adjuvant chemotherapy for fertility reasons have been studied (Zanetta et al. 1997) and recurrence rates are similar in those women having fertility sparing surgery and no chemotherapy (9%) and those having full FIGO staging surgery for early disease (12%).

Breast cancer and fertility

In women with breast cancer wishing to undergo assisted reproduction prior to cancer treatment, it is the standard practice to stimulate the ovaries using the short protocol during the interval between surgery and initiation of chemotherapy. A potential problem in these patients is the high levels of oestrogen in the IVF cycles, which may have an impact on the long-term survival in women with oestrogen sensitive tumours. In order to avoid the oestrogen surge, some centres offer natural cycle IVF, although the success rates are quite low at 7.2%, as only one egg is retrieved (Penlick et al. 2002). Tamoxifen, an anti-oestrogen, can be used to stimulate the ovaries with beneficial effects on the number of mature oocytes, as shown by Oktay et al. (2003). Recent work has shown that Letrozole (potent and highly selective third-generation SERM) could be introduced as a promising ovulation induction agent along with suppression of plasma estradiol and estrone levels (Mourisden et al. 2003).

The diagnosis of cancer in pregnancy is becoming more common as women are delaying childbirth, resulting in an increase in number of older mothers. The incidence of malignancies rises exponentially with age. Under the age of 25 the incidence is 25 per 100,000, rising to 261 per 100,000 in women aged 40–44. Invasive ductal carcinoma is seen most commonly in pregnancy, with high grade and lymphovascular infiltration, although the hormone receptor status is usually negative (Jemal et al. 2003). Women diagnosed with cancer during pregnancy are more likely to have metastatic disease, as seen in a recent case controlled study (Zemlickis et al. 1992). The prognosis of pregnancy associated breast cancer is poor and can be attributed to advanced stage at diagnosis or delays with treatment. The potential reasons for these are the masking of the pathological features of the tumour by the physiological changes in pregnancy and the reluctance to perform invasive and radiological investigations in pregnancy. The nature of the tumour is not necessarily more aggressive in pregnancy (Woo et al. 2003).

Pregnancy does not compromise the survival of women with a previous history of breast cancer and there are no reports of any deleterious effects on the foetus. It is recommended that pregnancy should be deferred for at least 2 years after treatment. A 5-year survival of 54% has been reported in women with a treatment pregnancy interval of less than 6 months, as compared to 78% in treatment pregnancy interval between 6 months and 2 years, and 100% in those who waited for over 5 years. Tamoxifen is a competitive oestrogen receptor antagonist with no adverse effects on the primordial follicles that is used in hormone dependent breast cancer treatment. However, the use of this medication mandates a 5-year delay in pregnancy, due to its presumed teratogenic potential. The subsequent delay in pregnancy compounded by chemotherapy induced depletion of ovarian reserve increases the risks of infertility (Bines et al. 2006).

Cervical cancer and fertility

Cervical cancer is the second-most common cancer in women worldwide and accounts for 6% of all malignancies in the UK (Luesely and Baker 2004). The incidence in 2004 was reported to be 8/100,000 in women between ages 30 and 40 years (Cooper and Westlake 2008). In many developing countries, cervical cancer continues to be the commonest cause of death in women belonging to the reproductive age group. The national cervical screening programme has reduced the incidence of cervical cancer by 80%, with a resultant decrease in mortality by 50% (Acheson 2008). However, there has been a 5-fold increase observed in the incidence of pre-invasive cancer (cervical intraepithelial neoplasia), as compared to invasive cancer (Blake et al. 1998).

Fertility issues regarding treatment of cancer of the cervix are related to the disruption of the function of the cervix as a passageway for the sperm to the uterine cavity and subsequently in retaining the foetus in the uterus until full maturity. The lack of cervical mucus to aid sperm migration can impair natural conceptions after cervical ablation or lesion excision.

Treatment of cervical precancerous lesions depends on the grade of cervical intraepithelial neoplasia (CIN) observed (Paraskevaidis et al. 2002, Lindeque 2005). While CIN 1 is managed conservatively with follow-up smears every 6 months, CIN 2 and 3 are usually treated by local ablation or excision. In those women who subsequently go on to conceive after LLETZ treatment, meta-analysis studies have demonstrated a 1.7 times higher incidence of pre-term births and a 2.69 times higher incidence of pre-term pre-labour rupture of membranes in subsequent pregnancies after LLETZ treatment (Kyrgiou et al. 2006). However, there is little data quantifying this risk, with different sizes of loops used or variations in the depth of cervical tissue excised. The current recommendation is that women undergoing LLETZ should be counselled regarding future pregnancy complications and therefore advised closer antenatal surveillance in the form of cervical length assessment by ultrasound. Cervical smears and colposcopy are both safe if indicated in pregnancy. For low grade lesions, conservative management with follow-up smears and colposcopic assessment every 3 months in the antenatal period and then 3 months after delivery is recommended. For high grade lesions or those with the possibility of micro-invasion, a loop excision biopsy is preferable, but is avoided in pregnancy with the higher risks of bleeding, incomplete excision and pre-term birth (Acharya et al. 2005; Crane 2003).

Treatment of cervical cancer in pregnancy presents a challenge to all – the woman, her family and the team of clinicians. Decisions involving a termination of the pregnancy or a possible delay in starting treatment until foetal maturity is reached, are very complicated issues and are best dealt with on an individual case basis through a multidisciplinary team approach. In women who do not wish to retain future fertility, the standard treatment for invasive cervical cancer would be a Wertheim's hysterectomy. However, when future fertility potential is desired, a radical hysterectomy is not appropriate and a radical trachelectomy (Kyrgiou et al. 2006) with lymph node dissection may be offered. This treatment was introduced in 1987. The operation involves removal of the cervix along with some parametrial tissue and a cuff of vagina, leaving behind the body of the uterus and ovaries for future fertility. The residual isthmus is sutured to the vaginal skin with a non-absorbable suture material. The operation can be preformed vaginally or abdominally, with a laparoscopic pelvic node dissection to exclude nodal metastasis.

Spontaneous conceptions have been reported after radical trachelectomy. As this is a highly specialised surgery, there are only a few centres reporting their experience. Worldwide, there have been 790 radical trachelectomies performed, with 302 pregnancies and 190 live births reported (Aust et al. 2007). Assisted reproduction with intrauterine insemination or *in vitro* fertilisation are used for couples with fertility problems. Embryo transfer during IVF can be very challenging due to stenosis, and a trial of catheter prior to actual transfer or a transmyometrial embryo transfer may be required. These pregnancies are at a risk of second trimester miscarriage or pre-term labour. The mode of delivery is always by a classical caesarean section, as there is no cervix to labour and no lower segment to incise.

Gestational trophoblastic neoplasia and fertility

Gestational trophoblastic neoplasia (GTN) comprises a spectrum of conditions, from the pre-malignant forms of partial and complete hydatidiform molar pregnancies to the more aggressive malignancies of choriocarcinoma and placental site trophoblastic tumours. GTN involves the proliferation of trophoblastic cell types and has maternal consequences during pregnancy and after delivery.

All of these conditions are rare, with molar pregnancy occurring at an incidence of 2–3 per 1000 live births (Alteiri et al. 2003) and gestational choriocarcinoma at an incidence of 1 per 20,000 to 1 per 50,000 pregnancies. Placental site trophoblastic tumours are very rare, with an incidence of 2–5 cases per million births (Sebire et al. 2003). In women who have had one molar pregnancy, the risk of a second molar pregnancy is raised 10-fold and increases to 10–26% in women who have had more than two molar pregnancies (Sebire et al. 2003).

Benign

Complete and partial molar pregnancies account for the majority of the cases of GTN. They arise from trophoblastic cells as a result of abnormal fertilisation, causing an imbalance in the genetic material. The benign moles produce trophoblastic cells, which are capable of rapid multiplication, production of high levels of human chorionic gonadotrophin and malignant potential, but are unable to produce a viable pregnancy. Only 1% of partial moles have malignant potential and would require additional treatment (Wielsma et al. 2006; Niemann et al. 2007), whereas, 8–20% of complete moles develop persistent disease after uterine evacuation (Parazzini et al. 1986).

Malignant

Choriocarcinoma is a highly malignant tumour that metastasizes widely to the liver, lungs and brain. It has been suggested that 50% of these tumours follow a molar pregnancy, 30% occur after a miscarriage and 20% arise after an apparently normal pregnancy. Placental site tumours are the rarest form of GTN and frequently follow a normal pregnancy (Papadopoulos et al. 2002), although it can complicate any form of conception. Commonly it is localised to the uterus, but could also present as metastatic disease.

There is no clinically effective method to accurately predict the need for additional treatment, hence all patients with molar pregnancy are required to take part in a structured follow-up programme where they are closely monitored. Uterine evacuation is the treatment for molar pregnancies, but approximately 10–15% of women with complete mole and 1% with partial mole will develop malignant disease, necessitating adjuvant chemotherapy. All of these malignant tumours are responsive to chemotherapy (Newlands et al. 1991). The low risk women are treated with Methotrexate and Folinic acid, whereas the high risk group receive etoposide/methotrexate/dactinomycin and cyclophosphamide/vincristine. In the majority of women in both groups, fertility is maintained and menstruation resumes within 6 months. Chemotherapy can cause some gonadal toxicity, advancing the menopause by 1 year in the low risk group and 5 years in the high risk group (Bower et al. 1998). Placental site tumours, although rare, are best treated by hysterectomy, which has future fertility implications. During the surveillance phase and following completion of chemotherapy, the standard recommendations are to postpone pregnancy for 12 months to minimise confusion between disease recurrence and a new pregnancy. The time interval also minimises the chemotherapy induced damaging effects on the oocytes.

Conclusion

As fertility preservation treatments have advanced over the past few years, young patients who survive their disease are now able to consider fertility options. It is a fascinating and a challenging field, with a growing number of options of treatment modalities made available. This can only be possible through a multidisciplinary team approach involving oncologists, nurses, fertility specialists, obstetricians, neonatologists, clinical psychologists and geneticists. With future developments in this field, it is certain that fertility preservation will be an integral part of all cancer treatments in young cancer survivors.

One woman's experience of infertility

I had wanted a baby for as long as I could remember. I had been trying to conceive for 4 years. I was 34. I was undergoing IVF treatment when the doctor saw that I had an abnormally thickened womb lining. I didn't know what that could mean, but she said that she would refer me to a specialist. Naively I thought the specialist would be able to explain why I hadn't been able to get pregnant and fix the problem. When I saw him in the hysteroscopy clinic it was all quite matter of fact – I would have a sample taken and then come back for the results.

My husband came with me that Friday in November for the results – it was cancer! The thought had never once crossed our minds. I was numb and heard very little of what was said; I didn't want to hear. I would need a hysterectomy; I would never be able to carry a baby. I just sat and cried the whole way through. My husband just sat silent. The specialist and the nurse tried to fill the gaps with words; I heard surrogacy, adoption, egg harvesting, phrases I couldn't make any sense of. I didn't want to leave the room, because that would make this all real – I just wanted to stay there not even thinking.

We were taken to the reception desk to make another appointment to discuss our 'options' another day. The next week just went by in a complete daze. My husband didn't want to talk about it; I went alone for a CT scan to check that the cancer had not spread. I wanted him to tell me everything was going to be alright. We had suddenly moved apart into parallel places, never quite reaching one another. Our relationship had stayed strong throughout the regimented 'must have sex' to conceive and the disappointment of not getting pregnant. We had become even closer through the IVF build-up and process. Now we seemed worlds apart. I felt so alone; not because I had cancer, but because the rest of the female population seemed capable of having babies, and I couldn't. I didn't care about having cancer; my world seemed to have come to an end as all of my future hopes and dreams of becoming a mother slipped away.

We went back to see the specialist again – this time the nurse specialist greeted us before we went in and asked us how we had been over the past week. It was good for me to be able to say the words out loud in front of my husband, in a safe environment. He was still very quiet, but held my hand tightly and put his arm around me when we went in to see the doctor. My cancer had not spread, but there would be the need for an MRI scan to give a clearer picture of the womb. The nurse and doctor talked about egg harvesting and fertilising embryos so that we could have the option of a surrogate baby. I knew as I had always known that this would not be the answer for me – I only wanted a baby if I could feel our baby grow in my own womb and give birth. The operation was explained, the date would be sent to me and my MRI would happen next week. I was on a horrible surreal treadmill that I couldn't get off.

I went through the next scan, blood tests, a pre-operative appointment to be told what to expect. I went to see the fertility doctor and counsellor, but was still clear that I did not want my eggs to be harvested. I went through the hysterectomy – it felt as if it was happening to someone else. The nurse specialist came to see me, I just cried, I couldn't think about the future, there was no point to it anymore. My husband tried so hard to reach out to me, but I kept rejecting him. After the operation, I didn't want to see anyone. My sister-in-law had recently had a baby; my family didn't know what to say or not to say to me, so I avoided them, I couldn't imagine being back at work, where some of the women I worked with talked about their families all of the time. My friends stopped calling me, because I never returned their calls. My husband tried to talk about us making love, but I just avoided him too – I avoided going to bed at the same time, I avoided his touch. There seemed no point in sex anymore; we couldn't make a baby, what was the point?

It's 5 years on now, but I remember it as though it were yesterday. My husband and I separated 2 years after my operation; we had lost the ability to understand one another. He and my GP wanted me to have counselling, but there was no point from my perspective, talking about it was never going to ease the pain. We just stopped talking to one another, stopped sleeping together, stopped eating together and lived separate lives.

I'm now working in a job that I love; less money but satisfying; I look after my niece after school 2 days a week, and have met a man who has teenage children. My life will never be what it should have been, but it's OK. My cancer hasn't come back and now I go for check-ups once a year.

I've been asked by the nurse specialist whether there's anything that I have learnt that I could share with a woman going through a similar experience. I wish that I had words of wisdom, that made it all seem less painful, but I don't. I think the only thing I know is that this is such an important issue, that it should not be taboo and that women in my position should be heard.

Reflective points

- A 29-year-old married nuliparous women has just been dianosed with ovarian cancer. What concerns might she have in relation to preserving her fertility?
- What are her information needs in relation to the effects of her cancer and cancer treatment in relation to her fertility?
- What are the supportive needs of both her and her husband?

References

Acharya, G., Kjeldbergs I., Hansens S.M., Sorheim, N., Jacobson, B.K. and Maltau, J.M. (2005) Pregnancy outcome after loop electrosurgical excision procedure for the management of cervical intraepithelial neoplasia. *Archives of Gynaecology and Obstetrics* **272**(2), 109–12.

Acheson, N. (2008) Cervical and endometrial cancer in relation to pregnancy. In: S. Kehoe, E. Jauniaux, P. Martin-Hirsch and P. Savage (Eds), *Cancer and Reproductive Health*, Chapter 12. London: Royal College of Gynaecology Press, pp. 113–46.

Alteiri, A., Franceschi, S. and Ferlay, J. (2003) Epidemiology and etiology of gestational trophoblastic diseases. *Lancet Oncology* **4**, 670–8.

Antoniou, A., Pharoah, P.D., Narod, S. et al. (2003) Average risks of breast and ovarian cancer associated with BRCA1 or BRCA2 mutations detected in case series unselected for family history: a combined analysis of 22 studies. *American Journal of Human Genetics* **72**, 1117–30.

Aust, T., Herod, J., MacDonald, R. and Gazvani, R. (2007) Infertility after fertility-preserving surgery for cervical carcinoma: the next challenge for reproductive medicine? *Human Fertility* **10**, 21–24.

Bines, J., Oleske, D.M. and Cobleigh, M.A. (2006) Ovarian function in premenopausal women treated with adjuvant chemotherapy for breast cancer. *Journal of Clinical Oncology* **14**, 1718–29.

Blake, P., Lambert, H. and Crawford, R (1998) *Gynaecological oncology – A guide to clinical management*. Oxford: Oxford University Press.

Bower, M., Rustin, G.J., Newlands, E.S. et al. (1998) Chemotherapy for gestational trophoblastic tumors hastens menopause by three years. *European Journal of Cancer* **34**, 1204–7.

Byrne, J., Fears, T.R., Gail, M.H. et al. (1992). Early menopause in long-term survivors of cancer during adolescence. *American Journal of Obstetrics and Gynaecology* **166**, 788–93.

Cooper, N. and Westlake, S. (2008) Cancer incidence and mortality: trends in the United Kingdom and constituent countries 1993–2004. *Health Statistics Quarterly* **38**, 33–46.

Crane, J.M. (2003) Pregnancy outcome after loop electrosurgical excision procedure: a systematic review. *Obstetrics and Gynaecology* **102(5)**, 1058–62.

Critchley, H.O., Wallace, W.H., Shalet, S.M., Mamtora, H., Higginson, J. and Anderson, D.C. (1992) Abdominal irradiation in childhood: the potential for pregnancy. *British Journal of Obstetrics and Gynaecology* **99**, 392–4.

Donnez, J., Dolmans M.M., Demylle. D. et al. (2004) Livebirth after orthotopic transplantation of cryopreserved ovarian tissue. *Lancet* **364**, 1405–10.

Fathalla, M.F. (1971) Incessant ovulation – a factor in ovarian neoplasia? *Lancet* **2**, 163.

Gruijters, M.J., Visser, J.A., Durlinger, A.L. and Themmen, A.P. (2003) Anti-mullerian hormone and its role in ovarian function. *Molecular and Cellular Endocrinology* **211**, 85–90.

Ives, A., Saunders, C., Bulsara, M. and Semmens, J. (2007) Pregnancy after breast cancer: population based study. *British Medical Journal* **334**, 194.

Jemal, A., Murray, T., Samuels, A., Ghafoor, A., Ward, E. and Thun, M.J. (2003) Cancer statistics, 2003. *Cancer Journal for Clinicians* **53**, 5–26.

Jensen, A., Sharif, H., Frederiksen, K. and Kjaer, S.K. (2009) Use of fertility drugs and subsequent risk for ovarian cancer: Danish population based cohort study. *British Medical Journal* **338**, b249.

Kuwayama, M., Vajta, G., Kato, O. and Leibo, S.P. (2005) Highly efficient vitrification method for cryopreservation of human embryos. *Reproductive Biomedicine Online* **11**, 300–8.

Kyrgiou, M., Koliopoulos, G., Martin-Hirsch, P., Arbyn, M., Prendiville, W. and Paraskevaidis, E. (2006) Obstetric outcomes after conservative treatment for intraepithelial or early invasive cervical lesions: a systematic review and meta-analysis of literature. *Lancet* **367**, 489–98.

Licciardi, F.L., Liu, H.C. and Rosenwaks, Z. (1995) Day 3 estradiol serum concentrations as prognosticators of ovarian stimulation response and pregnancy outcome in patients undergoing in vitro fertilization. *Fertility and Sterility* **64**, 991–4.

Lindeque, B.G. (2005) Management of cervical premalignant lesions. *Clinical Obstetrics and Gynaecology* **19(4)**, 545–61.

Luesley, D.M. and Baker P.N. (2004) *Obstetrics and Gynaecology. An evidence based text for MRCOG*. London: Arnold Publishers

Meirow, D. and Nugent, D. (2001) The effects of radiotherapy and chemotherapy on female reproduction. *Human Reproduction Update* **7**, 535–43.

Meirow, D., Levron, J., Eldar-Geva, T. et al. (2007) Monioring the ovaries after auto transplantation of cryopreserved ovarian tissue: endocrine studies, *in vitro* fertilization cycles and live birth. *Human Reproduction* **87**, 418.

Mourisden, H., Gershanowich, M., Sun, Y. et al. (2003) Analysis of survival and update efficacy from the International Letrozole Breast cancer Group. *Journal of Clinical Oncology* **21**, 2101–9.

Newlands, E.S., Baghshawe, K.D., Begent, R.H., Rustin, G.J. and Holden, L. (1991) Results with the EMA/CO regimen in high risk gestational trophoblastic tumors, 1979–1989. *British Journal of Obstetrics and Gynaecology* **98**, 550–7.

Niemann, I., Hansen, E.S. and Sundae, L. (2007) The risk of trophoblastic disease after hydatidiform mole classified by morphology and ploidy. *Gynaecological Oncology* **104**, 411–15.

Oktay, J., Buyuk, E., Davis, O. et al. (2003) Fertility preservation in breast cancer: IVF and embryo cryopreservation after ovarian stimulation with Tamoxifen. *Human Reproduction* **18**, 90–5.

Oktay, K., Buyuk, E., Libertella, N., Akar, M. and Rozenwaks. Z. (2004) Fertility preservation in breast cancer patients. A prospective controlled comparison of ovarian stimulation with tamoxifen and letrozole for embryo cryopreservation. *Human Reproduction* **82,** 51.

Papadopoulos, A.J., Foskett, M., Seckl, M.J. et al. (2002) Twenty-five years clinical experience with placental site trophoblastic tumors. *Journal of Reproductive Medicine* **47**, 460–4.

Parazzini, F., La Vecchia, C., Pampallona, S. (1986) Parental age and risk of complete and partial hydatidiform mole. *British Journal of Obstetrics and Gynaecology* **28**,101–10.

Paraskevaidis, E., Koliopoulos, S., Kalantaridou, S. et al. (2002) Management and evolution of cervical intraepithelial neoplasia during pregnancy and postpartum. *European Journal of Obstetrics, Gynecology Reproductive Biology* **5:104(1)**, 67–9.

Penlick, M.J., Hoek, A., Simpsons, A.H. and Heineman, M.J. (2002) Efficacy of natural cycle IVF: a review of the literature. *Human Reproduction Update* **8**, 129–39.

Sanchez, M., Novella-Maestre, E., Teruel, J., Ortiz, E. and Pellicer, A. (2008) The Valencia Programme for fertility preservation. *Clin. Transl. Oncol.* **10(7)**, 433–8.

Sebire, N.J., Fischer, R.A., Foskett, M., Rees, H., Seckl, M.J. and Newlands, E.S. (2003) Risk of recurrent hydatidiform mole and subsequent pregnancy outcome following complete or partial hydatidiform molar pregnancy. *British Journal of Obstetrics and Gynaecology* **110**, 22–6.

Seifer, D.B., Lambert-Messerlian, G., Hogan, J.W., Gardinier, A.C., Blazer, A.S. and Berk, C.A. (1997) Day 3 serum inhibin-B is predictive of assisted reproductive technologies outcome. *Fertil. Steril.* **67**, 110–4.

Seli, E. and Tangir, J. (2005) Fertility preservation options for female patients with malignancies. *Current Opinion in Obstetrics and Gynaecology* **17**, 299–308.

Singh, K.L., Davies, M. and Chatterjee, R. (2005) Fertility in female cancer survivors: pathophysiology preservation and the role of ovarian reserve testing. *Human Reproduction Update* **11(1)**, 69–89.

Sonmezer, M. and Oktay, K. (2006) Fertility preservation in young women undergoing breast cancer therapy. *The Oncologist* **11**, 422–34.

Thomson, A.B., Critchley, H.O., Kelnar, C.J. and Wallace, W.H. (2002) Late reproductive sequelae following treatment of childhood cancer and options for fertility preservation. *Best Practice Research in Clinical Endocrinological Metabolism* **18**, 311–34.

Wallace, W.H., Thomson, A.B., Sarah, F. and Kelsey, T.W. (2005) Predicting age of ovarian failure after irradiation to a field that includes the ovaries. *Human Reproduction* **62**, 738–44.

Wallace, W.H., Thomson, A.B. and Kelsey, T.W. (2003) The radiosensitivity of human oocyte. *Human Reproduction* **18**, 117–21.

Wang, C.B., Wang, C.J., Huang, H.J. et al. (2002) Fertility preserving treatment in young patients with endometrial adenocarcinoma. *Cancer* **94**, 2192–8.

Wielsma, S., Kerkmeijer, L., Bekkers, R., Pyman, J., Tan, J. and Quinn, M. (2006) Persistent trophoblast disease following partial molar pregnancy. *Australia and New Zealand Journal of Obstetrics and Gynaecology* **46**, 119–23.

Whitehead, E., Shalet, S.M., Jones, P.H.. Beardwell, C.G. and Deakin, D.P. (1982) Gonadal function after combination chemotherapy for Hodgekin's disease in childhood. *Archive of Disease in Childhood* **57**, 287–91.

Woo, J.C., Yu, T. and Hurd, T.C. (2003) Breast cancer in pregnancy:a literature review. *Arch. Surg.* **138**, 91–8.

Yang, D.S., Blohm, P.L., Cramer, L. et al. (2007) A successful human oocyte cryopreservation regime: survival, implantation and pregnancy rates are comparable to that of cryopreserved embryos generated from sibling oocytes. *Fertil. Steril.* **72**, S86.

Yong, P.Y., Baird, D.T., Thong, K.J., McNeilly, A.S. and Anderson, R.A. (2003) Prospective analysis of the relationships between the ovarian follicle cohort and basal FSH concentration, the inhibin response to exogenous FSH and ovarian follicle number at different stages of the normal menstrual cycle and after pituitary down-regulation. *Human Reproduction* **18**, 35–44.

Zanetta, G., Chiari, S., Rota, S. et al. (1997). Conservative surgery for stage 1 ovarian carcinoma in women of childbearing age. *British Journal of Obstetrics and Gynaecology* **104**, 1030–5.

Zemlickis, D., Lishner, M., Degendorfer, P. et al. (1992) Maternal and fetal outcome after breast cancer in pregnancy. *American Journal of Obstetrics and Gynecology* **166**, 781–7.

Chapter 15

Sexual Health and Dysfunction

Karen Donelly-Cairns

Learning points

At the end of this chapter the reader will have an understanding of:
- Sexuality and relationships
- Normal sexual function and sexual response
- The effects of cancer and treatments on sexuality and sexual function
- Therapeutic intervention

Introduction

Both gynaecological and breast cancers and their treatments may have profound implications, not only related to survival but also to sexual and psychosexual outcomes. With increasing numbers of women being cured, sexuality is becoming more important, particularly since health care professionals are beginning to appreciate the importance of open discussion as part of the patient assessment and treatment. Sexual history as part of the medical and nursing evaluation will go a long way to highlighting sexual issues, by normalising sexuality and the identification of patients and their partners who may require intervention. Solutions to mechanical aspects of sexuality after a cancer diagnosis are only one small part of the overall treatment approach to ensure healthy sexual outcomes (Quinn 2007). Although this topic has many dimensions, this chapter will aim to provide an overview of the definitions of sexuality and what it means to the woman's normal sexual function and response cycle and how this may alter with a cancer diagnosis and treatment, leading to a potential sexual dysfunction. The effects on relationships will be explored, as well as assessment tools and management of issues.

Women's Cancers, First Edition. Edited by Alison Keen and Elaine Lennan.
© 2011 Blackwell Publishing Ltd. Published 2011 by Blackwell Publishing Ltd.

Table 15.1   Common changes associated with sexuality (Hughes 2000; Katz 2003; Bruner and Berk 2004).

Loss of desire for sexual activity	Amenorrhoea
The inability to reach orgasm	Surgical removal of the breast, vulva
Vaginal dryness and stenosis, which contributes to dyspareunia	Depression
Changes in genital sensations due to pain or loss of sensation and numbness	Loss of self esteem
Premature menopause	Body image problems
Loss of body hair	Fears and anxieties
Increased fatigue	Change in family role, social role, relationships
Weight gain or loss	

Sexuality

Sexuality is a complex, multidimensional phenomenon that incorporates biological, psychological, interpersonal and behavioural dimensions (Anastasia 1998). It is important to recognise that a wide range of normal sexual functioning exists. Ultimately, sexuality is defined by each patient and his/her partner within a context of factors such as gender, age, personal attitudes, and religious and cultural values (National Cancer Institute 2009).

Emotional satisfaction, reproduction, physical attractiveness to others and formation of relationships are all aspects of sexuality (Herson et al. 1999). Sexuality includes feelings about one's body, the need for touch, interest in sexual activity, communication of one's sexual needs to a partner and the ability to engage in satisfying sexual activities (Wilmoth 1998). All cancers can impact on sexuality and intimacy, but having cancer does not eliminate sexual feelings (Thaler-DeMers 2001).

Many types of cancer and cancer therapies are frequently associated with sexual dysfunction. Across sites, estimates of sexual dysfunction after various cancer treatments have ranged from 40–100% (Derogatis and Kourlesis 1981). Cancer therapy, such as surgery, chemotherapy and radiotherapy, may have a physiological and psychological impact on sexual function (Anastasia 1998; Hughes 2000; Quinn 2003). The literature shows that 50% of women with breast or gynaecological cancers report some level of sexual dysfunction (Jenkins and Ashley 2002; McKee and Schover 2001; Rogers and Kristajanson 2002). An individual's sexual response can be affected in a number of ways by cancer and its therapies, which can affect the physical, psychological and social ability of the patient to maintain sexual health (Algier and Kav 2008).

The most common changes associated with sexuality are shown in Table 15.1.

Women may experience changes in genital sensations due to pain or a loss of sensation and numbness, as well as a decreased ability to reach orgasm. Loss of sensation can be as distressing as a painful sensation for some individuals. In women, premature ovarian failure as a result of chemotherapy or pelvic radiation therapy is a frequent antecedent to sexual dysfunction, particularly when hormone replacement is contraindicated because the malignancy is hormonally sensitive (Ganz et al. 1998).

Unlike many other physiological side effects of cancer treatment, sexual problems do not tend to resolve within the first year or two of disease-free survival (Ganz et al. 1998; Broeckal et al. 2002). Rather, they may remain constant and fairly severe or even continue to increase. Although it is unclear how much sexual problems influence a survivor's rating of overall health-related quality of life, these problems are clearly bothersome to many patients and may interfere with a return to normal post-treatment life.

Sexual function

It is important to have an understanding of the sexual response cycle, which represents the physiological process of sexual function, to then be able to understand when and why sexual function becomes impaired.

Four stages are used to describe the physical changes that happen when a woman is sexually excited. These changes may occur when a woman masturbates or when she is sexually active with another person. The sensations at each phase are unique to each woman. Some women are aroused when their breasts are fondled, whilst other women do not like this kind of touching. Women sometimes need to reflect the kind of physical contact they enjoy. When a woman has sexual intimacy with another person, there are also many emotional and social factors that may affect her physical experience.

Women may not experience all four stages each time they are sexually active. Most women find there are many times when sexual play involves only the first one or two stages. Some women never or rarely have orgasms.

Masters and Johnson (1966) first detailed the four phases of human sexual response as a linear progression from excitement to plateau to orgasm, followed by resolution (Figure 15.1).

Excitement

Activation of the central nervous system (CNS) causes specific changes in blood flow. Ovarian hormones also play essential roles in this process, encouraging vasodilation and

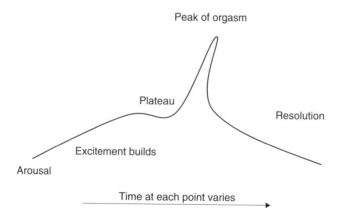

Figure 15.1   Sex cycle response.

increased blood flow. Uterine and internal mammary arteries contain some of the highest density of oestrogen receptors, hence their responsiveness in the excitement phase.

Genital vasocongestion occurs because of this increase in blood flow and smooth muscle relaxation. The vaginal wall becomes lubricated. The labia increase in size and spread open. The clitoris increases in size and the vagina expands whilst the uterus elevates. Other areas of the skin, including the face and breasts, demonstrate this increase in blood flow with the 'ex flush'.

Following Masters and Johnson, Kaplan (1974) replaced the excitement phase with two phases: desire, in which the neurological stimulus occurs; followed by arousal, in which blood flow produces the peripheral response leading up to orgasm.

Plateau

Masters and Johnson presented this as a separate phase, whilst Kaplan later blended it into the arousal phase. Actions associated with this phase include retraction of the clitoris and engorgement of the labia. Bartholin gland secretion occurs, as well as congestion of the outer third of the vagina and further expansion of the upper two-thirds of the vagina. Muscle tension builds.

Orgasm

In the orgasm phase, 8 to 12 muscular contractions of the levator ani muscles occur at precise intervals. Vaginal and uterine contractions occur followed by massive release of muscle tension. Regularly orgasmic women will achieve orgasm 50–70% of the time and a satisfying prolonged plateau phase other times.

Resolution

The final phase, or culmination, is often characterised by a gradual, pleasant diminishment of sexual tension and response, differing in the time it lasts amongst individuals.

As a largely biological model, the Masters and Johnson and Kaplan framework has been criticised, because it does not take into account non-biological experiences such as pleasure and satisfaction (Whipple and Brash-McGreer 1997) or place sexuality in the context of the relationship (Tiefer 2000).

The biopsychosocial sexual response

An alternative model has also been proposed to describe the female sexual response. Proponents believe that a large component of women's sexual desire is responsive rather than spontaneous. They maintain that the biopsychosocial nature of the female sexual response cycle is a result of the dynamic and mutable interaction of four components (Basson 2001, 2006) (Figure 15.2):

- Biology
- Psychology
- Sociocultural influences
- Interpersonal relationships

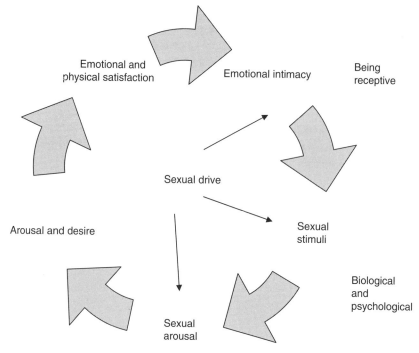

Figure 15.2   Cycle of female sexual response.

If only the biological or physiological component is addressed, as with the use of pharmacotherapy, successful treatment will frequently not be achieved. In this model, emotional intimacy of some kind motivates the woman to seek out or become responsive to sexual stimuli, which in turn leads to arousal. Once arousal is achieved, sexual desire is then accessed, allowing continuation of the experience for sexual reasons. Hence, sexual desire can be responsive to arousal instead of preceding it. Whilst spontaneous drive can occur, it is not essential. Thus, lack of spontaneous desire is not necessarily a dysfunction. In addition, satisfaction is the goal, which may or may not include orgasm.

Sexual dysfunction

In 1999, an international multidisciplinary panel of 19 experts in female sexual disorders was held by the Sexual Function Health Council of the American Foundation for Urologic Disease, to evaluate and revise the existing definitions for female sexual disorders from the *DSM-IV* and the *ICD-10*, in an attempt to provide a well-defined, broadly accepted diagnostic framework for clinical research and the treatment of female sexual problems (Basson et al. 2000). The Consensus-based Classification of Female Sexual Dysfunction (CCFSD) is based on the Masters and Johnson and Kaplan linear model of the female sexual response, which is problematic. However, the CCFSD classification represents an advance over the older systems, because it incorporates both psychogenical and organic causes of desire, arousal, orgasm and sexual pain disorders. The diagnostic system also has a 'personal distress' criterion, indicating that a condition is considered a disorder only if a woman is distressed by it (Parker Jones et al. 2005).

The four general categories from the *DSM-IV* and *ICD-10* classifications were used to structure the CCFSD system, with definitions for diagnoses as described as follows:

Sexual desire disorders

These are divided into two types. Hypoactive sexual desire disorder is the persistent or recurrent deficiency (or absence) of sexual fantasies/thoughts, and/or desire for or receptivity to sexual activity, which causes personal distress. Sexual aversion disorder is the persistent or recurrent phobic aversion to and avoidance of sexual contact with a sexual partner, which causes personal distress.

Sexual arousal disorder

This is the persistent or recurrent inability to attain or maintain sufficient sexual excitement, causing personal distress, which may be expressed as a lack of subjective excitement, or genital (lubrication/swelling) or other somatic responses.

Orgasmic disorder

Orgasmic disorder is the persistent or recurrent difficulty, delay in, or absence of attaining orgasm following sufficient sexual stimulation and arousal, which causes personal distress.

Sexual pain disorders

These are also divided into three categories: Dyspareunia is the recurrent or persistent genital pain associated with sexual intercourse. Vaginismus is the recurrent or persistent involuntary spasm of the musculature of the outer third of the vagina that interferes with vaginal penetration, which causes personal distress. Non-coital sexual pain disorder is recurrent or persistent genital pain, induced by non-coital sexual stimulation.

Disorders are further sub-typed according to medical history, laboratory tests and physical examination as lifelong vs acquired, generalised vs situational, and of organic, psychogenic, mixed or unknown origin.

Factors affecting sexual function in people with cancer

Sexual dysfunction may be multi-factorial; both physical and psychological factors contribute to its development. Physical factors include functional damage secondary to cancer therapies, fatigue and pain. In addition, cancer therapy such as surgery, chemotherapy, radiation therapy and bone marrow transplantation may have a direct physiological impact on sexual function (Watson et al. 1999). Medications used to treat pain, depression and other symptoms may contribute to sexual dysfunction. Psychological factors include misbeliefs about the origin of the cancer, guilt related to these misbeliefs, coexisting depression, changes in body image after surgery and stresses to personal relationships that occur secondary to cancer (Schover et al. 1997; Schover 1997). Increasing age is often believed to be associated with decreased sexual desire and performance; however, in one study, elderly men reported that sex remains important to their quality of life, that performance can be maintained into the 70s and 80s, and that altered sexual function is distressing (Helgasen et al. 1996).

Effect on relationships

The patient may or may not have an available partner at the time of diagnosis. Sexuality should be taken no less seriously by the clinician or the patient if there is no partner. For patients with a partner, the health care professional should consider and discuss the duration, quality and stability of the relationship before diagnosis. In addition, as many women fear rejection and abandonment, the health care professional should enquire about the partner's response to the illness and the woman's concerns about the impact of treatment on their partner (McNeff 1997; Stead 2004; Wimberly et al. 2005). Partners share many of the same reactions as the women, in that their most significant concerns typically relate to loss and fear of death. Moreover, the partner's physical, sexual and emotional health should be considered relative to his/her previous and current sexual status in a complete assessment. The health care professional should recognise that most couples experience difficulty discussing sexual preferences, concerns and fears, even under ideal circumstances and that sexual communication problems tend to worsen with illness and threat of death.

Assessment tools

There are no clear guidelines to address sexuality during the stages of cancer and its treatment (National Cancer Institute 2009). It has been well documented that most patients do not volunteer information about sexual problems, and that health care providers should incorporate at least a brief sexual assessment into routine health histories and medical evaluations. Whilst not every nurse can be a sexual counsellor, listening to concerns of patient and family, presenting factual information in a non-threatening manner, managing non-complex disease and treatment related symptoms, and providing appropriate referrals can be easily incorporated into routine care (Krebs 2007).

Health care professionals should assist women and their partners by asking specific open-ended questions to validate the importance of sexual health concerns. There are a number of articles and resources available to help address sexual assessment (Lamb and Woods 1981; Lamb 1996; Auchincloss 1989; Schover 1997). The Kaplan model provides a useful template to interview and assess women re sexual issues (Kaplan 1983). It focuses on:

- The chief complaint
- Sexual status
- Psychiatric status
- Family and psychological history
- Relationship assessment
- Summary
- Recommendations

The PLISSIT model (Annon 1975) is another model of assessment and intervention now widely used for sexual rehabilitation of cancer patients. Below are detailed the various elements of this model:

Permission

Permission to have or not have sexual thoughts, feelings or concerns begins at initial consultation. It is up to the oncology health care professional to initiate the discussion of sexual matters related to diagnosis and therapy. If the health care professional does not provide a safe and open environment for sexual discussion, it is unlikely that the patient will broach the subject.

Limited information

Specific factual information about the impact therapy will have on sexual function should be part of the treatment decision-making process. It should dispel myths about cancer or therapy (e.g. breast cancer is not caused by too much fondling, sex will not infect the partner with cancer, sex after radiation therapy will not cause the partner to become radioactive, etc.). This information should also begin with a general statement about available treatments for sexual dysfunctions that will be discussed in detail as therapy continues and as the next level of the model is reached.

Specific suggestion

A sexual history is necessary before providing specific suggestions. It is necessary to know if the sexual dysfunction the patient faces is related to sexual organ dysfunction, changes in body image, treatment related side effects or relationship discord. Once the problems are diagnosed, concrete methods of dealing with them should be presented in language the patient can understand.

This level of the model requires a comfort and knowledge of sexuality beyond the medical jargon that would be sufficient in the first two levels. It also requires a variety of approaches that includes teaching new sexual behaviours, new options for sexual expression, improved communication skills, and medical and surgical intervention.

Intensive therapy

When the patient's sexual function is severely prolonged, existed before cancer diagnosis or treatment, or is related to marital problems, intensive therapy is required. The patient should also be referred for more intensive therapy when sexual counselling is beyond the knowledge or comfort level of the health care professional. It has been estimated that only about 30% of cancer patients would require referrals at this level of the P-LI-SS-IT model (Yarbro 2004)

When a sexual problem has been identified, the most important assessment tool for the health care professional is the clinical interview with the woman or couple (Schover and Jensen 1988). The assessment should include:

- Current sexual status
- Pre-morbid sexual functioning
- Relationship status
- Psychological status
- Past medical history

(National Cancer Institute 2009)

The multidisciplinary team may be involved and are required to communicate effectively as they manage different aspects of sexual morbidity. It is important for the health care professional assessing the woman to be aware of a local psychosexual therapy service to refer the woman/couple to if required, rather than unearthing significant issues and then being unable to manage them.

Management of sexual issues

Although research is beginning to clarify the frequency and types of sexual problems women with cancer experience, few treatment programmes for sexual dysfunction in cancer patients have been designed or tested. Sexual rehabilitation programmes, which integrate medical and psychological modalities aimed at the treatment of sexual dysfunction in those who have had cancer, are required to enhance and improve this quality of life area. In addition, these programmes must be cost-effective and accessible to women (National Cancer Institute 2009).

Women are often apprehensive about the first sexual experience after treatment and can often begin a pattern of sexual avoidance. Mixed signals are often sent to their partners that can lead to avoidance of general intimacy and touch. The partner may also contribute to the generalised avoidance of intimacy through his or her reluctance to initiate any behaviour, which may be perceived as pressure to be more intimate or may contribute to any potential physical discomfort from greater expression of physical intimacy. It is often this lack of communication between partners that can lead to relationship issues. A health care professional has a role to reassure women and their significant others that even when intercourse is difficult or impossible, their sexual activity is not necessarily over. They may need to look at new ways to give and receive pleasure and satisfaction by expressing their love and intimacy with their hands, mouths, tongues and lips. Providers should encourage the couple to express affection in alternative ways (e.g. hugging, kissing, non-genital touching) until they feel ready to resume sexual activity. The couple should be encouraged to communicate honest feelings, concerns and preferences.

Each woman is assessed individually and may have a number of physical, psychological and emotional issues that impact on their sexuality or relationship. Often a combination of medical treatments and sexual rehabilitation programmes may be required to provide full sexual rehabilitation for the woman.

Listed below are some specific treatments for various sexual dysfunctions; however, no two cases are identical and for some women with sexual issues following cancer treatment a simple intervention may be all that is required, whereas for others the issues may be complex and require various other health/psychological professionals.

Sexual desire disorders

These have the lowest rate (25–35%) of successful treatment amongst sexual dysfunctions. Aetiological complexity, the importance of relationship issues, frustration at a lack of intimacy or poor interest in improving sexual relations with the current partner may explain why the response to treatment is generally so disappointing, particularly in unmotivated patients (Plaut et al. 2004).

Therapy may involve:

- HRT
- A hypoprolactinemic drug. if a high prolactin level was found
- Thyroxine if hypothyroidism was diagnosed
- A low dose antidepressant. if a mood disorder is a cofactor
- Better glycaemic control in diabetics
- Review of medication. which may lead to loss of libido
- Lifestyle improvement, e.g. reduce alcohol and smoking
- Weight control
- Regular exercise
- Better diet
- Sleep improvement, to improve fatigue
- Appropriate counselling and medical support following cancer treatment
- Refer to psychosexual counsellor or Relate, if problem more likely psychological, relationship or partner related factors

Sexual arousal disorders

Therapy may involve:

- HRT
- Rehabilitation of the pelvic floor
- Non-hormonal drugs in those that cannot have hormones, e.g. hormone dependant cancers (e.g. sildenafil)
- EROS clitoral therapy device to improve vascular response

Orgasmic disorders

These can either be primary or secondary orgasmic disorders.

A health care provider for women who have a cancer diagnosis is more likely to find a woman who has acquired orgasmic difficulties.

The therapy may involve:

- managing urge or mixed incontinence, which may lead to inhibition of orgasm
- treating any hormonal imbalance with systemic and/or local HRT
- treating pelvic floor inadequacies
- review medication that may lead to orgasm inhibition
- address relationship issues
- address partner issues

Sexual pain disorders

These may be multi-factorial in nature, especially if the problem becomes chronic.

Dypareunia therapy may involve:

- Addressing psychological and or organic cause, collaborating with colleagues
- Treat recurrent infections, e.g. bacterial vaginosis
- Restore normal pH
- Teach relaxation techniques
- Refer to physiotherapists re pelvic floor disorders
- Analgesia as to the nature of the pain
- Use of lubricants
- Dilator therapy

Vaginismus therapy may involve:

- Depending on the anxiety/phobia level, treat with anxiolytics or low-dose SSRI
- Address underlying negative affects
- Encourage self contact, massage and awareness through sexual education
- Teach the role of pelvic floor exercises
- Dilator therapy
- If in a relationship, encourage foreplay
- Discuss contraception if relevant
- Encourage sharing of control in intimacy
- Psychosexual therapist referral may also be required

Hormones

Although ovarian hormones play an important role in the maintenance of sexual health in women, a large body of evolving information about sexual functioning (and dysfunction) suggests that these hormones may be necessary but not sufficient to overcome disorders of desire and arousal in women (Basson 2003). The long-term safety of oestrogen supplementation has been challenged by the results of the Women's Health Initiative hormone studies (Rossouw et al. 2002), and there is limited long-term safety data for androgen supplementation in healthy women (Wierman et al. 2006).

Management of vaginal dryness with non-oestrogen or low-dose vaginal oestrogen preparations may be an important first step that all clinicians can institute in their symptomatic patients (Ganz et al. 2000).

Conclusion

Managing sexual issues is becoming more acceptable amongst health care professionals and with additional advice and training this important issue will hopefully continue to develop, so that women who have undergone cancer treatment can feel comfortable and confident to discuss their sexual concerns and know they will be addressed.

Effective management of diminished sexual desire in women with a cancer history must take a comprehensive approach (Basson 2006). Health care professionals, who wish to assist their female cancer survivors who complain of diminished sexual desire, should pay careful attention to the partner relationship and its quality, the woman's body image and mental health, as well as vaginal dryness and dyspareunia, which can provide aversive conditioning for engaging in sexual activity and thus decrease desire. Identification and modification of medications that are known to contribute to low desire can also be very helpful in these situations (e.g. opiates, selective serotonin reuptake inhibitors). Although not all clinicians will be prepared to provide counselling for all of the issues associated with sexual functioning, at a minimum they can identify the patient's needs and provide appropriate referrals.

The success of treatment for female sexual dysfunction depends on the underlying cause of the problem. The outlook is good for dysfunction that is related to a treatable or reversible physical condition. Mild dysfunction that is related to stress, fear or anxiety often can be successfully treated with counselling, education and improved communication between partners.

Reflective points

- Most women will not ask health care professionals questions about sexual function; plan a standard question or assessment that could be used in your clinical setting that ensured that sexual function is offered up for discussion to patients.
- Discuss with your team the information and support available for the patients being treated in your care with regard psychosexual services.

References

Algier, L. and Kav, S. (2008) Nurses' approach to sexuality-related issues in patient receiving cancer treatments. *Turkey Journal of Cancer* **38(3)**, 135–41.

Anastasia, P.J. (1998) Altered Sexuality. In: R.M. Carroll-Johnson, L.M. Gorman and N.J. Bush (Eds) *Psychosocial Nursing Care along the Cancer Continuum*. Pittsburgh: Oncology Nursing Press Inc, pp. 227–40.

Annon, J.S. (1975) *The Behavioral Treatment of Sexual Problems.* Vol. 1. Honolulu, Hawaii: Enabling Systems, Inc.

Auchincloss, S.S. (1989) Sexual dysfunction in cancer patients: issues in evaluation and treatment. In: J.C. Holland, and J.H. Rowland (Eds) *Handbook of Psychooncology: Psychological Care of the Patient with Cancer.* New York: Oxford University Press, pp. 383–413.

Basson, R., Berman, J. and Burnett, A. (2000) Report of the International Consensus Development Conference on female sexual dysfunction: definitions and classifications. *Journal of Urology* **163.** 888–93.

Basson, R. (2001) Female sexual response: the role of drugs in the management of sexual dysfunction *Obstetric Gynecology* **98(2)**, 350–3.

Basson, R. (2003) Biopsychosocial models of women's sexual response: applications to management of 'desire disorders'. *Sexual Relationship Therapy* **18**, 107–15.

Basson, R. (2006) Sexual desire and arousal disorders in women. *New England Journal of Medicine* **35**, 1497–506.

Broeckel, J.A., Thors, C.L. and Jacobsen, P.B. (2002) Sexual functioning in long-term breast cancer survivors treated with adjuvant chemotherapy. *Breast Cancer Research and Treatment* **5(3)**, 241–8.

Bruner, D.W. and Berk, L. (2004) Altered body image and sexual health. In: C.H. Yarbro, M.H. Frodge and. M. Goodman (Eds) *Cancer Symptom Management.* Sudbury, MA: Jones & Bartlett, pp. 597–623.

Derogatis, L.R. and Kourlesis, S.M. (1981) An approach to evaluation of sexual problems in the cancer patient. *Cancer Journal of Clinicians* **31(1)**, 46–50.

Ganz, P.A., Rowland, J.H. and Desmond, K. (1998) Life after breast cancer: understanding women's health-related quality of life and sexual functioning. *Journal of Clinical Oncology* **16(2)**, 501–14.

Ganz, P.A., Greendale, G.A., Petersen, L., Zibecchim, L., Kahnm, B. and Belin, T.R. (2000) Managing menopausal symptoms in breast cancer survivors: results of a randomized controlled trial. *Journal of National Cancer Institute* **92**, 1054–64.

Helgason, A.R., Adolfsson, J. and Dickman, P. (1996) Sexual desire, erection, orgasm and ejaculatory functions and their importance to elderly Swedish men: a population-based study. *Age Ageing* **25(4)**, 285–91.

Herson, L., Hart, K.A. and, Gordon, M.J. (1999) Identifying and overcoming barriers to providing sexuality information in the clinical setting. *Rehabilitation Nursing* **24**, 148–51.

Hughes, M.K. (2000) Sexuality and the cancer survivor: a silent coexistence. *Cancer Nursing* **23**, 477–82.

Jenkins, M. and Ashley, J. (2002) Sex and the oncology patient. *American Journal of Nursing* **102(Suppl 4)**, 13–5.

Kaplan, H.S. (1974) *The New Sex Therapy.* New York: Brunner/Mazel Inc.

Kaplan, H.S. (1983) *The Evaluation of Sexual Disorders: Psychological and Medical Aspects.* New York: Brunner/Mazel Inc.

Katz, A. (2003) Sexuality after hysterectomy: a review of the literature and discussion of the nurses' role. *Journal of Advanced Nursing* **42**, 297–303..

Krebs, L. (2007) Sexual assessment: research and clinical. *Nursing Clinics of North America* **42(4)**, 515–29.

Lamb, M.A. and Woods, N.F. (1981) Sexuality and the cancer patient. *Cancer Nursing* **4(2)**, 137–44.

Lamb, M.A. (1996) Sexuality and sexual functioning. In: R. McCorkle, M. Grant, M. Frank-Stromborg, et al. (Eds) *Cancer Nursing: A Comprehensive Textbook*, 2nd edn. Philadelphia, PA: WB Saunders Co, pp. 1105–27.

Masters, W.H. and Johnson, V.E. (1966) *Human Sexual Response.* Boston, MA: Little, Brown.

Mckee, A.L. and Schover, L.R. (2001) Sexuality rehabilitation. *Cancer* **92(Suppl 4)**, 1008–12.

McNeff, E.A. (1997) Issues for the partner of the person with a disability. In: M.L. Sipski and C.J. Alexander (Eds) *Sexual Function in People with Disability and Chronic Illness*. Gaithersburg, MD: Aspen Publishers, Inc, pp. 595–616.

National Cancer Institute (2009) *US National Institutes of Health Sexuality and Reproductive Issues* http://www.cancer.gov

Parker Jones, K., Kingsberg, S. and Whipple, B. (2005) *Nurture your Nature*: *Inspiring Women's Health Sexual Wellness Initiative*. A collaboration between the National Women's Health Resource Center and the Association for Reproductive Health Professionals. Funded by an educational grant from Proctor & Gamble.

Plaut, S.M., Graziottin, A. and Heaton, J. (2004) *Sexual Dysfunction Fast Facts*. Oxford: Health Press Ltd.

Quinn, B. (2003) Sexual health in cancer care. *Nursing Times* **99**, 33–4.

Quinn, M. (2007) Sexual Function after treatment of gynaecological cancer sexologies. *Cancer and Sexual Function* **16(4)**, 286–91.

Rogers, M. and Kristjanson, L.J. (2002) The impact on sexual functioning of chemotherapy induced menopause in women with breast cancer. *Cancer Nursing* **25**, 57–65.

Rossouw, J.E., Anderson, G.L., Prentice, R.L., LaCroix, A.Z., Kooperberg, C. and Stefanick, M.L. (2002) Risks and benefits of estrogen plus progestin in healthy postmenopausal women: principal results from the Women's Health Initiative randomized controlled trial. *JAMA* **288**, 321–33.

Schover, L.R. and Jensen, S.B. (1988) *Sexuality and Chronic Illness*. Philadelphia: Guilford Publications.

Schover, L.R., Montague, D.K. and Lakin, M.M. (1997) Sexual problems. In: V.T. DeVita, S. Hellman and S.A. Rosenberg (Eds) *Cancer: Principles and Practice of Oncology*, 5th edn. Philadelphia, PA: Lippincott-Raven Publishers, pp. 2857–72.

Schover, L.R. (1997) *Sexuality and Fertility after Cancer*. New York: John Wiley & Sons.

Stead, M.L. (2004) Sexual function after treatment for gynecological malignancy. *Current Opinion Oncology* **16(5)**, 492–5.

Thaler-DeMers, D. (2001) Intimacy issues: sexuality, fertility and relationships. *Seminars Oncology Nursing* **17**, 255–62.

Tiefer, L. (2000) Working Group on *A New View of Women's Sexual Problems*. *Electronic Journal of Human Sexuality* 2000: 3. www.ejhs.org/volume 3/newview.htm.

Yarbro, C. (2004) Response cycle and sexual dysfunction. *Clinical Journal of Oncological Nursing* **8**, 84–6.

Watson, M., Wheatley, K. and Harrison, G.A. (1999) Severe adverse impact on sexual functioning and fertility of bone marrow transplantation, either allogeneic or autologous, compared with consolidation chemotherapy alone: analysis of the MRC AML 10 trial. *Cancer* **86(7)**, 1231–9.

Whipple, B. and Brash-McGreer, K. (1997) Management of female sexual dysfunction. In: M.L. Sipski and C.J. Alexander (Eds) *Sexual Function in People with Disability and Chronic Illness. A Health Professional's Guide*. Gaithersburg, MD: Aspen Publishers, Inc, pp. 509–34.

Wierman, M.E., Basson, R., Davis, S.R., Khosla, S., Miller, K.K. and Rosner, W. (2006) Androgen therapy in women: an endocrine society clinical practice guideline. *Journal of Clinical Endocrinology and Metabolism*. **91**, 3697–710.

Wilmoth, M.C. (1998) Sexuality. In: Burke CC (Ed) *Psychological Dimensions of Oncology Nursing Care*. Pittsburgh: Oncology Nursing Press Inc, pp. 103–27.

Wimberly, S.R., Carver, C.S. and Laurenceau, J.P. (2005) Perceived partner reactions to diagnosis and treatment of breast cancer: impact on psychosocial and psychosexual adjustment. *Journal of Consulting Clinical Psychology*. **73(2)**, 300–11.

Chapter 16

Women and Cancer: Rehabilitation and Survivorship

Alison Keen

Learning points

At the end of this chapter the reader will have an understanding of:
- The concepts of rehabilitation and survivorship
- The impact of a cancer diagnosis and treatment on women
- Policy and health care plans for cancer rehabilitation

Introduction

The aim of this chapter is to describe the experience of rehabilitation and survivorship by discussing relevant and recent research and papers on these concepts. Supporting the theory will be the lived experience of women with cancer. Therefore, it is from the backdrop of women coping with the continuing effects of the diagnosis and treatment of cancer that form the themes for this chapter. The impact of living with cancer and the way in which rehabilitation can improve that experience will be discussed, with reference to the concept of coping and living with uncertainty and its affect on survivorship. Women with breast and gynaecological cancers share many of the physical, psychological and psychosocial problems experienced by other oncology patients. These may not be seen as unique to this group of patients, if seen as individual effects of their cancer. However, there are frequently multiple problems faced by these women that as a whole *can* be seen as unique, a view supported by Corney et al. (1992) and Hamilton (1999). Qualitative data reviewed by Ersek et al. (1997) shows that for many women dealing with cancer it is not just about themselves, but that the impact on the family is the main cause for concern. Many studies (Cain et al. 1983; Corney et al. 1992; Ersek et al. 1997) have shown that women with cancer are often faced with many losses all at the same time, which can include loss of fertility, sexual function, sexual desire, identity as a woman, self-esteem and role (see also Chapter 14 on Fertility and Chapter 15 on Sexual Health and Dysfunction).

Women's Cancers, First Edition. Edited by Alison Keen and Elaine Lennan.
© 2011 Blackwell Publishing Ltd. Published 2011 by Blackwell Publishing Ltd.

There are many detailed qualitative papers describing the prolonged phase of chronic cancer (Andersen 1992; Body et al. 1997; Doyle 2008, Fallowfield 1990; Quigley 1989), where patients experience symptoms from disease, side effects from treatments and live with the emotional burden of the uncertainty of surviving the disease. In addition to the many complex emotional responses, Ersek et al. (1997) report some positive outcomes of post-treatment survival for women with ovarian cancer that include an appreciation of life, an improvement in some relationships and the taking up of healthier lifestyles. However, many women describe continual anxiety, a fear for the future and depression, and this highlights the heterogeneous nature of survivorship (Andersen 1992). The patients' experience of survivorship and their perspective on rehabilitation will be highlighted, with the aim to interpret the cancer experience and coping mechanisms used by women with cancer.

Rehabilitation

Rehabilitation could not be discussed fully without quality of life (QoL) being explored; as Fallowfield (1990) stresses 'Failure to attempt to monitor QoL is neither good medicine, nor is it good science.' p. 647.

Ferrel et al. (2003) reminds us that social well-being is one vital aspect of patients' overall QoL. This for women with cancer predominately means being able to fulfil roles, and for women with advanced cancer this translates into a prevalent concern being for the welfare of family and friends and the worry about burdening them with their own care (Houck et al. 1999). Kornblith et al. (2001) show the importance of social support in women with breast cancer, in that a lack of support increases stress and psychological morbidities. All of these studies show that the impact of cancer on women affect not only the physical, but also manifest into all areas of QoL.

Rehabilitation is described by Wells (1990) and detailed in the NHS Cancer Reform Strategy (2007), as not being simply a process, but also a philosophy of care that provides an attitude of hope and encouragement, the goal being to ensure that the control remains with the patient. This interpretation means that rehabilitation is not about doing things for people, but about enabling them to do things. Graham Pole (2000) describes recovery and rehabilitation in refreshingly unconventional terms. He says that the factors that empower us to recover from illness are poorly understood and that medical treatment is only one component and may not be the dominant one. It is the patient who must be a partner in the process of healing, by building on inherent resources. Women often have an incredible capacity to find these resources to enable them to continue functioning in their roles as carers, mothers and partners. Rehabilitation is recommended by many authors to start at diagnosis (David 1998; Lehman et al. 1988: DOH 2007; Wells 1990). Ersek et al (1997) discovered that rehabilitation is an important factor in enhancing the QoL in cancer survivorship. He asked women with ovarian cancer what QoL meant to them. The majority of the responses were being happy, being able to enjoy life and the ability to sustain good relationships. Quigley (1989) describes a period that she calls 're-entry', as a time when the cancer survivor resumes roles and functions that were previously disrupted. Survivors are confronted by the possibility of long-term or permanent functional and psychological losses, even when cured of cancer (Dudas and Carlson 1988). Gambosi and Ulreich (1990) believe that there are interventions that can help people surviving cancer to rehabilitate. They found that health care professionals could influence the quality of cancer survival by providing opportunities for discussion, education, information and perceived support, and benefit the cancer survivor by helping to identify coping methods to aid rehabilitation. As part of the Cancer Reform Strategy, the National Cancer Survivorship has been launched to provide supportive measures for 'people living with and beyond cancer' (p. 33). These measures include psychological support, the planning of supportive care by allied health care professionals (e.g. physiotherapists and occupational therapists); and continuity of care. The role of the Clinical Nurse Specialist in providing these supportive measures is stressed. More work needs to be done on incredibly important issues arising from surviving cancer, which include post-treatment care, managing progressive and recurrent disease, late effects of treatment, childhood and young people who survive cancer, work and financial issues, and self care.

Rehabilitation specific to women with cancer

Hamilton (1999) reports on women struggling with the change of role imposed on them by illness, meaning that commonly the role changes from being that of caregiver to being dependent on others. She discusses poignantly the complex needs of women with ovarian cancer. She highlights that some women are afraid to 'reconnect' with their children and partners as a result of their fears of recurrence; feeling that they could not risk the closeness as they might have to 're-distance' themselves before letting go again. Ersek et al. (1997) finds that there is a strong link between gender and perceptions of cancer survivorship. This supports the notion that many women with cancer have identified relationships with partners and children as having a significant effect on QoL. This is blamed on feelings of guilt due to hurt and pain being experienced by significant others, and being unable to fulfil one's role and needing to accept help.

> *The worst thing I've ever had to do in my life was to sit my kids Jeremy and Gail down (they were 8 and 6 at the time) and tell them that I had cancer. They wanted to know what was going to happen to me and who was going to look after them.*
>
> Mary, a 51-year-old single parent with ovarian cancer

Psychosocial reactions to the diagnosis of cancer were measured by Cain et al. (1983) and described in terms of mood changes and functional difficulties following diagnosis. Data was compared with women from the normal population and women who were attending psychiatric outpatient centres. Levels of anxiety and depression were observed to be much higher than in the normal population and equal to that of women who were attending a psychiatric outpatient centre. This study goes on to demonstrate the effectiveness of psychological intervention for women; anxiety and depression levels were lowered compared with those in the control group. This notion is further validated by Gordon (1980), who describe education, counselling and advocacy as strategies to help women resume daily activities.

Taking control by strength of personality

Many women cite that by regaining a sense of control and equilibrium, through sheer force of will and strength of character, is a positive coping mechanism. This was highlighted by one woman who had been treated twice for her cancer, as she was clear that one of the things that helped her was 'my own personality and will to survive and stubbornness'.

Believing in one's own ability to fight the cancer and win is a theme very much related by women with cancer and linked to remaining positive. A representative comment from a woman who had been diagnosed twice with cancer was:

> *...because I think personality is 90% of it, because I think if you believe, you have to believe that you are going to get well. I thought I might die. A year on here I am, fine and if you believe that you will be alright ... do all the stuff that makes you feel good about yourself and believe it. Then you will get well.*
>
> Pam, a 65-year-old teacher with endometrial cancer

Making positive lifestyle changes

Lifestyle changes reported by women include taking homeopathic medicines, exercise, avoiding food and drink that they believe might be linked to their particular cancer, eating organic produce and regular massage. A comment from a woman who had completed treatment for ovarian cancer 2 years previously was:

> *I am trying really hard to do everything I possibly can for it not to come back again. I feel as if I have been given another chance. So my chance was to give something back. So that's why we're going to run this cancer stall.*

Support

Many women talk about the support that they receive in helping them to cope with cancer. The most common forms of support mentioned come from partners, family and friends on both a practical and emotional level. Women with cancer often describe a sense of 'aloneness' that the diagnosis carries with it. This can sometimes be remedied by the perceived support of other patients and involvement in support groups. Sharing the experience can dispel the sense of isolation that women can feel, by making them realise that they are not the only one faced with this experience. This includes support from health care professionals, doctors, nurses and other allied health care professionals. This is described as showing kindness, normalising the situation and going out of their way to be helpful and also giving information at just the right time.

Commonly, women cope by actively supporting and helping others. Examples of kindness and helpfulness are offering to 'mentor' new patients and fund-raising for cancer units or charities.

Cancer survivorship

Doyle (2008) in her paper on survivorship tells us that '…cancer survivorship in adults is a process beginning at diagnosis and involving uncertainty. It is a life-changing experience with a duality of positive and negative aspects.' (p. 1).

A 44-year-old woman, who had yearly follow-up for breast cancer 5 years after treatment said:

> *Having cancer was in an odd way one of the best things that ever happened to me. I gave up my job in management and applied for a job on a stud farm. My salary is half of what it used to be, but I was brought up with horses and I want to spend the rest of my life doing a job that I enjoy.*

With improvements in diagnosis and treatments for cancer, the numbers of people surviving are increasing (Macmillan Cancer Support 2008). Whether the person is cancer-free for life, or lives with cancer, they are still survivors, however long their period of survivorship (Quigley 1989). Who qualifies as a survivor still remains a concept for debate (Rose 1989; Ganz 2005). As Mullan (1985), a physician who developed cancer, reminds us, there is no moment of cure; this means that however long or short the period of survivorship, the person should be armed with the resources and supportive means to survive well. Resources, be they external to the patient or the resourcefulness the person finds from within as a result of previous experiences, are integral to the concept of coping with the disease and treatment. Kagawa-Singer (1993) finds when examining the coping mechanisms of 50 patients with cancer, in order to cope well people need to 'broaden the concept of health'. She describes patient's health concept not as being influenced by their cancer diagnosis, but as being inherent to the person's sense of self-integrity and capabilities.

A woman with recurrent endometrial cancer was a marathon runner and incredibly fit. She said that she felt healthy despite having cancer. It is a belief supported by Wells (1990), who suggests that viewing health and illness at opposite ends of a continuum is archaic and has hampered the success of many health promoting strategies. Frank-Stromburg (1986) reinforces this perspective by advocating that health seen as an absence of illness has made it … 'impossible to discuss healthy aspects of the sick individual.'(p. 38). This matters when focusing on the rehabilitation and survivorship of people with cancer means focusing on the whole person, and optimising their wellness by promoting their good health. This contributes to the patient regaining a sense of control, which in turn can have a positive impact on how they cope with their disease, treatment and rehabilitation.

Jenny, a 50-year-old woman, diagnosed 2 years ago with stage IV ovarian cancer, discussing the impact of living with cancer said:

> *I think I took my health for granted. Because I was one of those uniquely healthy people, who don't get ill … I have changed, I feel very differently about life. I don't get so worried about things that aren't important, I don't work to such pressure. I feel well*

as a part of my lifestyle changes. With regards my health, I eat more healthily now, mainly fruit and vegetables and carrots. Lots of fresh fruit and vegetables. I always have three meals a day. Whereas before I used to skip lunch or eat on the move. From the very beginning of my day, when I wake up in the morning, I very consciously wake and greet the day. I wake with a real sense of the night being over and the days started; I am more conscious, I do things more consciously, I live more consciously.

Surviving well – despite the fear of recurrence

Fear of recurrent disease is a very common concern for many people diagnosed with cancer. This is often expressed in terms of living with uncertainty of survival, with the disruption this causes to everyday peace of mind. One woman who had finished treatment for cervical cancer 2 years previously, still worried about recurrence whenever she was reminded by a media report, attending a follow-up clinic or experiencing the odd ache or pain:

> *…now the slightest pain and I think oh, oh, no please God no. God knows what I would be like if one day I was told it had come back.*

Uncertainty is a part of life after cancer (Dow 2003; Doyle 2008). Women with early stage gynaecological cancer often express as much concern and fear as women with later stage disease (Keen 2000). The women reported a heightened awareness of the possibility of recurrence, particularly before 'follow-up' appointments. This is being addressed in some cancer centres by offering telephone follow-up to some patients, rather than hospital visits, to minimise the psychological stress. Also, there is evidence that follow-up appointments rarely coincide with disease recurrence (Auchincloss 1995) and need to be re-evaluated nationally as part of the Cancer Reform Strategy (DOH 2009).

The essence of applying the Cancer Reform Strategy (DOH 2009) to the lived experience of people after completion of their primary cancer treatment will be facilitated through the Cancer Intelligence Initiative. The strategy does focus on patient experience and survivorship, identifying a broader deeper support that needs to be developed nationally. Before this can be developed, there are many unanswered questions, a fundamental one being the number of cancer survivors. Cancer Relief Macmillan has an awareness-raising initiative called '2 million reasons to. …', based on the calculation that there are 2 million people surviving cancer. However, more accurate data needs to be assimilated to calculate the prevalence, so as to be clearer about the 'burden of care' (Corner 2009).

Some strategic models looking at survivorship compare living life after cancer with the lives of people living with a chronic illness (Hewitt et al. 2003; Macmillan Cancer Survivorship Survey 2008). These studies compared the experiences of three groups: people with cancer' people with a long-standing chronic illness, and people who had neither cancer nor a chronic illness. The needs, issues and experiences were documented and showed that people surviving cancer gave similar accounts as people with chronic illness, the most obvious link between the two, being that both groups are always 'potentially ill'.

There continues to be a dearth of information on the short-, medium- and long-term effects of cancer treatment; the financial costs of cancer in terms of loss of income, loss of working hours, loss in household income and career prospects. Added to those burdens, there are also the insurance and mortgage implications.

A transformative framework is to being developed by The National Cancer Action Team (NCAT) in collaboration with other organisations, including the Department of Health, Macmillan Cancer Relief, National Workforce Review Team, Royal Colleges, Commissioners and Cancer Networks. Rehabilitation is now very politically appealing. Currently, the emphasis is to support self-management and promote recovery, thereby optimising well-being: this is a philosophy of care that is gathering momentum. At last the very special needs of people surviving cancer are being addressed. Despite many years of authors championing the case for rehabilitation, it is the politically powerful word…'survivorship' that has ensured that this ongoing area of care and support is being developed strategically and will eventually mean that people with cancer not only have optimal care and support during treatment, but as a vital part of their ongoing life. These essential areas of ongoing care have been researched, documented and recommended since the late 1980s and now, almost 30 years on, we are finally seeing political ownership and understanding of the needs of people after cancer treatment. It will be interesting to see how these reforms will be applied to enhance the experience of cancer survivors.

Gender health inequities

The issues of health disparities with relation to gender are receiving more attention; this is vital in ensuring that there is a continuing drive toward equity. The National Cancer Institute (NCI) in the USA is focusing their attention on understanding the causes of health inequalities and is developing strategies to overcome them. Research includes establishing the influences that social status and education have on cancer related interventions. This is important because many inequalities still exist. An example of this is in the USA, mortality rates have shown an encouraging decline and cancer survival rates have improved in the general population. However, in the black, Hispanic white and American Indian populations, women with breast cancer have higher mortality rates. Also noted is the fact that these poorer population groups have limited access to cancer screening. From the disparity in gender perspective, Ferrell et al. (2003) report in their analysis of women with ovarian cancer, that '…a diagnosis of ovarian cancer requires a woman to revaluate her interactions with family, friends and employers and cope with the unexpected and unwanted changes in areas spanning from financial stability to sexuality and fertility' (p. 647). Sherwin (1992) reminds us of inequities by stating that '…women represent half of the global population and one-third of the (paid) labour force, they receive only one-tenth of the world income and own less than 1% of world property' (p. 224).

In the UK, Andersen (2000) is clear that health inequity needs to be addressed by nurse scientists by placing…'focus on gender, racialisation and health, especially on how gender and race intersect to put racialised women at a disadvantage' (p. 220). The National Cancer Survivorship Initiative will aim to provide the resources necessary to provide the appropriate aftercare for cancer survivors. The focus of care will undoubtedly shift and services will need to be reconfigured accordingly.

Conclusion

Women with cancer have so many issues to cope with, and need the resources and support to optimise their health and survival. Cancer advocacy associations, charitable organisations, policy-makers, health care professionals and survivors themselves are all essential participants in recognising and facilitating this. The future for rehabilitation in cancer care is being forged ahead in the UK by a national review of rehabilitation services to provide a toolkit for mapping service provision, a 'best practice' approach for providing accurate commissioning of services; workforce provision assessment and peer review assessment will all play their part in ensuring a robust future for this essential aspect of ongoing care.

Reflective points

- Reflect back on a patient in your care who has had more than one mode of cancer treatment. What measures could be put in place to assess and provide that patient with access to relevant rehabilitation services?
- Discuss with women following cancer treatments the impact of their diagnosis and treatment on them and their family.

References

Andersen, B.L. (1992) Psychological interventions for cancer patients to enhance quality of life. *Journal of Consulting and Clinical Psychology* **60(40)**, 552–68.

Andersen, J.M. (2000) Gender, race, poverty, health and discourses of health reform in context of globalization: a postcolonial feminist perspective in policy research. *Nursing Inquiry* **7**, 220–9.

Auchincloss, S.S. (1995) After treatment. Psychosocial issues in gynaecological cancer survivorship. *Cancer Supplement* **76(10)**, 2117–24.

Body, J.J. (1997) The concept of rehabilitation in cancer patients. *Current Opinion in Oncology* **9(4)**, 332–40.

Cain, E.N., Kohorn, E.I., Quinlan, D.M., Schwartz, P.E., Latimer, K. and Rogers, L. (1983) Psychological reactions to the diagnosis of gynaecological cancer. *Obstetrics and Gynaecology* **62(5)**, 635–41.

Corney, E., Everett, H., Howells, A. and Crowther, M (1992) The care of patients undergoing surgery for gynaecological cancer: the need for emotional support and counselling. *Journal of Advanced Nursing* **17**, 667–1.

Department of Health (2007) Cancer Reform Strategy.

David, J. (Ed.) (1998) *Rehabilitation, Adding Quality to Quality of Life in Cancer Care Prevention, Treatment and Palliation*. London: Chapman Hall.

Dow, K.H. (2003) Challenges and opportunities in cancer survivorship research. *Oncology Nursing Forum* **30(3)**, 445–69.

Doyle, N. (2008) Cancer survivorship: evolutionary concept analysis. *Journal of Advanced Nursing* **10(1111)**, 1365–2648.

Dudas, S. and Carlson, C.E. (1988) Cancer rehabilitation. *Oncology Nursing Forum* **15(2)**, 183–8.

Ersek, M., Ferrel, B.R. and Dow, K.H. (1997) Quality of life in woman with ovarian cancer. *Western Journal of Nursing Research* **19**, 334–50.

Fallowfield, L. (1990) *The Quality of Life: The Missing Measurement in Healthcare*. Human Horizon Series. London: Souvenir Press.

Ferrell, B.R. et al. (2003) A quality analysis of social concerns of women with ovarian cancer. *Psycho-Oncology* **12**, 647–63.

Frank-Stromburg, M. (1986) Health promotion behaviours in ambulatory cancer patients:Facts or fiction. *Oncology Nursing Forum* **13(4)**, 37–43.

Gambosi, J.R. and Ulreich, S. (1990) Recovering from cancer: a nursing intervention program recognising survivorship. *Oncology Nursing Forum.* **17(2)**, 215–19.

Ganz, P.A. (2005) A teachable moment for oncologists: cancer survivors, 10 million strong and growing. *Journal of Clinical Oncology* **23(24)**, 5458–60.

Gordon, R.L. (1980) *Interviewing: Strategy, Techniques and Tactics*. New York: Dorsey Press.

Graham Pole, J. (2000) The marriage of art and science. *Society of Gynaecological Nurse Oncologists Annual Symposium*, Florida, USA.

Hamilton, A.B. (1999) Psychological aspects of ovarian cancer. *Gynaecological Oncology* **50**, 202–7.

Hewitt, J. et al. (2003) Cancer Survivors in us. *Journal of Gerontology* **58(1)**, 82–91.

Houck, K., Avis, N.E., Gallant, J.M. et al. (1999) Quality of life in advanced ovarian cancer: identifying specific concerns. *Journal of Palliative Medicine* **2**, 397–402.

Kagawa-Singer, M. (1993) Redefining health: living with cancer. *Society of Scientific Medicine* **37**, 295–304.

Keen, A.E. (2000) Rehabilitation in Gynaecological Cancer: The Patient's Perspective. Unpublished Dissertation as part of MSc – Southampton University.

Kornblith, A.B., Herdon, J.E. and Zuckerman, E. et al. (2001) Social support as a buffer to the psychological impact of stressful life events in women with breast cancer. *Cancer* **91(2)**, 443–54.

Lehman, J., Dehisa, J., Warren, G. et al. (1988) Cancer rehabilitation: assessment of need development and evaluation of a model of care. *Archives of Physical Medicine and Rehabilitation* **59(9)**, 410–9.

Macmillan Cancer Support (2008) *Health Well-being Survey.*

Macmillan Cancer Support (2008) *Cancer Prevalence in the UK*. Kings College London, Macmillan Cancer Support and National Intelligence Network.

Mullan, F. (1985) Seasons of survival: reflections of a physician with cancer. *New England Journal of Medicine* **313(25)**, 270–3.

Quigley, K.M. (1989) The adult cancer survivor: psychological consequences of cure. *Seminars in Oncology Nursing* **5(1)**, 63–9.

Rose, M.A. (1989) Health promotion and risk prevention: application for cancer survivors. *Oncology Nursing Forum* **16(3)**, 335–40.

Sherwin, S. (1992) *No Longer Patient: Feminist Ethics and Health Care*. Philadelphia: Temple University Press.

Wells, R.J. (1990) Rehabilitation: making the most of time. *Oncology Nursing Forum* **17(4)**, 503–7.

Chapter 17

Palliative Care

Jane Grant and Carol L. Davis

Learning points

At the end of this chapter the reader will have an understanding of:
- The scope of palliative care
- Organisational aspects of palliative care
- Psychological factors influencing care interventions
- Social and cultural factors
- The importance of spirituality to the concept of total care
- The management of a wide range of physical problems and symptoms in women with advanced cancer
- Ethical dilemmas in palliative care

Introduction

Palliative care has been defined as 'the active, total care of patients whose disease is not responsive to curative treatment'. Control of pain, of other symptoms and of psychological, social and spiritual problems is paramount. The goal of palliative care is achievement of the best quality of life for patients and their families. Many aspects of palliative care are also applicable earlier in the course of the illness in conjunction with anti-cancer treatments (WHO 1990). The primary aim of palliative care is to make the life that remains as comfortable and meaningful as possible, rather than to prolong life. It encompasses attention to detail in several domains:

- physical
- psychological
- social
- cultural
- spiritual

Women's Cancers, First Edition. Edited by Alison Keen and Elaine Lennan.
© 2011 Blackwell Publishing Ltd. Published 2011 by Blackwell Publishing Ltd.

As such, palliative care is practised, to a varying extent at any given time, by all health care professionals in a wide range of health care settings. The principles of palliative care are an integral part of good clinical practice.

The scope of palliative care

Optimal control of physical and psychological problems are vital aspects of palliative care, but they are not the only ones. Palliative care aims to allow the patient and their family to focus on issues that are important to them, which may include coping with changing roles, including issues around sexuality, emotional adjustment to progressive disease and death, and dealing with 'unfinished business', as well as best possible relief of their symptoms.

Many lay people and some doctors regard palliative care and terminal care as synonymous. This is not the case; terminal care is one part, albeit an important one, of palliative care, which may also include bereavement support if necessary. Most adults (but not children) with cancer will die of this disease. It has been argued, therefore, that in some patients, palliative care should begin at diagnosis. In general, as the role of specific anti-cancer treatments diminishes, that of palliative care increases, but this relationship is not linear and can vary at different stages of the disease process (Figure 17.1). Indeed, in some women's cancers with a good prognosis, such as ovarian germ cell tumours, the woman may have specialist palliative care needs, particularly relating to symptom control, at diagnosis. These needs will resolve with anti-cancer treatment and there is a high rate of cure. In such situations, specialist palliative care involvement should be short-term only. If relapse occurs, then fast-track referral back to specialist palliative care services may be appropriate (see variable model in Figure 17.1).

Although it is easy for a patient to see their need for palliative care in a negative light, it frequently engenders hope; hope for relief of pain, hope for adequate relief of other symptoms, and hope for a peaceful death (Herth 1990). Furthermore, rehabilitation is an important aspect of palliative care. Its remit is wider than that of physical rehabilitation and also encompasses psychological, spiritual and social rehabilitation of the patient and their family and friends.

Organisational aspects

Palliative care and end of life care are part of the remit of many health care professionals. The semantics of palliative care do not always seem straightforward. Those health care professionals who deliver palliative care and end of life care as part of their clinical role but who do not specialise in palliative care are usually termed palliative care generalists.

In the UK, several important Department of Health initiatives to improve end of life care delivered by palliative care generalists have been successfully rolled out over the last few years. In the recent National Audit Office Report on end of life care, 54% of general nurses and a third of doctors reported being trained in the use of at least one of the three National Institute for Health and Clinical Excellence (NICE) recommended approaches

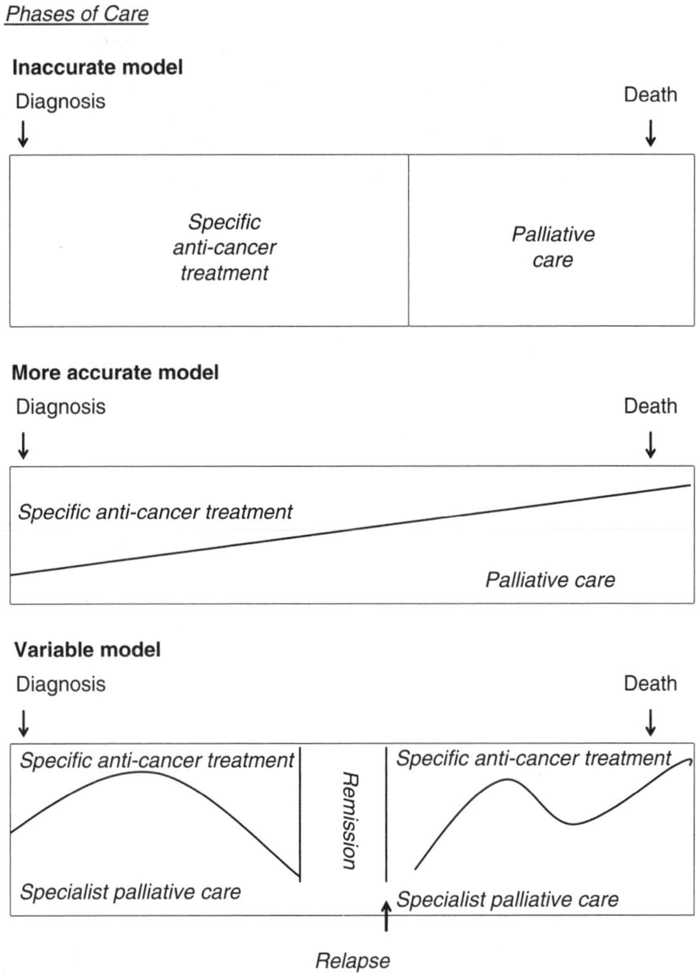

Phases of Care

Inaccurate model

Diagnosis   Death

↓   ↓

Specific anti-cancer treatment

Palliative care

More accurate model

Diagnosis   Death

↓   ↓

Specific anti-cancer treatment

Palliative care

Variable model

Diagnosis   Death

↓   ↓

Specific anti-cancer treatment   *Remission*   *Specific anti-cancer treatment*

Specialist palliative care   *Specialist palliative care*

Relapse

Figure 17.1   Depictions of the relationship between palliative care and specific anti-cancer treatment.

to end of life care (Gold Standards Framework, Liverpool Care Pathway or Preferred Priorities of Care). For those specialising in palliative care, the figures were 91% of nurses and 95% of doctors.

The National end of life care strategy was published in July 2008, with the aim of improving the provision of care for all adults approaching the end of their life, including support for their families and carers. The strategy sets out recommendations for both generalists and specialists in palliative care.

Specialist palliative care services are those services with palliative care as their core speciality, whose staff have developed a specific interest and expertise in the subject, and have additional qualifications relevant to the speciality. Such services provide care for patients with advanced cancer. Most also care for patients with HIV disease and motor neurone disease, whilst many provide a service that extends to those with other chronic non-malignant diseases. Worldwide, there is increasing disease and detection earlier in the course of the disease (NICE Guidance on Cancer Services, 2004 www.nice.org.uk/ nicemedia/pdf/osgspmanual.pdf, last accessed 21 September 2008). The general principles of palliative care apply to all these patients, but the detail and choice of therapeutic interventions vary. For specialists in palliative care, the challenge is to facilitate the provision of appropriate palliative care for all who need it, without becoming 'Jacks of all trades and masters of none'.

There is no single model for the provision of specialist palliative care services, which may include some or all of the following aspects:

- Specialist Domiciliary Care/Advice
  - Nursing
  - Medical
  - Occupational Therapy; Physiotherapy; Social Work
  - Some 'hospice at home' services
- Inpatient Care
  - Hospice/in-patient unit
  - Designated beds/ward within a general/specialist hospital
  - Occupational Therapy; Physiotherapy; Social Work
- Outpatient Clinics
- Day Care
- Hospital palliative care team providing advice/support for inpatients, and occasionally outpatients, in general/specialist hospitals
- Support Groups for Carers
- Bereavement Support
- Education
- Research

These services are provided by a multi-disciplinary team, often supplemented by trained volunteers. A multi-disciplinary specialist palliative care team usually includes nurses, doctors, physiotherapists, occupational therapists, chaplains and social workers (NICE Guidance on Cancer Services, 2004 www.nice.org.uk/nicemedia/pdf/osgspman-ual.pdf, last accessed 21 September 2008). People with advanced cancer are usually based at home and so the focus of care must be in the community. The patient remains under the care of their general practitioner/family doctor and the rest of the primary health care team. The palliative care team provides advice and support for the patient, their family and the primary health care team, and works alongside appropriate health care professionals in both secondary and tertiary care, including interventional radiologists, site specific clinical nurse specialists, clinical and medical oncologists, and surgeons.

Psychological factors

It is almost impossible to separate the psychological aspects of cancer from the physical, social, cultural and spiritual aspects, even in the same person. They are closely inter-related and influence each other (Figure 17.2).

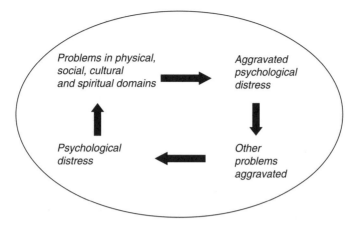

Figure 17.2   The inter-relationship of psychological and other factors in patients with advanced cancer.

Receiving bad news can generate a wide range of feelings including fear, sadness, horror and anger. Uncertainty fuels anxiety. A person can react to the news of a diagnosis of cancer, recurrence, incurable disease, impending death or to living with cancer, in more than one way, and the balance of feelings and reactions varies across time. It is important to remember that, in general, there is no right or wrong way to face up to these situations and each person will have their own individual concerns (Jeffrey 2006).

A simple question such as 'How does this leave you feeling?' encourages a person to ventilate their feelings. The old adage 'A problem shared, is a problem halved' often holds true; feelings do not need answers, they need listening to.

A wide range of coping strategies might be employed by a patient. Different patients employ different coping strategies at different times and so do their families and close friends. It is important, although not always easy, to recognise when such coping mechanisms become maladaptive. Persistent anger, pathological anxiety or depression must be addressed. It can be particularly difficult to delineate appropriate sadness from clinical depression.

Assessment of psychological problems and psychological care must be an integral part of the overall care of patients with malignant disease. Such psychological care should always be individualised and should be aimed at facilitating and strengthening that person's adaptive and coping mechanisms. To achieve this, those involved in the delivery of cancer care need to:

- Think of the patient as a person within a family unit
- Employ good listening skills
- Communicate openly and honestly
- Have a caring attitude and be alongside the patient and their problems
- Adequately assess problems in all the domains of care
- Negotiate realistic goals with the patient
- Recognise that a patient's problems and their needs change over time, and review and revise plans and goals accordingly.

Some patients will require more formal psychological intervention, for example, relaxation therapy, counselling or psychotherapy.

Social factors

A basic tenet of palliative care philosophy is that the patient is regarded as part of a unit, which also includes his or her family, friends and carers (Sheldon 1997). These people are linked by a series of complex relationships, which may be strengthened, weakened and/ or changed by the challenge of incurable disease. The response of an individual to the knowledge that, say, their partner is going to die will, in turn, affect that partner. Problems encountered include not only the distress and anxiety that such news will cause, but also the need to change roles and to adopt new ones. The patient is often distressed for their partner. Palliative care extends beyond the patient and includes all those close to them. Specific physical problems related to both local and distant disease spread can have a profound effect on the patient, her family/carers and their relationships. Examples of this include the problem of dyspareunia in women with locally advanced cancers of the lower gynaecological tract and of personality change in patients with brain metastases, particularly frontal lobe metastases. Palliative care social workers have specific skills to enhance care by exploring the social and relationship problems that arise when someone is dying (Hearn et al. 2008). Their involvement can enhance the resilience of patients' families and carers (Monroe and Oliviere 2007).

Caring for a terminally ill family member can be both physically and psychologically exhausting. Provision of some form of 'respite' in the form of a day or night sitter, or a short admission of the patient, perhaps to a nursing home, can be invaluable for both the patient and their carer. It is not unusual for one or both parties to feel guilty that such support is needed and they may need reassurance that this is a common need and not one that just pertains to them.

Financial and legal worries can have a devastating effect on the ability of a patient and their family to cope with terminal illness. These can be easily overlooked, particularly as people may be embarrassed to raise the topic themselves (Sheldon 1997). Once a possible problem has been identified, input from a medical social worker can be invaluable.

Risk factors for abnormal grief in bereavement include the sudden, unexpected loss of a loved one and the loss of a partner with whom the bereaved had an ambivalent relationship. These and other risk factors can often be identified before the patient dies and this facilitates the design of a proactive, individualised counselling programme for the carer aimed at preventing abnormal grief.

Bereaved children form a special group. The value of helping children express their feelings in a variety of ways, including through drawing and painting, is now well recognised. Specialised programmes for the children of ill parents and bereaved children have been developed in several countries, and many employ innovative techniques for helping children cope with these situations.

Consideration of and attention to social factors and needs is another crucial component of good palliative care and part of the role of all professionals involved in that woman's care.

Cultural factors

In the UK, it is recognised that patients from ethnic minorities are under-represented in the hospice population. The reasons for this are probably complex, but cultural issues must be a factor. Some cultural groups may not agree with the philosophy of palliative care or be wary of it for other reasons. Problems may arise if a health care professional and a woman are from different cultural backgrounds. In modern societies, which are increasingly mobile, views about cultural norms vary within any one cultural group, particularly across different generations (Neuberger 2004). There may be no easy solution to these dilemmas, but awareness of cultural differences together with a sensitive and flexible approach to care will help to prevent and resolve problems.

Many societies are increasingly multi-cultural. Cultural factors may exert a very marked influence on an individual's attitude to illness, pain, other disease-related problems, treatment measures, death and bereavement. They must be considered and respected. Assessment of any symptom or problem in a woman with cancer should include consideration of the effect of culture. Information is not always volunteered and it is often necessary to ask a woman and her family/carers about their culture and related beliefs and needs. The following case history demonstrates the point.

Case history

A 66-year-old Chinese woman, who understands only a few words of English, is an inpatient with sub-acute bowel obstruction and advanced ovarian cancer.

You are summoned to the ward to see Mrs Tsung and her son. He seems very agitated and is shouting in Cantonese and shaking his mother. The ward sister, who looks flustered, explains that Mrs Tsung's son is very upset that his mother has been administered strong analgesics and insists that his mother should be allowed to suffer pain. He shakes his fist at you repeatedly. The ward sister suggests that she will manage the situation initially and will report back to you when things seem calmer.

A bit later, you and she sit down with the hospital chaplain who was visiting the ward to see other patients. It has become apparent that Mrs Tsung's son feels that his mother's cultural and religious needs are being overlooked. He says that she needs to suffer to atone for her sins. The chaplain explains that this may be the case, but it is difficult to know what the patient wants. It is decided to contact an 'official' interpreter. Mrs Tsung's son is adamant that his mother must not receive an analgesic infusion, but eventually agrees to administration of analgesics on an 'as required' basis. He says he will take his mother home again if the morphine infusion is continued. After further discussion, you change the drug regimen and add corticosteriods.

The following day, the interpreter establishes that Mrs Tsung has a strong Buddhist faith and does not want to receive regular analgesics if conscious. She wants to fly home to China. You agree to continue the current treatment and to investigate the feasibility of air travel. That night, she deteriorates suddenly, developing severe abdominal pain and delirium. The family are called in. They realise that she is actively dying and agree to whatever treatment is required to treat her symptoms.

Mrs Tsung dies 12 hours later with her extended family at her bedside. Her symptoms appeared well controlled. Her body was flown back to China. Her son sent a thank-you letter.

Spiritual care

Even in some modern dictionaries, the terms 'spirituality' and 'religion' are defined in very similar ways. These words have often been used interchangeably, but they are now increasingly distinguished from each other. Spirituality encompasses the purpose and meaning of one's life and is the basis for an individual's attitudes, values, beliefs and actions. It is usually grounded in cultural, religious and family traditions, but is influenced by life experience; spiritual beliefs may change with time, particularly when a person is faced with a life crisis.

Religion is a system of faith and worship, often of God or God-like figures, characterised by specific rites, rituals and texts. Followers of a certain religious faith often do not form a homogenous group. It is important to make no assumptions about the meaning of a declared religious faith to a person, but to explore what it means to them, as an individual.

Everyone faced with a life-threatening disease will have spiritual needs and spiritual issues will influence the way that they cope with the problems of having that disease. In some people, but not all, religious beliefs will be central to their spirituality. Spiritual needs are very individual and questions about spirituality do not, usually, have clear-cut answers. The recognition that a person has spiritual needs, and perhaps spiritual distress, can be very comforting to them. However, one should not impose one's own spiritual beliefs on others. Signs of spiritual distress can vary greatly, but may include persistent severe pain, hopelessness, fear of sleep, recurrent dreams and questions like 'Why me?'

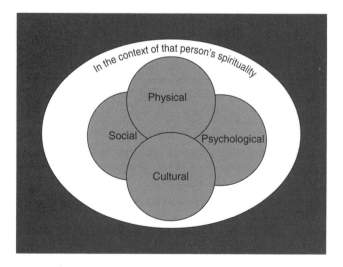

Figure 17.3   The importance of spirituality to the concept of total care.

'What have I done to deserve this?' In many ways the spiritual dimension brings together the physical, psychological, social and cultural dimensions of suffering (Figure 17.3).

Any professional involved in a woman's care can address spiritual issues with her and her family. Chaplains have special expertise and are often regarded by the patient as being separate from the clinical team. Their input is not restricted to patients with strong religious beliefs, but patients often see them as such until they meet them.

Physical problems

A wide range of physical problems and symptoms can be caused by advanced women's cancers. Gynaecological cancers tend to spread locally and distant metastases are a less frequent problem. Advanced breast cancer, however, causes widespread metastases most commonly to bone, lung, liver and brain. In addition to the effects of local and metastatic disease, systemic effects including fatigue and anorexia are common in women with advanced cancer.

The mechanisms and effects of the local spread of gynaecological cancers are detailed in Table 17.1.

Problems caused by the local spread of breast cancer include lymphoedema, brachial plexopathies, painful lumps that may ulcerate and bleed, en curasse disease and local infiltration of muscles, bone, pleura and pericardium.

For any solid tumour, the most common sites of distant metastatic spread are lung, bone, liver and brain. Of the women's cancers, cancer of the breast and gynaecological sarcomas are particularly likely to metastasize to these sites. Specific symptoms relate to the site of metastases (Table 17.2) and are often accompanied by non-specific symptoms of fatigue, poor appetite, weight loss and general debility.

Table 17.1 Mechanisms and effects of local spread of gynaecological cancers.

Mechanisms	Effects
Venous and lymphatic obstruction	Thrombosis and lymphoedema, body image issues
Involvement of lumbo-scaral plexus/cauda equina	Neuropathic pain, loss of motor and sensory function in perineum/legs, compromised bladder/bowel function
Urinary tract obstruction	Obstructive nephropathy
Local infiltration of bladder, bowel and abdominal wall	Enterovaginal/vesico-vaginal fistulae, bowel obstruction, ascites
Local infiltration of musculo-skeletal system, e g. psoas muscle/pelvic bones	Pain including muscle spasm
Mucosal/cutaneous ulceration	Pain, bleeding, odour, discharge, psycho-sexual and body image issues, psychological distress
Local lymph node involvement	Pain, venous obstruction, lymhoedema, ulceration, bleeding

Table 17. 2   Effects of distant metastases.

Bone Metastases	Liver Metastases
Bone pain	Abdominal discomfort
Neuropathic pain	Pain
Spinal cord compression	Liver capsule pain
Pathological fractures	Splinting of diaphragm
Hypercalcaemia	Gastric outflow obstruction
	Pain from bleeding into tumour
	Jaundice
	Vomiting
Chest Metastases	**Brain Metastases**
Parenchymal masses	Headache
Lymphadenopathy (mediastinal and hilar)	Confusion
Lymphangitis	Visual disturbance
Pericardial effusions	Fits
Pleural effusions	Cranial nerve palsies
	Motor and sensory deficits
	Personality change

Clinical decision-making for patients with advanced disease needs to take into account the following:

- Performance status
- Extent of disease
- Anti-cancer options
- Potential side effects of disease specific treatment
- Patient wishes
- Health economic considerations, including the funding of anti-cancer drugs

The principles of palliative care can be employed whilst clinical decision-making is underway. If a woman has specialist palliative care needs, then involvement of specialist palliative care services can run alongside active anti-cancer management and can be discontinued when no longer required. Conversely, if/when there are no active treatment options, the remit of palliative care can be increased both from a general perspective and when required, from a specialist palliative care perspective (Figure 17.1).

General principles of symptom management

- Good communication with a woman and her family/carers, as well as with all professionals involved in her care is essential for effective symptom management and palliative care.
- Thorough assessment of the problem is required with attention to detail, so that an appropriate plan can be formulated, instigated, monitored and evaluated.
- Reassurance and explanation are always appropriate.

- An individual approach is essential.
- Effective symptom management usually requires both pharmacological and non-pharmacological intervention.
- Treatment should be as simple as possible.
- Avoid polypharmacy whenever possible.
- Persistent symptoms warrant regular medication.
- Recognise that advanced cancer is a dynamic changing situation; review effectiveness and appropriateness of intervention frequently and revise management accordingly.

Space precludes a thorough review of the possible interventions for all potential symptoms that women with cancer might develop. Rather, we have chosen to review the management of pain, nausea and vomiting, and constipation in detail. Other symptoms specific to women with breast or gynaecological cancers are considered, but in less detail.

Pain

Pain is one of the most common and most feared symptoms of cancer. Most lay, and indeed professional people, have a particular fear of dying in pain. One-third of patients with cancer have pain at diagnosis and over two-thirds of those with advanced cancer suffer pain. It has been calculated that patients with advanced cancer have an average of four different pains simultaneously (Bruera and Portenoy 2003). Worldwide, it has been estimated that several million people with cancer die in pain every year.

The physical component of the suffering caused by cancer pain and other symptoms is undoubtedly important but, nonetheless, it is only one component. Psychological, social, cultural and spiritual factors also contribute to the totality of cancer pain (Saunders and Sykes 1993).

Good communication with the patient, their family and other health care professionals is vital to good pain control. Attention to detail, a collaborative interdisciplinary approach to assessment and management and frequent review of the situation and revision of the management plan are essential.

Pain needs to be recognised and assessed promptly in patients with cancer. Adequate assessment requires skills in taking a history from both the patient and their carers, physical examination, psychosocial assessment and the appropriate use of carefully selected diagnostic investigations. Blood tests, plain X-rays, radiosotopic bone scans, ultrasound scans, CT and MRI scans can all be invaluable in some instances. Their use must be governed, however, by the physical condition and likely prognosis of the patient, as well as consideration of whether the result of the investigation is likely to affect management.

Causes of pain in a woman with cancer include:

- Direct effect of primary or secondary tumour
- Treatment related
- Related to the debility caused by cancer
- Unrelated to cancer (e g. osteoarthritis)

Approaches to management include:

- Modification of disease process
- Elevation of pain threshold
  - pharmacological
  - non-pharmacological
- Interruption of pain pathways
- Modification of way of life and environment
- Attention to psychological, social, cultural and spiritual factors (see first sections of this chapter)

Frequently, more than one approach is employed at any one time, but they should be used in a systematic, consistent way. All of these interventions should be carried out within a person-centred framework with explanation and reassurance, and due attention to the contribution of other, non-physical factors to the pain.

It is well established that cancer pain can be controlled in the majority of patients by simple, cheap pharmacological interventions. Such treatment should be based on the World Health Organisation guidelines, which advocate a step-wise or ladder approach to the pharmacological management of cancer pain (Figure 17.4) (Zech et al. 1995). If pain is not controlled on maximum dosage at one step, then a move up to the next step is required. There is no maximal dose of strong opioids. Variations to this model are sometimes employed, but they are all grounded in the same principles:

- 'By the mouth' (the oral route is the preferred route of administration)
- 'By the clock' (chronic cancer pain requires treatment with regularly administered analgesics)
- 'By the ladder' (treatment should be approached in a logical, stepwise manner)

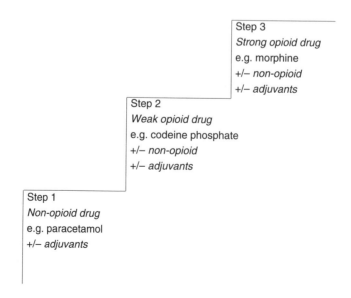

Figure 17.4   The World Health Organisation three-step analgesic ladder (Zech et al. 1995).

Nociceptive pain, such as caused by bone or liver metastases, usually responds well to opioid drugs, either alone or in combination with adjuvant drugs such as non-steroidal anti-inflammatory drugs or corticosteroids. On the other hand, neuropathic pain often responds less well to opioids and usually requires the addition of adjuvant analgesics such as anti-depressant or anti-convulsant drugs.

Pain can often lead to decreased mobility and abnormal position, and careful positioning, simple exercises and physiotherapy can all be helpful. Other non-pharmacological measures include transcutaneous electrical nerve stimulation (TENS) and acupuncture. The use of appropriate appliances and aids can reduce pain and minimise disability. Psychological, social, cultural and spiritual factors should be considered and addressed.

In some patients with cancer, pain is particularly difficult to control. The reasons for this can be complex and include problems in all the domains of care, as illustrated by the following case history.

Case history

Susan, a 50-year-old, married nurse with advanced metastatic breast cancer involving her bones (lumbo-sacral spine) and liver was admitted to hospital with a short history of increasing lower back and bilateral leg pain. She had already received a range of anticancer therapies, including maximal radiotherapy to her lumbo-sacral spine. She was distressed and had signs of nerve root compression at L4-S1. Her pain took several days to control. Measures used included reassurance, explanation, oral opioids, a non-steroidal anti-inflammatory drug, an anti-depressant as an adjuvant analgesic, high dose corticosteroids and, eventually, an epidural infusion of local anaesthetic and morphine. Her pain and distress improved considerably, but not totally. She was now well enough to talk freely and explore the components of her pain and distress, which included fear of dying in pain, worry about her children, and recognition that her nursing expertise raised specific fears of spinal cord compression with paralysis, incontinence and pressure sores. A multi-disciplinary approach to her care included input from not only nurses and doctors, but also the chaplain, physiotherapist and pharmacist. A pressure relieving mattress was used. She became pain-free and, once the amount of local anaesthetic in the epidural was reduced, more mobile. Susan was discharged home with an epidural infusion and was supported in the community by her family, friends, the primary health care team, the local palliative care team and her minister. She remained pain-free until her death, 6 weeks later.

In conclusion, a multi-faceted, interdisciplinary approach to the management of cancer pain is essential. The appropriateness of different interventions varies with time. In women whose cancer responds to anti-cancer therapy, pain may resolve and their analgesic requirements need constant review. It is much easier to start new drugs than to remember to reduce the dose and stop them!

Nausea and vomiting

In general, nausea and vomiting tend to be symptoms that are poorly controlled. Our experience suggests that this is due to both a lack of assessment of the cause of the

Table 17.3 Causes and treatments of nausea and vomiting in women with cancer.

Chemically mediated	Specific treatment options	Anti-emetic
Hypercalcaemia	Hydration and bisphosphonates	Dopamine antagonist, e.g. haloperidol, phenothiazine, levomepromazine
Uraemia	Rehydration/catheterisation/ nephrostomies depending on cause	
Chemotherapeutic agents		5HT$_3$ Antagonist, e.g. ondansetron ± steroids
Drugs, e.g. opioids	Review need for drug and renal function	Dopamine antagonist, e.g. haloperidol
Raised intercranial pressure from cerebral metastases	Steroids and radiotherapy	Antihistamine, e.g. cyclizine

Mechanically mediated	Specific treatments	Anti-emetic
Gastric stasis/outflow obstruction	1. Incomplete obstruction	Prokinetic agent, e.g. metoclopramide
	2. Complete obstruction – NG tube and consider gastroenterostomy and if surgery inappropriate a venting gastrostomy. Oncology review and opinion. Consider further anti-cancer treatments. Consider the use of steroids	Haloperidol and/or cyclizine. Avoid prokinetics
Small bowel obstruction	Naso-gastric tube – rehydration and consider surgery? ileostomy. Consider anti-spasmodics, e.g. hyoscine butylbromide	Haloperidol and/or cyclizine. Avoid prokinetics
Large bowel obstruction	Rehydration and consider surgery? defunctioning colostomy and/or stenting. Consider anti-spasmodics, e.g hyoscine butylbromide	Haloperidol and/or cyclizine. Avoid prokinetics
Constipation	Laxatives – (see next section) Rectal assessment and intervention if appropriate	Haloperidol or levomepromazine

problems, and an apparent lack of knowledge of the mechanisms of action and side-effect profiles of anti-emetic drugs.

Women's cancers can cause nausea and vomiting through both chemical and mechanical mechanisms. It is important to establish the cause of the symptoms through careful history-taking and examination, combined with knowledge of the disease process. The choice of anti-emetic and other treatments depends on the cause. Sometimes there may be several

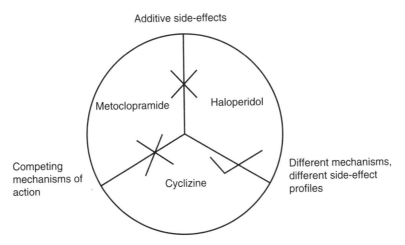

Figure 17.5 Pragmatic guide to choice of anti emetic drug.

different causes of nausea and vomiting concurrently. Careful assessment combined with pattern recognition usually facilitates recognition of the different concurrent causes although, on occasion, stepwise use of anti-emetics from different classes is required (Mannix 2006).

Chemically mediated nausea tends to be constant and unrelieved by retching or vomiting. The vomit is often of small volume and contains bile. This pattern is very different to that of mechanically induced nausea and vomiting. For example, gastric outflow obstruction causes bouts of nausea followed soon after by a large volume vomit that does not contain bile and which relieves the nausea. It is important to remember that both mechanisms can co-exist. In patients with large bowel obstruction, there is usually a chemically medicated cause of the nausea (due to stagnant faeces), as well as the more obvious mechanical cause.

In every case the approach to a patient complaining of nausea and/or vomiting needs to include not only the appropriate choice of anti-emetic but also measures to address the cause of the problems. Further anti-cancer treatments may be appropriate but, if not, the appropriateness of palliative interventions such as a gastroenterostomy or corticosteroids should be considered. The approaches to management of nausea and vomiting of different causes are described in Table 17.3 and Figure 17.5.

Attention needs to be given to the choice of route of administration of the anti-emetic(s). Often a non-oral route is needed. Some patients require more than one anti-emetic and it is important to consider their side-effect profiles as well as their mechanisms of action when prescribing:

It is important to remember that both cyclizine and ondansetron are very constipating. A broad spectrum anti-emetic, for example levomepromazine, is appropriate if there is no clear cause for the symptoms or if different mechanisms co-exist. A much lower dose of levomepromazine, such as 6.25 mg/24 hours, should be prescribed when treating nausea and vomiting, than when using the drug as an anti-psychotic and sedative.

Constipation

Constipation can be defined as the infrequent and difficult passage of small hard faeces. There is no such thing as normal bowel habit for a population of patients. Patients' symptoms need to be rated against their own definition of constipation and what they consider to be a normal or acceptable bowel habit for them. Physical illness is a risk factor for constipation, and constipation is more common in terminally ill people with cancer than in those who are terminally ill with other diseases.

Constipation can cause other symptoms including anorexia, nausea and vomiting, abdominal pain, confusion and diarrhoea. In addition, it can exacerbate other symptoms such as breathlessness or back pain. It can have a marked adverse effect on quality of life and some patients find it as distressing as pain.

Many women find constipation embarrassing, whether at home or in hospital. Treatment can cause urgency and incontinence, which can be particularly distressing for women from some cultural groups. The economic consequences of constipation include the cost of nursing and medical time, sometimes including hospitalisation as well as the cost of oral and rectal laxatives.

It is a common and important problem in women with advanced cancer and in those with gynaecological cancer, and it can be caused by both local disease infiltration of the bowel and/or the nervous system. There may be multiple causes in any one patient. Causative factors are shown in Table 17.4.

Whatever the cause, the same general principles of management should be followed:

(1) Take a detailed history, including details of normal bowel habit for that patient and use of laxatives.
(2) Palpate abdomen and check bowel sounds.
(3) Perform rectal examination.
(4) Identify and treat any underlying correctable cause(s) if appropriate.
(5) Encourage fluid intake.
(6) Increase dietary fibre in fitter patients, unless bowel obstruction present. Patients with advanced cancer are unlikely to be able to tolerate enough fibre and fluid to make any significant difference to the problem.
(7) Consider use of regular oral laxatives, choose laxative according to individual circumstances, including age, urinary continence and cause of constipation (Table 17.5).
(8) Consider rectal intervention if oral measures ineffective, or hard stool in rectum.
(9) Nurses are usually more expert in the management of constipation than doctors!

Table 17.4 Causes of constipation in patients with advanced cancer.

Specific	General
Gastro-intestinal and gynaecological malignancy Spinal cord compression Metabolic (e.g. hypercalcaemia, uraemia) Iatrogenic (e.g. vincristine, opioids, iron, tryclic antidepressants, antispasmodics such as hyoscine)	Reduced mobility Anorexia Dehydration Shortness of breath

Table 17.5   Treatment options for constipation.

Type	Action	Example
Bulk Forming Agents	Increase mass and water content of stool and thus stimulate peristalsis. Need to maintain/increase fluid intake. Avoid if risk of intestinal obstruction.	Ispaghula husk (e.g. Fybogel) Methylcellulose (e.g. Celevac) Stercula (e.g. Normacol)
Osmotic Laxatives	Attract water into the bowel lumen and thus increase stool output. Some also have a stimulant action (e.g. magnesium salts).	Magnesium salts (e.g. magnesium hydroxide, magnesium sulphate, liquid paraffin and magnesium hydroxide) Macrogols (e.g. Movicol)
Stimulant Laxatives	Stimulate the colon, increase peristaltic movement and reduce water absorption from gastrointestinal tract. May cause abdominal cramps. Avoid in patients with intestinal obstruction.	Senna danthron-containing laxatives (e.g. Codanthramer suspension, Codanthrusate capsules), bisacodyl sodium picosulphate

Laxatives

The choice of laxative depends on several factors, including the nature of the stools, acceptability to the patient and cost (Sykes et al. 2006).

Bulk laxatives are used infrequently in palliative care, because patients are often unable to maintain the necessary high fluid intake. Danthron-containing laxatives should be avoided in patients with urinary or faecal incontinence and those with a urinary catheter (in case of leakage around catheter), because danthron can cause superficial skin burns. Patients and carers should be warned that danthron containing laxatives cause discoloured (red/brown) urine. Lactulose can cause hiccoughs, excessive wind and discomfort and can exacerbate symptoms of bowel obstruction.

Rectal interventions are indicated if there is hard stool in the rectum and/or appropriate oral measures have been ineffective. The first choice rectal intervention for uncompli- cated constipation is glycerine suppositories. If these are ineffective then a stimulant enema such as a high phosphate enema should be administered.

Oral and rectal stimulant laxatives should be avoided in patients with possible or proven bowel obstruction. Softening rectal measures can sometimes be effective in emptying the rectum and lower colon. Oral softening agents are useful if the obstruction is incomplete. It should be remembered that constipation can cause bowel obstruction, which is usually referred to as a pseudo-obstruction.

Opioid induced constipation

Opioids cause constipation through several different effects on the gastrointestinal tract, namely:

- Increased water absorption from gut (they also cause dry mouth for this reason)
- Decreased gastric, biliary and pancreatic secretions
- Decreased gastrointestinal mobility
- Decreased rectal sensitivity to faecal load

Thus, a combination of a stool softener and a stimulant laxative is usually required for the prevention and treatment of opioid induced constipation. Regular prophylactic laxatives should be prescribed for almost all patients on strong opioids, the exception being those with profuse diarrhoea such as caused by a carcinoid tumour or Clostridium difficile infection. The choice of drugs is often dictated by local practice.

Opioid induced constipation should be managed by adhering to the general principles detailed above. Laxative drugs will need to be used in higher doses than when used prophylactically. The regimen should be reviewed regularly, at least every few days, and be adjusted if necessary. If ineffective, then rectal interventions should be added and a change in the regimen or choice of oral laxatives should be considered. There is some evidence that some patients become tolerant to the constipating effects of opioids over time.

Ascites

One of the commonest causes of ascites in women with cancer is peritoneal metastases from a primary ovarian cancer. However, there are many other causes including:

- Peritoneal metastases from other primary cancers
- Hypoalbuminaemia, usually associated with extensive liver metastases
- Venous compression or thrombosis of inferior vena cava or hepatic vein
- Tumour blocking diaphragmatic lymph ducts
- Other concurrent disease, e.g. heart failure, cirrhosis

Management of Ascites

Cytotoxic chemotherapy, administered either intraperitoneally or systemically, may be appropriate, especially for primary carcinomas of the ovary, breast or colon. Alongside such anti-cancer therapy or for those in whom such treatment is inappropriate, therapy aimed at symptomatic control is usually required, although if the symptoms are minor, explanation and reassurance may be sufficient.

Paracentesis is the treatment of choice for rapid symptom control. Local guidelines vary, but it is good practice to drain only up to 5 litres of ascites per day, because the sudden release of abdominal tension may lead to venous decompression, hypotension and collapse. Repeated paracentesis is appropriate in patients with an expected prognosis of only a few weeks but in other selected patients, a pleuro-peritoneal shunt may be considered. In some oncology centres, permanent indwelling peritoneal cannulae are inserted, allowing intermittent drainage of ascites.

A therapeutic trial of diuretics is appropriate in patients with symptomatic ascites. Spironolactone is usually regarded as the diuretic of choice and doses between 100 and 400 mg daily are used. However, it can take up to 7 days to improve symptoms and 28 days for full effect. If required, the addition of frusemide often helps achieve a more rapid response, or may help in those women whose ascites fails to respond to spironolactone.

Fistulae

Fistulae are defined as abnormal openings between two epithelial lined surfaces. They can be external draining from a skin site, for example an entero-cutaneous fistula, or internal with no communication to the surface of the skin, for example a vesico-vaginal fistula. Malignancies of the female reproductive tract are more likely than most other cancers to cause fistulae because of their propensity for local spread and the anatomy of the pelvis. Radiotherapy and surgery are other pre-disposing factors.

The assessment and management of fistulae is a particularly good example of inter-professional, multi-speciality teamwork. If a fistula develops, discussion with the gynae-cological cancer surgeons is required. The cause should be assessed and investigation and management decided upon, in the context of that woman's disease, performance status and her wishes.

Fistula management should incorporate the following principles:

- Protection of the surrounding skin
- Collection and containment of fistula output, depending on the fistula site, the volume, consistency and type of effluent drainage
- Control of odour
- Attention to psychological, sexual and social consequences

The choice of possible intervention depends on many factors, including the type of fistula, the site and the output (Naylor et al. 2001). If radiotherapy induced, then the radiation field needs to be considered because of the risk of further fistulae and the con-traindication for surgery. A high output enterocutaneous fistula could be treated with octreotide, initially 300 mcg per day, by subcutaneous infusion. This drug promotes fluid re-absorption from the small bowel, thus reducing the output, which should make the fistula easier to manage and may encourage healing of the fistula. Occasionally, surgical excision of the fistula tract is possible.

Enterovesical fistulae are bound to cause urinary tract infection, which will require treatment. Most women with such fistulae require prophylactic antibiotics and microbiology advice should be sought.

Fistulae that drain externally are often distressing because of their output and odour and the effect they have on a woman's body image and sexuality. There are numerous appliances that can be used in fistula management on the advice of a specialist stoma nurse. Depending on the site and skin contours, adherence of any collecting device may be difficult and leakage can be a risk causing further distress.

Fungating women's cancers

A fungating wound occurs when the tumour invades the epithelium breaking through the skin surface. The wound can either be ulcerative, forming ulcerative craters or proliferative, forming raised nodules. Fungating wounds may develop at the site of the primary cancer, such as the breast or the vulva, or at affected lymph nodes in the axilla or groin. In these cases, anti-cancer treatments must be considered. Alongside this, the wounds must be actively managed and skin care is a priority (Grocott 1995).

It has been estimated that up to 10% of patients with metastatic cancer will develop a fungating lesion, 62% of which are accounted for by patients with breast cancer (Haisfield-Wolfe and Rund 1997).

Between 2 and 5% of women with breast cancer develop malignant, fungating wounds and it is a particular problem in women who have either neglected their disease or chosen not to seek medical advice and present with advanced local disease.

Many women with fungating breast wounds will suffer lymphoedema.

General principles in the management of fungating wounds

- Assess wound and the woman's overall condition
- Seek the advice of a tissue viability team to ensure the optimal dressing
- Be alert for infection – the appropriate use of antibiotics may reduce the problems of both odour and exudate
- Ensure adequate analgesia, especially during dressing change
- Radiotherapy ± laser treatment can reduce bleeding and discharge. Occasionally surgery and skin grafting may need to be considered
- Address related problems, e.g. pruritis around the wound area

The problems associated with fungating breast disease are likely to have a profound effect on a woman's quality of life. Disfigurement caused by the wound will have an effect on a woman's body image and can be viewed sometimes as an assault on her womanhood and sexuality.

These problems can be further exacerbated when there are issues with bleeding, exudate and infection. The latter can cause an unpleasant odour, which is hard for a woman to escape from; the breast is only inches away from one's nose! Fungating disease may compromise a woman's choice of clothing; loose garments to cover dressings are sometimes essential. It can also preclude the continued wearing of a breast prosthesis.

Local infiltration does not just affect the skin. Muscles, ribs, plus the pleura and pericardium, can all be involved.

Ethical issues

Ethical dilemmas can arise at any stage of a patient's disease process and in any health care setting. Particular dilemmas that may arise in palliative care for women with breast and gynaecological cancers include issues around nutrition and hydration, patient autonomy and the role of the patient's relatives in decision-making and requests for euthanasia. Further detailed discussion of these issues is outside the remit of this chapter.

It is important to remember that dilemmas arise when a situation or plan is not 'black and white'. There is never a perfect answer to a dilemma. An ethical dilemma must be considered from the woman's point of view, within an ethical and legal framework. Decisions need to be balanced and to achieve this it is usually necessary both to think widely and to discuss the issue widely, but appropriately and to maintain confidentiality throughout. The patient, family and other health care professionals, particularly nurses, should all contribute to this process. Others' views must be respected. Ethical decision-making should always be individualised and relate to the individual circumstances of that patient. Particularly complex dilemmas can be referred to the local clinical ethical committee.

We are required always to act in the patient's best interests. A relative's contribution to a discussion, which is aimed at identifying what is in the patient's best interests, is always important. Nonetheless, consideration of their views needs to be tempered by the fact that the agenda of the relatives may be different from that of the patient. In the UK, the relatives should not be asked to make proxy decisions for the patient, unless the patient has signed an enduring Power of Attorney. In the UK, practice has changed since the introduction of the Mental Capacity Act 2005 (HMSO Mental Capacity Act 2005).

Conclusion

The care of women with cancer in the twenty-first century should be delivered by an inter-disciplinary, cross-speciality team. Whilst specialist palliative care services are bound to be mainly involved in the care of women with advanced disease, they also have a role in selected patients earlier in their disease process. Furthermore, just because a woman has metastatic disease does not mean her disease is terminal, or that the symptoms/problems she has cannot be addressed. Palliative care specialists need to be aware of all the resources available for patients these days and gynae/oncology specialists need to remember that palliative care is not just about terminal care.

Ten years ago, if palliative care services were asked to see a woman with ovarian cancer and bowel obstruction, the referral would have been for terminal care. Now palliative care services plan to work alongside the gynae/oncology surgeons, the non-surgical oncologists, the gynaecological cancer nurse specialists and sometimes the interventional radiologists, to improve the woman's general physical well-being and fitness, with a view to proceeding to further anti- cancer treatments.

This chapter will have achieved its aim if it has acquainted the reader with the philosophy and basic principles of palliative care, and the role of modern specialist palliative care services for women with cancer, as well as the correct approach to the management of constipation!

Reflective points

- Consider the organisational policies and guidelines in your workplace that support the philosophy of palliative care.
- Reflect on the practical and supportive services available in your setting.
- Think of a patient who you have cared for recently at the end of their life – what were their psychological and symptom management needs?

References and Bibliography

Booth, S. and Bruera, E. (Eds) (2004) *Palliative Care Consultations in Gynae-oncology*. Oxford: Oxford University Press.

Bruera, E. and Portenoy, R.K. (2003) *Cancer Pain*. Cambridge: Cambridge University Press.

Doyle, D., Hanks, G., Cherny. N. and Sir Kenneth Calman (Eds) (2005) *The Oxford Textbook of Palliative Medicine*, 3rd edn. Oxford: Oxford University Press.

Fallon, M. and Hanks, G. (Eds) (2006) *ABC of Palliative Care*, 2nd edn. Oxford: Blackwell Publishing Ltd.

Grocott, P. (1995) The palliative management of fungating malignant wounds. *Journal of Wound Care* **4(5)**, 240–2.

Haisefield-Wolfe, M.E. and Rund, C. (1997) Malignant cutaneous wounds: a management protocol. *Ostomy/Wound Management* **43(1)**, 56–66.

Harmer V. (Ed.) (2011) *Breast Cancer Nursing Care and Management*. Oxford: Wiley-Blackwell.

Hearn, F. et al. (2008) Re-emphasising The social side: a new model of care. *European Journal of Palliative Care* **15(16)**, 276–8.

Herth, K. (1990) Fostering hope in terminally ill people. *Journal of Advanced Nursing*. **15**, 1250–9.

HMSO – *Mental Capacity Act 2005* www.opsi.gov.uk/ACTS/acts2005/ukpga_20020009_en_1

Jeffrey. D. (2006) Communication. In: M. Fallon and G. Hanks (Eds) *ABC of Palliative Care*, 2nd edn, Oxford: Blackwell Publishing Ltd, pp. 52–5.

Lawton F., Friedlander M. and Thomas G. (Eds) (1998) *Essentials of Gynaecological Cancer*. Chapman & Hall.

Mannix. K. (2006) Nausea and vomiting. In: M. Fallon and G. Hanks (Eds) *ABC of Palliative Care*, 2nd edn) Oxford: Blackwell Publishing Ltd, pp. 25–8.

Monroe, B. and Oliviere, D. (Eds) (2007) *Resilience in Palliative Care: Achievement in Adversity*. Oxford: Oxford University Press.

National Institute for Clinical Excellence. *Guidance on Cancer Services. Improving Supportive and Palliative Care for Adults with Cancer: The Manual*. NICE 2004 www.nice.org.uk/nicemedia/pdf/osgspmanual.pdf (last accessed 21 September 2008).

Naylor, W., Laverty. D. and Mallett. J. (Eds) (2001) *The Royal Marsden Hospital Handbook of Wound Management in Cancer Care*. Oxford: Blackwell Science Ltd.

Neuberger, J. (2004) *Caring for Dying People of Different Faiths*, 3rd edn. Oxford: Radcliffe Medical.

Randall, F. and Downie, R.S. (1999) *Palliative Care Ethics. A Companion for all Specialities*, 2nd edn. Oxford: Oxford University Press.

Saunders, C. and Sykes, N. (1993) *The Management of Terminal Malignant Disease*, 3rd edn. London: Edward Arnold.

Sheldon, F. (1997) *Psychosocial Palliative Care*. Cheltenham: Stanley Thornes (Publishers) Ltd.

Speck. P. (2005) In: D. Doyle, G.W.C. Hanks and N. MacDonald (Eds) *Oxford Textbook of Palliative Medicine*. Oxford: Oxford University Press.

Sykes, N. et al. (2006) Constipation, diarrhoea and intestinal obstruction. In: M. Fallon and G. Hanks (Eds) *ABC of Palliative Care*, 2nd edn. Oxford: Blackwell Publishing Ltd, pp. 29–35.

Twycross R. (1997) *Symptom Management in Advanced Cancer* 2nd edn. Oxford Radcliffe Medical Press.

WHO (1990) *Cancer Pain Relief and Palliative Care*, report of WHO Expert Committee. Vol. 804, WHO Technical Report Series. Geneva. WHO 1–75.

Zech, D.F.J., Grond, S., Lynch, J., Hertel, D. and Lehmann, K.A. (1995) Validation of World Health Organisation guidelines for cancer pain relief. A 10-year prospective study. *Pain* **63**, 65–7.

Index

Page numbers in *italics* denote figures and tables.

Women's Cancers, First Edition. Edited by Alison Keen and Elaine Lennan.
© 2011 Blackwell Publishing Ltd. Published 2011 by Blackwell Publishing Ltd.